# THE HANDBOOK
## OF
# ERICKSONIAN PSYCHOTHERAPY

# THE HANDBOOK OF ERICKSONIAN PSYCHOTHERAPY

*edited by*

Brent B. Geary & Jeffrey K. Zeig

The Milton H. Erickson Foundation Press
Phoenix, Arizona
2001

Library of Congress Cataloging-in-Publication Data

The handbook of Ericksonian psychotherapy / edited by Brent B. Geary &
    Jeffrey K. Zeig.
        p.  cm.
    Includes bibliographical references and index.
    ISBN 0-9716190-1-8 (alk. paper)
        1. Psychotherapy — Handbooks, manuals, etc.  2. Erickson, Milton H.
    I. Geary, Brent B.  II. Zeig, Jeffrey K., 1947–
    RC480.H2844  2002
    616.89'14--dc21                                        2002017300

Published by
The Milton H. Erickson Foundation Press
3606 North 24th Street
Phoenix, AZ  85016


Manufactured in the United States of America


10  9  8  7  6  5  4  3  2  1

# Table of Contents

# Contributors

**Brian M. Alman**, Ph.D., Senior Vice-President of Clinical Strategies, LifeStar Corporation, is also Medical Hypnosis Consultant for Kaiser Permanente and has a private practice in San Diego, California.

**Daniel L. Araoz**, Ed.D., Professor, Long Island University at C.W. Post, is also Coordinator of the U.S. Army Technical Officers Training Program at the U.S. Military Academy, West Point, New York.

**Terry L. Argast**, Ph.D., is Clinical Director for the Southern California Society for Ericksonian Psychotherapy and Hypnosis.

**Joseph Barber**, Ph.D., is with the Department of Rehabilitation Medicine, University of Washington School of Medicine, Seattle, Washington.

**Norma Barretta**, Ph.D., an Approved Consultant for the American Society of Clinical Hypnosis, is in private practice in the Los Angeles–Palos Verdes Peninsula area. She is also an invited faculty member for the Erickson Foundation Congress.

**Philip F. Barretta**, M.A., an Approved Consultant for the American Society of Clinical Hypnosis, is a frequent faculty member of the Erickson Foundation Congress. "Mostly retired" from private practice, he teaches Ericksonian hypnosis and neurolinguistics.

**Cheryl Bell-Gadsby**, M.A., is a Program Coordinator with the Social Services and Community Safety Division at the Justice Institute of British Columbia, Canada. A feminist therapist, clinical supervisor, and educator, she has special expertise in trauma, family violence, sexual exploitation, and hypnotherapy.

**Pennie Dexter Carrell**, Ph.D., is in private practice in Santa Barbara and Anaheim, California.

**Susanne T. Coleman**, M.S., is a doctoral candidate in the Department of Family Therapy at Nova Southeastern University, Fort Lauderdale, Florida.

**Yvonne M. Dolan**, M.A., is a psychotherapist and consultant in private practice with The Solution Group, Denver, Colorado. She also teaches workshops on solution-focused therapy and Ericksonian hypnosis.

**Barry L. Duncan**, Psy.D., an educator, trainer, and therapist, is Associate Professor in the Department of Family Therapy, Nova Southeastern University,

Fort Lauderdale, Florida. He is an Approved Supervisor of the American Association for Marriage and Family Therapy.

**Betty Alice Erickson**, M.S., in private practice in Dallas, Texas, has served as an Editor of the Milton H. Erickson Foundation *Newsletter* since 1993. She established, and now supervises, a pain-management program for an HIV/AIDS center. A daughter of Dr. Erickson, she teaches hypnosis, brief therapy, and Ericksonian psychotherapy.

**Helen Erickson**, Ph.D., is Professor Emeritus, The University of Texas at Austin, and the Chair, Center for the Advancement of Modeling and Role Modeling, Austin, Texas. She is a daughter of Dr. Erickson.

**Brent B. Geary**, Ph.D., is President, Behavioral Health Systems, Inc., Phoenix, Arizona, and Coordinator of Training for the Milton H. Erickson Foundation.

**Stephen Gilligan**, Ph.D., is in private practice in Encinitas, California.

**Eric Greenleaf**, Ph.D., is in private practice in Berkeley, California. He is Director of the Milton H. Erickson Institute of the Bay Area, and was the first recipient of the Milton H. Erickson Award for Scientific Writing in Hypnosis.

**Ronald A. Havens**, Ph.D., is Professor of Psychology, Department of Psychology, University of Illinois at Springfield, and is in private practice part-time with the Maher Psychiatric Group, also in Springfield, Illinois.

**Harriet H. Hollander**, Ph.D., is a Director of the Milton H. Erickson Institute of New Jersey and Professor Emeritus of the Clinical Hypnosis Society of New Jersey.

**Lynn D. Johnson**, Ph.D., is Director, Brief Therapy Center, Salt Lake City, Utah. He is also Adjunct Professor of Education Psychology, University of Utah.

**Carol Kershaw**, Ed.D., is Co-Director, Milton H. Erickson Institute of Houston, Texas. She also has a private practice in Houston.

**Richard E. Landis**, Ph.D., is Training Director, Southern California Society for Ericksonian Psychotherapy and Hypnosis.

**Carol Lankton**, M.A., is a marriage and family therapist in private practice in Pensacola, Florida. An Approved Consultant for the American Society of Clinical Hypnosis, she also teaches Ericksonian approaches.

**Stephen R. Lankton**, M.S.W., is a licensed marriage and family therapist in Pensacola, Florida, and a corporate consultant. He is a recipient of the Milton H. Erickson Foundation's Lifetime Achievement Award for his outstanding contributions to the field of psychotherapy, and is President, American Hypnosis Board for Clinical Social Work.

**William J. Matthews**, Ph.D., is a Professor in the School Psychology Program, University of Massachusetts at Amherst.

**Robert B. McNeilly**, M.B.B.S., was in general medical practice in Melbourne, Australia, until, inspired by meeting Dr. Erickson, he established a hypnotherapy and psychotherapy practice 22 years ago. He also teaches the Ericksonian approach to health professionals.

**Scott D. Miller**, Ph.D., specializes in treating the homeless mentally ill and other traditionally underserved populations. He also conducts workshops and training sessions on client-directed, outcome-oriented clinical work.

**Joyce C. Mills**, Ph.D., is a Supervisor and Professor of Play Therapy in Kauai, Hawaii. She also serves on the Board of Directors of the Turtle Island Project and is on the Advisory Board of *Shape Magazine*.

**Jane A. Parsons-Fein**, C.S.W., is Director of the Parsons-Fein Training Institute for Psychotherapy and Hypnosis, which integrates the hypnotic approaches of Milton Erickson and Virginia Satir, and directs a training program in Stockholm, Sweden. She is President Emeritus and cofounder of the New York Milton H. Erickson Society of Psychotherapy and Hypnosis.

**Maggie Phillips**, Ph.D., in private practice in Oakland, California, is Director of the California Institute of Clinical Hypnosis and National Secretary of the American Society of Clinical Hypnosis. She is a member of the faculties of the Esalen Institute and the University of California at Santa Cruz Extension.

**Dirk Revenstorf**, Ph.D., teaches at the Insititute of Clinical Psychology, University of Tübingen, Germany.

**Michele K. Ritterman**, Ph.D. is Adjunct Professor, California School of Professional Psychology, as well as in private practice.

**Teresa Robles**, Ph.D., is President of the Mexican Society of Hypnosis and Director of the Ericksonian Center of Mexico. She has taught at the National University and Metropolitan University in Mexico City, and conducts workshops on Ericksonian hypnosis and psychotherapy and on family therapy, both in Mexico and internationally.

**Ernest L. Rossi**, Ph.D., is a diplomate of the American Board of Examiners in Clinical Psychology. He is a recipient of the Milton H. Erickson Foundation's Lifetime Achievement Award for his contributions to psychotherapy.

**Alan W. Scheflin**, J.D., Professor of Law at the Santa Clara University School of Law in California, received the American Psychiatric Association's Manfred S. Guttmacher Award in both 1991 and 1998.

**Dan Short**, M.S., is Editor-in-Chief of the Milton H. Erickson *Newsletter* and School Psychologist for Highland Park ISD in Dallas, Texas. He is a Ph.D. candidate at the University of Massachusetts at Amherst.

**Sandra M. Sylvester**, Ph.D., is the founder of the WarriorHeart Program in Sacramento, California, a nonprofit organization that works with the chronically ill.

**Bernhard Trenkle**, Dipl.Psych. is President of the Milton Erickson Society of Germany and Director of the Milton Erickson Institute of Rottweil, Germany. He also has a private practice in Rottweil. He is a recipient of the Milton H. Erickson Foundation's Lifetime Achievement Award.

**Catherine Walters**, M.A., is in private practice with the Maher Psychiatric Group, Springfield, Illinois.

**R. Reid Wilson**, Ph.D., is Associate Clinical Professor of Psychiatry at the University of North Carolina School of Medicine, and Clinical Director of anxieties.com.

**Michael D. Yapko**, Ph.D., is Director of the Milton H. Erickson Institute of San Diego, California, and is in private practice.

**Jeffrey K. Zeig**, Ph.D., is Director of the Milton H. Erickson Foundation, Phoenix, Arizona.

# PRINCIPLES

# 1

# Assessment in Ericksonian Hypnosis and Psychotherapy

*Brent B. Geary*

L ike all other aspects of the Ericksonian approach, assessment is in-
extricably tied to utilization. This is the fabric of the Ericksonian
model—utilization interwoven with assessment. The therapist is a design-
er, tailoring the treatment to fit the particular circumstances of the
patient. Assessment provides the measurements from which interventions
are fashioned. It allows the clinician to decide what to utilize and how to
utilize it.

## ASSESSMENT AS A PROCESS

Erickson blurred the boundaries between assessment and other aspects of
treatment. He demonstrated that assessment is a process, not a static stage.
Assessment is ongoing; it occurs throughout therapy. Ericksonian practitioners are mindful of assessment from the initial contact with a patient
to termination. The utilization perspective promotes a continuous sorting
of information (e.g., feedback from the patient, changes in the social
network, the therapist's own associations) and evaluating those items that
are to be discarded and those that are to be incorporated to attain therapeutic ends.

## Key Principles

Assessment in the Ericksonian framework rests on two guiding axioms.

### Everything Can Be Utilized

Erickson, of course, was the exemplification of this proposition. He utilized aspects of his own character and background, dynamics in the therapeutic relationship, and multitudinous variables associated with his patients. Even supposedly undesirable factors (e.g., resistance, lack of insight, previous treatment failures) were fodder for Erickson's techniques (Haley, 1973). His work illustrated the multiple dimensions in each person's life and every therapeutic encounter that can be utilized: time, space, the real and imagined, hopes, fears, accomplishments, skills. So, an important facet of assessment is to maintain an open and broad perspective regarding the myriad possibilities that exist for utilization.

### Not Everything Will Be Utilized

There are simply too many data, too much experience to track and use in a particular session or overall treatment process. Therefore, the second crucial task of assessment is that of winnowing out those aspects of the therapeutic context that offer the most promise for having an impact when utilized. This is the artistry of assessment; in an individualized treatment approach, each therapist will discover an array of things that can be utilized and from these create a therapy suited to a particular patient.

## TRADITIONAL ASSESSMENT

Traditional hypnosis has customarily employed standardized methods—susceptibility or hypnotizability tests to assess the degree to which individuals can or will respond to suggestions for alterations in perception, memory, and behavior (Kihlstrom, 1985; Weitzenhoffer & Hilgard, 1959, 1962). This owes to the proposition that hypnotizability is a relatively stable characteristic among people (Hilgard, 1965). Other methods of psychological assessment are often advocated as valuable in directing the manner in which hypnosis is incorporated into psychotherapy, including objective psychometric instruments, projective devices, structured diagnostic interviews, and third-party reports. Practitioners from various orientations might also use measurement methodologies to evaluate specific theoretical constructs (e.g., ego strength, regression, dissociation, developmental level) viewed as salient from their perspective. From this standpoint, the philosophy of assessment is somewhat different from that of the Ericksonian model. Here, assessment is more "front-loaded," that is, it is conceived of as an initial stage in the therapeutic process, followed by treatment and outcome measurement.

Ericksonians do not necessarily eschew information derived from standardized sources. However, measures of hypnotizability, personality, and other variables do not occupy a central place in the Ericksonian approach. The premise is that everyone with intact mental processes can benefit from hypnosis to some degree. The extent to which this is possible is tested through clinical intervention rather than by the administration of a set procedure that yields a quantifiable result. As self-report tools, objective and projective methods can provide valuable information, and no doubt there are many Ericksonian practitioners who utilize such instruments. But the primary context for assessment in the Ericksonian approach remains the patient's ongoing narrative and responsiveness in the psychotherapeutic relationship.

## DIMENSIONS OF ASSESSMENT

A number of areas provide valuable information in helping practitioners to answer the difficult question, "If I can't utilize everything, what do I utilize?" They span a broad range of patient, therapist, and relationship variables and together form a comprehensive package to draw upon in considering the endeavor of assessment.

### Treatment Readiness

Motivation for treatment has long been acknowledged as one of the most critical variables in psychotherapy (Mann, 1973; Prochaska, DiClemente, & Norcross, 1992). Two conceptualizations of treatment readiness are particularly cogent in organizing this complex variable. Fisch, Weakland, and Segal (1982) classified patients who present for therapy as "window-shoppers," "complainants," or "customers." Determination of the level of motivation derives from the manner in which patients (overtly or covertly) answer two questions: (1) "Is there a problem?" (2) "Are you willing to work on the problem?" The window-shopper responds "No" to both questions; the complainant says "Yes" to the first, but

"No" to the second; and the customer replies in the affirmative to both questions. The authors outline various strategies and procedures for working with all levels of motivation.

Prochaska and his colleagues (Prochaska, 1991; Prochaska & DiClemente, 1992; Prochaska, DiClemente, & Norcross, 1992) have identified five stages that people typically traverse when engaging in personal change. The first stage, Precontemplation, is marked by unawareness or underawareness of problems and individuals in this stage have no intention of changing their behavior in the near future. Contemplation is characterized by "knowing where you want to go but are not quite ready yet" (Prochaska, DiClemente, & Norcross, 1992, p. 1103), being aware that a problem exists, and thinking about change, but without committing to action. Persons in the third stage, Preparation, start to institute behavioral measures for change but not to the extent of taking effective action. The Action stage involves commitment of time and energy to the modification of behavior and experience with the firm intention of conquering the problem(s). The final stage, Maintenance, entails consolidation of progress and stabilization of behavior to avoid relapse. Prochaska (1995) later added a sixth and final stage, Termination, during which "there is zero temptation to engage in the problem behavior, and there is a 100 percent confidence (self-efficacy) that one will not engage in the old behavior regardless of the situation" (p. 253). These researchers advocate "the need to assess the stage of a client's readiness for change and to tailor interventions accordingly" (Prochaska, DiClemente, & Norcross, 1992, p. 1110). There is abundant research to support their recommendation, and treatment readiness is a variable of which all therapists should be mindful.

## Expectancy

Expectancy is a tremendously powerful factor in the manner in which patients respond to treatment and this is especially true of hypnosis (see Chapter 3 by William Matthews for more about expectancy theory). However, patients' expectations regarding hypnosis present a double-edged sword. On the positive side, favorable impressions regarding the possibilities that hypnosis can reveal in one's life add tremendous leverage to a patient's responsiveness to hypnotic interventions. On the other hand, unrealistic expectations are the worst enemies of hypnosis. Patients often dream that essential character change, single-session modification of long-standing behavioral patterns, and other magical solutions will ensue from the application of hypnosis. In his 22 years of practicing hypnosis, this author has heard requests for hypnosis to, for example: "Make me stop eating," "Make me able to stop my husband from using cocaine," and "Help me to elicit an ego state that was present before I learned to talk so that I can learn a new language without interference from the language I already speak." It is incumbent on practitioners to ascertain the expectations that patients have of hypnosis and to modify them, if necessary, to be realistic and attainable. Failure to do so almost certainly dooms the therapy to disappointment, if not outright failure.

## Hypnotic Phenomena

A number of clinicians (Geary, 1994, 1996; Gilligan, 1987; Wolinsky, 1991) have noted similarities between hypnotic states and the processes involved in psychological and interpersonal problems. Specifically, the focused awareness that is characteristic of trance is a cardinal feature of the difficulties that bring patients to psychotherapy. Examples are abundant: the brooding and rumination of depression, fixation on fear and avoidance in anxiety disorders, the repetitive replaying of disputes in relationships, and so on. It follows that the behavioral and perceptual underpinnings of therapeutic trance states, the hypnotic phenomena, would also be present in other trancelike situations, such as those that are found in emotional and interpersonal disorders.

Geary (1994) proposes a system in which the trance phenomena that are involved in the maintenance of presenting problems can be assessed and utilized. From this perspective, hypnotic phenomena are viewed as existing on continua of experience (Table 1.1).

**Table 1.1**

**Continua of the Trance Phenomena**

Age regression - - - - - - - - - - - - - - - - - - - - - - - - - - Age progression

Amnesia - - - - - - - - - - - - - - - - - - - - - - - - - - - - - - - - Hypermnesia

Anesthesia - - - - - - - - - - - - Analgesia - - - - - - - - - - - Hypersensitivity

Catalepsy - - - - - - - - - - - - - - - - - - - - - - - - - - - Flexibility/movement

Dissociation - - - - - - - - - - - - - - - - - - - - - - - - - - - - - - Association

Positive hallucination - - - - - - - - - - - - - - - - - Negative hallucination

Time expansion - - - - - - - - - - - - - - - - - - - - - - - Time condensation

Posthypnotic suggestion - - - - - - - - - - - - - - - Prehypnotic suggestion

The various hypnotic phenomena represent the extreme poles of most of these continua. However, not all hypnotic phenomena have complements that are also hypnotic phenomena. In these cases, appropriate labels for the opposite of the particular hypnotic phenomenon have been added (e.g., age progression, hypersensitivity, flexibility/movement). The behavioral and perceptual markers of the respective hypnotic phenomena (and their complements) are used figuratively in this system. For instance, because positive hallucination is the creation of perceptual experience that is not actual, the fantasies found in jealousy can be metaphorically considered to represent positive hallucinations. It is clear that a strict, psychiatric definition of positive hallucinations would not include such internal experiences. Thus, definitions of the hypnotic phenomena must be "loosened" somewhat in order for these classifications to have clinical usefulness. An examination of trance phenomena with a figurative eye allows one to consider problems in a new light. Patients often present in "stuck" (cataleptic) states, angry (hypersensitive), apprehensive (age progression), and otherwise unable to access (are dissociated from) the resources that would help them to accomplish their goals in life.

An advantage of this system is that the elements of problems are immediately translated into hypnotic processes. In clinical utilization, the practitioner decides which phenomena (there will always be multiple trance phenomena involved in any problem) offer the most potential for change when targeted for intervention. Sometimes a specific phenomenon that is involved in a problem will be utilized isomorphically, that is, in its same form. For example, the jealous individual might be encouraged to continue to generate positive hallucinations but be instructed to modify them into more benign scenarios. At other times, the complements of problem phenomena hold more promise for effecting change in the symptom(s). One might use action-oriented metaphors that encourage movement, for instance, in the treatment of a withdrawn, inactive depressed patient. This approach ties assessment and utilization together from the outset of therapy.

## Patient Variables

All patients bring strengths, limitations, and unique stylistic expression to the therapeutic encounter. The Ericksonian method generally seeks to identify and utilize resources while circumventing or accommodating limitations. Hence, both capabilities and restrictions must be assessed to formulate a realistic treatment plan.

Zeig (in Robles, 1991) offers a comprehensive set of criteria for assessment that focuses on patients' ways of interacting with both internal and external environments. For example, some individuals tend to prefer linear or mosaic information-processing styles, and some enhance experience whereas others reduce it. Zeig recommends that interviews be conducted to evaluate these variables, as well as others, such as whether people are focused or diffused in their attentional style, whether they tend to be intropunitive or extropunitive, and whether they absorb or emit in relational contexts. Information gained from this "action assessment" is designed to "focus the therapist, providing information on how the patient 'does' the problem."

Erickson seemed to be particularly mindful of skills that patients possessed, seeking to transfer existing talents into potential solutions for problems. He also probed for experiential referents, instances from the patient's past that could be reprised in memory and/or action to overcome contemporary difficulties. Haley (1973) also pointed out Erickson's adroitness at assessing developmental levels, transitions, and obstacles in his patients' lives. Another area for assessment, discerning the function of a symptom, has been most refined in family therapy but is certainly also germane to individual and couple therapeutic processes.

### Therapist Variables

Assessment is often presented as a unilateral concern, with scrutiny of the patient the sole focus. However, since at least two people are involved in the therapeutic relationship, assessment should be a two-way street. A therapist must engage in self-assessment to determine whether or not he or she is qualified to treat a particular patient, what forms of reactions the patient elicits, and which skills at the therapist's disposal are most salient for a specific case. Therapists can recall past patients who presented similar problems and styles to stimulate thinking about what might be beneficial or effective in a current situation. Associations that are generated in therapists during therapeutic conversations can be exceedingly valuable. One can listen for themes (e.g., struggle, hope, holding on/letting go), symbols (e.g., "This pit in my stomach"), and metaphors (e.g., "It's like I'm on this runaway train and I can't find the brake handle") to stimulate ideas about approaches that might be valuable for the patient. Continuous mindfulness of the therapist's professional experiences and personal reactions should be an integral part of any assessment process.

## The Therapeutic Relationship

The importance of continuously assessing dynamics in the therapeutic relationship cannot be overstated. Prominent practitioners of every psychotherapeutic persuasion emphasize the critical role that a positive therapeutic alliance plays in providing a foundation upon which the effectiveness of techniques rests. A wealth of research lends strong support to this contention (Orlinsky, Grawe, & Parks, 1994). As hypnosis often hastens and intensifies relationship processes, the practitioner who employs hypnotic methods must keep tabs on the manner in which relationship variables arise and develop. For instance, trust of the therapist is extremely important if the patients are to absorb and utilize hypnotic processes to their fullest extent. So, before initiating hypnosis, it is wise for therapists to pay heed to the level of trust that is present in the therapy. Conveyance of empathy, respect, and genuineness, those qualities that Rogers so long ago identified as essential for fostering change, are as salient today and it is vital that the Ericksonian practitioner assess them during the therapeutic process.

## Values

Recent research by Shalom Schwartz and his colleagues (Schwartz, 1992, 1994; Schwartz & Bilsky, 1987) has systematized the study of values and made them more available for use in psychotherapy. Because values "guide selection or evaluation of behavior and events" (Schwartz & Bilsky, 1987, p. 551), they are exceedingly important in the genesis and maintenance of problems and are powerful forces in bringing about change. Erickson's work is replete with examples of ways in which he discerned patient values and utilized them toward therapeutic ends (Geary, 1998). The assessment of values allows the therapist to delve into motivations and meanings that are evident in patients' lives. Consideration of values provides vital information regarding ways in which the therapy can be geared toward that which is most important for a particular individual. For instance, hypnotic strategies for a person who is hedonistically oriented will be drastically different from those designed to help someone who places greater emphasis on tradition and conformity. Sherman (1988) discussed ways in which Erickson incorporated social psychological principles into his therapy. The comprehensive study of values exhibits another way in which social psychology has lent valuable knowledge that practitioners can use to their patients' benefit.

## Direct and Indirect Methods

Since clinical assessment is oriented toward the formulation of therapeutic interventions, from the beginning of contact with the patient, the Ericksonian practitioner is gathering information with which to decide what approaches to take in that person's therapy. Erickson employed both direct and indirect techniques, although the latter have been stressed in writings about his approach. Indeed, the Ericksonian field has been somewhat remiss in providing clear guidance regarding the contexts in which the various methods under the direct and indirect categories are most therapeutically appropriate. This author believes that the following guidelines for the use of direct and indirect methods are useful in the evaluation of alternative approaches. It should be noted that direct and indirect suggestions have been found to be equally effective in hypnosis research (Lynn, Neufeld, & Maré, 1993) and that Ericksonian practitioners will, in reality, use a combination of these techniques. Also, the reader should remember that the guidelines are based on clinical experience and anecdotal evidence rather than on well-controlled studies. Moreover, since they are necessarily general in nature, there will be specific instances in which they do not entirely hold.

### *Attributional Style of the Patient*

Some people view the external environment as the determinant of their behavior. They see themselves as responding to forces that impinge upon them from without. Other people have a different perspective, maintaining that they are active agents, in control of what they decide to do at any given time. The manner in which a patient attributes control and influence can be an important consideration in choosing the approach to take. Since the therapist is part of the outside environment, individuals with an external style might respond better to clear and direct methods whose aim is to influence them in positive directions. Conversely, those who consider that it is their prerogative to decide what to do and when to do it might better adapt to an indirect approach in which the therapist offers possibilities for action rather than edicts regarding ways to behave.

### *Cognitive Style of the Patient*

People who are concrete in their thinking will generally respond better to communication that is more direct with regard to expectation and purpose, whereas those with an abstract style are better at gleaning messages that may be embedded within more metaphorical communication. Therapy should be designed to address particular needs and to enhance the motivation of a patient at whatever level is best for his or her understanding. Therapists can evaluate how their patients process information in order to convey therapeutic meanings in ways that are best suited to their preferences.

### Style of the Therapist

In the spirit of self-assessment, clinicians should be cognizant of the styles that they find the most comfortable. Some practitioners are not adept at taking a direct stance with their patients; others find abstract, anecdotal, and metaphorical communication difficult. Although particular methods can be learned and it is wise for therapists to develop as large an armamentarium of therapeutic techniques as possible, they should remain true to stylistic preferences that will allow them to maintain essential human contact rather than only apply techniques.

### The Role the Patient Wants the Therapist to Play

Patients come to therapy for a variety of reasons and desire different forms of interaction with therapists. Some people want guidance, others need advice, and still others seek the warmth of a caring relationship. At a symbolic level, patients look for therapists who will be parents, teachers, friends, companions, and a host of other figures. Because, above all, psychotherapy is the provision of a service, it is appropriate for practitioners to ascertain the role that patients want them to play. This can help to guide the stance that the therapist takes in the relationship. If a patient wants the therapist to act as a consultant, indirect methods that offer possibilities are consistent with the patient's desire. In other cases, more direct methods might be relevant if a client seeks advice and direction.

### Fearful/Apprehensive Patients

Hypnosis is rife with myths and misconceptions. Many patients who are candidates for hypnotic procedures are nervous about what might happen. It is sensible and respectful to be relatively direct with such patients in the initial stages of hypnotic therapy. Providing clear messages regarding hypnotic processes can help to alleviate fears and allow suggestions to be more effective. After apprehension is quelled, other variables assume more importance in fashioning the approach to therapy.

*Crisis Situations*

Indirect methods are essentially contraindicated for situations in which patients present or experience overwhelming circumstances. Individuals in crisis are in an enhanced state of responsiveness and respond quite readily to direct communication. As the overwhelming nature of the situation subsides, indirect methods may become more helpful.

*The Degree of Resistance Anticipated or Encountered*

Indirect methods have customarily been advocated as particularly useful with resistant patients (Zeig, 1980). However, Ericksonians have often ignored the fact that many patients are resistant to indirect methods as well. During assessment, a clinician can probe for responsiveness and/or resistance to both direct and indirect methods. In this way, resistance to interventions can be minimized or circumvented through subsequent choices regarding which method to use.

*Maintaining Leverage in the Therapeutic Relationship*

If a subject is told during hypnosis that something will happen and it does not, the failure will be attributed to the inadequacy of either the patient or the therapist, and thus direct methods are often risky from this standpoint. If there is uncertainty regarding whether or not a response will occur, it is better to offer it as a possibility, that is, through an indirect suggestion. On the other hand, a therapist's credibility is enhanced if he or she tells the hypnotic subject that something will happen and it does. Hence, in situations in which there is a high expectation that an experience will occur, direct suggestions generally work well. High-probability occurrences in hypnosis include relaxation (changes in breathing, muscle tone, and so on), perceptual alterations (e.g., enhanced vividness, analgesia and anesthesia), and catalepsy and spontaneous amnesia for portions of the hypnotic session. Less reliably elicited are specific amnesia, arm levitation, targeted recall, and hallucinations. The therapist enhances his or her opportunities to maintain therapeutic leverage by suggesting that lower-probability occurrences *might* or *can* occur and that alterations with a high likelihood of happening *will* happen.

## Goals of Treatment

As information about the nature and history of the problem, its meaning to the patient, and other relevant facets of information are elicited, the therapist and patient together begin to identify goals for the therapy (although, of course, the patient might express such goals very early in the proceedings). Similar to expectations for hypnosis, patient goals often have to be clarified, restated, and/or negotiated. Patients often state understandable but nonetheless unrealistic objectives for their psychotherapeutic encounters (e.g., "I never want to feel this anxiety again"). Therapists remain oriented to the existence of two goals. Each session has a particular objective that is incremental in satisfying the overarching goal for the entire therapeutic process. Both must be realistic and attainable. It is incumbent upon the therapist to formulate outcome objectives that can be satisfied and promote the types of changes that patients desire.

### Other Variables

The foregoing considerations do not constitute an exhaustive list of factors that can be assessed in the psychotherapeutic process. Some Ericksonian practitioners consider family-of-origin variables (e.g., birth order, family rules and roles, family secrets) highly influential in the origin and maintenance of problems and, therefore, of use in treatment. Erickson was interested in whether his patients grew up in urban or rural environments, utilizing the respective temperaments that he believed resulted as a backdrop for his therapy (Zeig, 1985). Valuable data can be obtained by asking patients about ways in which they typically change, how they believe their problem(s) will be solved, times in the past when they have overcome hardship, and what personal strengths and resources they believe will be most helpful in accomplishing that which they seek. Any area tapped during assessment is grist for utilization and so should be considered.

### CASE EXAMPLE

Rhonda, a 36-year-old married woman with two children, sought help with depression. She described her dysphoria in terms of being "stuck, not getting anywhere." Rhonda said that she felt "displaced" from her life, her family, and her job. "I just don't seem to feel things anymore like I used to," she complained. She presented a sequential, chronological account of a series of events she had encountered during the past six years that resulted in a worsening mood. Rhonda admitted that she had a tendency to "take things hard," that she was prone to interpreting remarks from others as criticism and brooding about them "for days on end." Asked what was most disturbing about her depression, she replied, "I think it's just my general lack of enjoyment, the lack of energy that I feel. I don't even seem to have the same kind of motivation to be as involved with my children and help them as I used to." She had participated in psychotherapy previously, she said, "But we just talked. I'm talked out. I want to experience something, feel something." Rhonda was taking medication and found it "somewhat" helpful but was interested in hypnosis, because: "Maybe it can help me feel more energy, feel more alive. I want to stay focused on what's good for me, what I need to do for myself. I want to feel better about how the future can be. I would consider this successful if I were able to move from a 5 to a 7 [on a 10-point scale] in my mood."

From this brief synopsis of Rhonda's first session, a number of the assessment areas outlined in this chapter can be highlighted for their influence on the manner in which the hypnosis was conducted. This patient's description of her depression as being "stuck" and "not getting anywhere" is a classic representation of catalepsy. Further, Rhonda was experiencing dissociation (the displacement from her life, family, and job) and analgesia at the emotional level, as shown in her lament about "not feeling the same anymore." Age regression was also involved in Rhonda's recounting of the events that had occasioned the decline in her mood. She seemed to have a favorable and realistic expectation of hypnosis; all of her objectives were certainly within the purview of the method. Rhonda exhibited a linear and absorbing style (per Zeig's criteria), and she was especially disturbed by the manner in which depression had interfered with her ability to derive enjoyment ("hedonism" in the Schwartz values system) from life and remain loving and helpful ("benevolence") to her children. Rhonda's attributional style tended to be external; her cognitive style was mildly abstract. Her request of the therapist seemed to be to play the role of a facilitator and there was no identifiable resistance. Rhonda seemed to be ready for treatment.

The initial hypnotic session employed an approach that involved complementary interventions for the catalepsy, dissociation, analgesia, and age regression. A blend of direct and indirect methods was used to accommodate, respectively, her external attributional style and her ability to abstract from analogies and anecdotes. The induction of hypnosis was accomplished in a sequential manner (utilizing the linear processing style), moving through the sensory systems, with progressive relaxation in the body. Suggestions were offered that Rhonda fully enjoy the array of sensations and images in "this place," slurred somewhat to sound like "displace," a play on one of the words she used to describe her experience with depression. Rhonda was reminded that many of the things that she heard and experienced would "stay with her for days" so that she could consider them and personalize the material in her life. In utilizing age progression, Rhonda was asked to imagine herself at some point in the future admiring the accomplishments of her children and acknowledging her vital role in their development. It was also suggested that her unconscious mind "can move you from a 5 to a 6; that's something the unconscious can readily do. And if it can move you from a 5 to a 6, certainly it can help you to move from a 6 to a 7."

Posthypnotic suggestions were offered that would allow Rhonda to feel increasingly connected with her life, family, and job, and permit the enjoyment that she had derived during hypnosis to expand into her daily activities. Several brief analogies on the subject of "connection" were interspersed (e.g., cars of a train, the energy of attracting magnets). Rhonda listened to the audiotape of the hypnosis almost every day. She reported great satisfaction with the results and, over the next six months, steadily improved. Subsequent hypnotic sessions built on the information derived from the initial assessment and incorporated comments that Rhonda offered in the time that followed.

## PROCESS ASSESSMENT

Assessment never really ends. The initial assessment provides the launch-pad for the psychotherapy. But clinicians continue to assess responsiveness on the part of their patients, both in the consulting room and through reports of between-session experiences. Because therapy is generally composed of multiple encounters, a consistent focus is maintained upon the extent to which treatment is facilitating change in the desired direction. Whether hypnotic or other methods are utilized, assessment of the therapeutic process promotes ongoing adjustments and refining of utilization. The ultimate assessment occurs, of course, when patients decide whether or not they have achieved their therapeutic ambitions. If they have, evaluation leads to termination. If not, the assessment cycle begins anew.

## CONCLUSION

Utilization is the fuel that drives Ericksonian psychotherapy, a vehicle that allows therapists and patients to navigate great distances of personal change and evolution. Assessment is the mechanism by which the often dismaying range of possibilities for utilization can be narrowed and individualized. Assessment and utilizing are in a reciprocal relationship: thorough assessment refines that which is utilized, and this, in turn, fosters more material to be assessed. Erickson's revolutionary principle of utilization continues to reverberate throughout the psychotherapeutic world. It promotes a conceptualization of assessment as a perpetual theme in the process of psychotherapy. It is as essential to utilization as is the melody to a song.

---

**Key Points**

- Assessment begins with the first therapist–patient contact.
- Assessment does not end until therapy ends.
- Anything can be utilized; anything can be assessed.
- Self-assessment by the therapist is as important as is assessment of the patient.
- Assessment and utilization are inseparable.

---

### References

Fisch, R., Weakland, J. H., & Segal, L. (1982). *The tactics of change*. San Francisco: Jossey-Bass.

Geary, B. B. (1994, December). *Systematic utilization of the hypnotic phenomena in Ericksonian hypnosis and psychotherapy*. Presented at the Sixth International Congress on Ericksonian Approaches to Hypnosis and Psychotherapy, Century City, CA.

Geary, B. B. (1996, May). *Guidelines in the utilization of direct and indirect methods in hypnotic psychotherapy*. Presented at the International Congress on Hypnosis and Modified States of Consciousness, Rome, Italy.

Geary, B. B. (1998, November). *Utilization of values in Ericksonian hypnosis and psychotherapy*. Presented at the Third European Congress on Ericksonian Hypnosis and Psychotherapy, Venice, Italy.

Haley, J. (1973). *Uncommon therapy: The psychiatric techniques of Milton H. Erickson, M.D.* New York: Norton.

Hilgard, E. R. (1965). *Hypnotic susceptibility.* New York: Harcourt, Brace & World.

Kihlstrom, J. F. (1985). Hypnosis. *Annual Review of Psychology, 36,* 385–418.

Lynn, S. J., Neufeld, V., & Maré, C. (1993). Direct versus indirect suggestions: A conceptual and methodological review. *International Journal of Clinical and Experimental Hypnosis, 41* (2), 124–152.

Mann, J. (1973). *Time-limited psychotherapy.* Cambridge, MA: Harvard University Press.

Orlinsky, D. E., Grawe, K., & Parcs, B. K. (1994). Process and outcome in psychotherapy—*Noch einmal.* In A. E. Bergin & S. L. Garfield (Eds.), *Handbook of psychotherapy and behavior change* (4th ed.). New York: Wiley.

Prochaska, J. O. (1991). Prescribing to the stages and levels of change. *Psychotherapy, 28,* 463–468.

Prochaska, J. O. (1995). Common problems—common solutions. *Clinical Psychology: Science and Practice, 2,* 101–105.

Prochaska, J. O., & DiClemente, C. C. (1992). Stages of change in the modification of problem behaviors. In M. Hersen, R. M. Eisler, & P. M. Miller (Eds.), *Progress in behavior modification* (pp. 184–214). Sycamore, IL: Sycamore Press.

Prochaska, J. O., DiClemente, C. C., & Norcross, J. C. (1992). In search of how people change. *American Psychologist, 47,* 1102–1114.

Robles, T. (Ed.). (1991). *Terapia cortada a la medida. Un seminario Ericksoniano con Jeffrey K. Zeig.* Mexico: Alom Editores.

Rogers, C. (1951). *Client-centered therapy: Its current practice, theory, and implications.* Chicago: Houghton-Mifflin.

Schwartz, S. H. (1992). Universals in the content and structure of values: Theoretical advances and empirical tests in 20 countries. *Advances in Experimental Social Psychology, 25,* 1–65.

Schwartz, S. H. (1994). Are there universal aspects in the structure and contents of human values? *Journal of Social Issues, 50,* 19–45.

Schwartz, S. H., & Bilsky, W. (1987). Toward a psychological structure of human values. *Journal of Personality and Social Psychology, 53,* 550–562.

Sherman, S. J. (1988). Ericksonian psychotherapy and social psychology. In J. K. Zeig & S. R. Lankton (Eds.), *Developing Ericksonian therapy: State of the art.* New York: Brunner/Mazel.

Weitzenhoffer, A. M., & Hilgard, E. R. (1959). *Stanford Hypnotic Susceptibility Scale, Forms A and B.* Palo Alto, CA: Consulting Psychologists Press.

Weitzenhoffer, A. M., & Hilgard, E. R. (1962). *Stanford Hypnotic Susceptibility Scale, Form C*. Palo Alto, CA: Consulting Psychologists Press.

Wolinsky, S. (1991). *Trances people live*. Falls Village, CT: Bramble.

Zeig, J. K. (1985). *Experiencing Erickson*. New York: Brunner/Mazel.

# 2

# Hypnotic Induction

*Jeffrey K. Zeig*

## INTRODUCTION

Initiating hypnotic induction is a little like fostering love. One cannot elicit an emotional state, such as love, by intoning, "Go deeply into love." Similarly, one does not elicit hypnosis by commanding a passive patient, "Go deeply into trance."

Note a key word in the previous sentence, *elicit*. Hypnosis is elicited, not induced (despite the label "induction"). Ernest Rossi (1976) cogently expounded the elicitation model in a number of the books that he coauthored with Milton Erickson, including *Hypnotic Realities*. The word "induction" conjures up images of implanting suggestions in a passive patient. Elicitation speaks to the essence of the matter. The hypnotherapist establishes conditions that allow the patient to bring forth previously dormant trance components.

## TRADITIONAL HYPNOSIS

Before describing the advances of the Ericksonian approach, I will investigate the traditional model, which is based on five stages that are accomplished linearly: *preinduction, induction, deepening, therapy,* and *termination*. Direct suggestions are a favored technique. Following is a reductionistic description.

In the *preinduction* stage, the operator establishes rapport, diagnoses the problem, demystifies hypnosis, and uses classic suggestibility tests to ascertain the patient's hypnotic capacity.

In the *induction* stage, the operator generally uses a preferred hypnosis script based mostly on suggestions of relaxation and fascination.

In the *deepening* stage, the hypnotist intensifies the experience through such techniques as direct suggestion ("Go deeper and deeper"); counting ("As I count from 1 to 10, you will go one tenth the way deeper with each count."); and imagery (e.g., "the beach scene" or "staircase method.") Also, there may be a challenge suggestion, such as, "Your eyes are glued shut, try to open them; you will find you can't."

In the *therapy* stage, the hypnotist offers direct suggestions, usually positive ("You will relax in an airplane") or negative ("Cigarettes will taste bad").

In the *termination* stage, the hypnotist reorients the patient, gives ego-building suggestions ("You are a great person capable of doing many things on your own behalf"), and reestablishes rapport. In the induction, deepening, and therapy stages, it was implied that rapport was with the unconscious mind.

The traditional induction is linear. It is a means of establishing trance.

The Ericksonian model is patient-based and flexible. It is more mosaic and multileveled than linear. To understand the Ericksonian advantage, we should understand the phenomenology of trance.

## The Characteristics of Trance

Continuing with the previous analogy, when a lover wishes to elicit feelings of love in a partner, he or she does so by setting a stage and decorating it with "props." For example, a man might offer his loved one flowers, poems, and other romantic gestures. In response, the object of his affection might access tender feelings toward the lover.

Love can be considered a compilation of specific phenomenological components, including respect, admiration, lust, luminance, and attachment. To elicit the phenomenology of love, the lover both establishes a setting and acts in ways in which phenomenological components of love can be experienced.

Similarly, one can conceive of the job of the hypnotist as being that of a "stage director," setting up props in the patient's psychosocial theater in order to elicit target phenomenological components.

## THE PHENOMENOLOGY OF HYPNOSIS

What are the phenomenological characteristics of hypnosis? Hypnotized patients, asked to dissect their experience, report a number of phenomenological components, including:

- Alterations in attention
- Modifications in intensity
- Sensations of dissociation
- Changes in responsiveness (cf. Zeig, 1988)

The four categories are not comprehensive. Hypnotized patients often report other experiences, such as mild feelings of mystification and unreality. An additional characteristic of trance is a social injunction, which includes defining the particular situation as "hypnotic" (Barber, 1969). Defining the situation in this manner can change the way in which the hypnotic subject experiences the hypnotist's offerings.

Because the aforementioned four categories predominate, they could be considered primary phenomenological characteristics of hypnosis. The additional factors (and more) can be considered secondary phenomenological factors. What experientially constitutes primary and secondary characteristics of hypnosis depends on the interaction between the orientation of the patient and that of the clinician.

It is incumbent upon a clinician to understand the patient's phenomenology of hypnosis in order to structure the most effective induction. Therefore, the four primary characteristics will be described in detail.

### Alterations in Attention

Attention is customarily altered in two dimensions: it is directed internally, and it is focused. There are clinical situations in which hypnosis is best effected by eliciting diffuse and external attention, but they are beyond the scope of this chapter. Although it is more accurate to speak of alterations in attention, thereby allowing the possibility for diffuse and external attention, most patients, when asked to describe their attentional process in hypnosis, specifically indicate that they directed their attention internally, and that their attention was riveted rather than wandering.

### Modifications in Intensity

There are two directions in which intensity can be altered—it can be increased or decreased. Hypnotized patients often report an increased vividness, as, for example, vivid relaxation. They also may report other vivid sensory experiences, including changes in tactile, visual, auditory, proprioceptive, and the chemical senses (taste and smell). Body sensations may be more vivid, sounds may be more vivid, the experience of time passing may be more vivid, and so forth.

Hypnotized patients also may report that experiences are notably absent in any sensory sphere. A patient may describe being unaware of sights, sounds, odors, tastes, touch or the position of limbs in space. Moreover, there can sensory distortions. Limbs may feel larger or smaller. Sounds may seem closer or more distant.

## Dissociation

There are two aspects to dissociation: sensations of being "part of and apart from" the experience, and sensations of automaticity, whereby experiences "just happen." Hypnotized patients commonly report, "I was here in the office, but I was *there* absorbed in my fantasy." Hypnotized patients also may experience automaticity mentally or physically. For example, images or memories may "just happen," as may movements, such as arm levitation.

## Changes in Response

Hypnotized patients commonly respond to a more nuanced suggestion—they respond to innuendo and implication. This type of behavior has been characterized as response to minimal cues. For example, if the hypnotherapist offers, "You can head forward into trance," hypnotized subjects might move their heads forward in response to the couched suggestion.

Also, hypnotized patients often engage in a refined search for meaning, activating an internal search to find personal and experiential meaning in the hypnotist's offerings. If, for example, the therapist tells an ambiguous story, hypnotized subjects tend to personalize more than would be common in the waking state.

It is difficult to know for any particular patient the exact phenomenology that would lead the patient to report, "I am hypnotized." It can be assumed that in a hypnotic situation, if the patient reports all four of the primary phenomenological characteristics, the patient will agree that he or she is hypnotized. Some patients, however, may accomplish just one of the phenomenological characteristics and report hypnosis. They may merely focus their attention internally and say that they were in a hypnotic trance. One of the arts of the hypnotist is to determine which phenomenological characteristics are sufficient for a given patient to indicate the existence of trance.

As previously indicated, the job of the hypnotherapist is to place props on a patient's psychosocial stage so that the patient, by "playing" with these "props," can elicit his or her unique hypnotic phenomenology. In initiating trance with a new patient, the therapist can place all four hypnotic props on the patient's stage by making suggestions that cover each of the four areas and observe which toys the patient finds especially compelling. Indirect methods can be used to offer the hypnotic phenomenology because they best facilitate the experience of some of the phenomenological components.

## INDIRECT METHODS

We can note the essential importance of indirect methods to hypnosis, especially as they relate to the goal phenomenology. The first two phenomenological characteristics, altered attention and modified intensity, can be evoked through direct suggestion. For dissociation and responsiveness to minimal cues, however, indirect suggestion is most effective. One cannot tell a patient, "Lift your hand," and expect the movement to be involuntary. It is best to use some degree of indirection to promote automaticity.

In building responsiveness, the hypnotist can use direct suggestion— "Close your eyes." But, because the hypnotherapist fosters responses to minimal cues during the elicitation process, indirect suggestions are increasingly offered, ranging from embedded commands, such as, "You can ... *lift* your hand," to telling a series of anecdotes that imply lifting one's hand, such as describing a pupil asking a question in a classroom or a child wanting cookies up on a shelf, until the response of arm levitation follows.

Indirect suggestions empower the trance by fostering phenomenological goals. Erickson championed indirect suggestions, and his collaborators, such as Rossi (1976), have categorized the types of indirect suggestion that Erickson used. Following are four examples of indirect suggestions, each of which can be used to invoke a specific phenomenological response.

## Examples of Indirect Suggestion

- The "yes set"
- Embedded commands
- Dissociation statements
- The implied causative

Consider how each is structured and why it is valuable in inducing hypnotic phenomenology.

*The Yes Set*
The "yes set" is created by sequencing a series of truisms, for example:

"You can hear the sounds outside."
"You can listen to my voice."
"You can hear your own breathing."
"And, you can notice the sound changes that occur as you focus inside."

The "yes set" is especially useful for eliciting the phenomenological response of *guiding attention*. In the above example, the "yes set" guides attention to the auditory sphere, progressively, from external to internal reality.

*Embedded Commands*
Pausing (and inflecting) after a permissive auxiliary verb can create embedded commands because, in English, the subsequent verb is in the imperative form. The sentence, "You can go into trance," thus can be made into an embedded command: "You can ... *go* into trance." The verb *go* can be under- or overemphasized to highlight the command.

Embedded commands are mildly confusing because they simultaneously address two levels: It is not immediately apparent whether the clinician is giving information or commanding a response.

Among other goals, embedded commands can be used to address the phenomenology of *increasing intensity*, for example, "You can ... really experience the vivid sensations of comfort."

*Dissociation Statements*

Dissociation statements come in many forms, such as: "Your conscious mind can listen to my voice while your unconscious mind can float, because it is so interesting to realize different experiences."

Dissociation statements can be used to address the phenomenology of *dissociation*, whereby things "just happen" and/or the person feels "part of and apart from" the experience.

*The Implied Causative*

The "implied causative" is in the form, "When $X$, then $Y$," where $X$ can be a behavior and $Y$ can be a state, or vice versa; for example, "When you take a deep breath, then you can go into a trance," or "When you go into a trance, you can take a deep breath." The implied causative is used to *promote responsiveness*, one of the four primary phenomenological characteristics.

These four examples of indirect suggestion represent some of the language of hypnosis. They are commonly used within the "induction" structure as props that stimulate into play (elicit) phenomenological goals. Indirect suggestions also result in a multilevel induction that fosters activation in the patient, who must search for personal meaning.

So that we may better understand how the language of hypnosis is used, let us examine the induction structure used at the Erickson Foundation.

## THE ARE MODEL

At the Intensive Training Program offered by the Milton H. Erickson Foundation, Brent Geary and I have developed a general model influenced by Milton Erickson. We teach a three-step procedure for placing hypnotic props on the patient's stage. The "induction" procedure is called the ARE model: A for absorb, R for ratify, and E for elicit.

Clinicians can use the ARE model in a sequential manner. Absorption is elicited through the use of specialized techniques, many of which are indirect. Ratification is accomplished in a more direct manner. The elicitation, again, is indirect.

### Absorption

There are both *absorption devices* and *absorption techniques*. An absorption device might involve engaging the patient in a sensation, perception, hypnotic phenomenon, fantasy, or memory. An experienced clinician will not leave the choice of an absorption device to chance; rather, the selection of the device will depend on the characteristics of the patient and the goal to be accomplished by both the induction and the therapy. The choice of induction devices is beyond the scope of this chapter.

Numerous primary and secondary techniques are available to accomplish absorption. Primary techniques include speaking in the present tense, using possibility words, and providing comprehensive details. Among secondary techniques are changes in tone of voice, pauses, and alterations in voice locus. The distinction between primary and secondary absorption techniques is artificial and is a matter of the frequency of application.

Consider an example: Say that the hypnotist chooses as an absorption device a sensation, namely, warmth. Subsequently, the hypnotherapist can describe warmth, speaking about details and possibilities in the present tense.

> As you close your eyes, and go inside, you may be able to notice sensations of warmth. And I do not know if you will notice these sensations of warmth in the front or the back of your body. Perhaps the sensations of warmth seem large or small ... Perhaps, as you realize those sensations of warmth, it can seem to you as if somehow there is a cushion of warmth. And it may feel as if you can begin to rest easily into that very pleasant cushion of warmth. And those sensations of warmth can be so interesting. And you might notice how the sensations of warmth can begin to change. They may begin to move. They may begin to develop inside. They may begin to alter in shape ... And you do not need to notice all the sensations ...

During absorption, while describing details and possibilities in the present tense, the hypnotherapist stresses phenomenological experiences. Again, it is as if the hypnotherapist puts props on the patient's psychosocial stage. Through the absorption patter, the patient is encouraged to focus attention, direct attention internally, and experience sensations more or less vividly. As will be seen, dissociation suggestions also can be interjected. Note that it is not the commands of the hypnotherapist that are operative, but rather that the hypnotherapist suggests possibilities from which the patient can choose. As the patient activates in order to experience the suggested phenomena, hypnosis is accomplished.

*Additional Absorption Strategies*

The absorption stage provides an opportunity for the accomplishment of additional operations. For example, during absorption the therapist can seed the intended therapy by indirect allusions to the interventions to come. Such foreshadowing increases the response to the intended therapeutic target. (For further information about seeding, see Zeig, 1990 and Geary, 1994.)

During absorption, the clinician can tailor the absorption technique and device to the unique style of the patient, thereby creating rapport. Also, the hypnotherapist can use a technique such as linkage, whereby conjunctions—such as "and" or "or"—join phrases to create an interwoven flow of ideas, which mirrors actual internal experience.

Absorption, moreover, provides an opportunity to offer therapeutic directives unexpectedly. The absorption stage is not merely a means to establish trance, but also serves as a method of therapy. By "doubling up" on techniques and using "condensed communication," the clinician offers a rich multilevel matrix that can accomplish both induction and therapy goals. This is in contradistinction to traditional induction, which is solely a linear vehicle used to establish the trance state.

*The Language of Hypnosis*

Indirect techniques that compose the language of hypnosis can be inserted into the induction patter further to facilitate phenomenological goals. For example, the "warmth induction" can be modified as follows:

> As you close your eyes, and go inside, you may be able to notice sensations of warmth. And I do not know if you will notice these sensations of warmth in the front or the back of your body. Perhaps the sensations of warmth seem large or small ... Perhaps, as you realize those sensations of warmth, it can seem to you as if somehow there is a cushion of warmth. And it may feel as if you can begin to rest easily into that very pleasant cushion of warmth. *And you can notice the warmth in your feet. And you can notice the warmth in your legs. And you can notice the warmth in your body. And you can ... notice the developing warmth.* (**Yes set and embedded command**) And those sensations of warmth can be so interest-

ing. And you might notice how the sensations of warmth could begin to change. They may begin to move. They may begin to develop inside. *And your conscious mind can notice the warmth while your unconscious mind can attend to the developments.* (**Dissociation statement**) They may begin to alter in shape ... And you do not need to notice all the sensations. *But when you begin to realize the sensations of warmth, you can take a deep breath and really experience the developing comfort.* (**Implied causative**)

Notice how the inclusion of the language of hypnosis makes the "induction" multilevel and adds other possibilities for achieving the goal phenomenology. Interspersing the language of hypnosis places new phenomenological props on the patient's stage. Therapeutic directives also can be interspersed in the induction by using direct and indirect language forms.

## Ratification

During the ratification stage, the hypnotherapist uses a series of simple declarative sentences to ratify the trance by reflecting back changes that took place in the patient subsequent to the initiation of the elicitation process. Note that in ratification, the hypnotherapist no longer describes possibilities, but, rather, describes facts. For example, during the ratification stage, the hypnotist may say:

As I have been talking with you, certain changes have occurred: Your breathing rate has changed; your pulse rate has changed; your swallowing reflex has changed; your body's sensations may feel different.

The implication of the ratification statements is that the patient is responding, that these responses are "hypnotic" alterations, and that these changes mean that the patient is experiencing hypnotic alterations correctly.

## Elicitation

Elicitation has three aspects:

- Eliciting dissociation
- Eliciting responsiveness
- Eliciting resources

*Dissociation*

Dissociation can be elicited through suggestive techniques, such as dissociation statements. It also can be elicited through hypnotic phenomena, such as arm levitation, catalepsy, and positive and negative hallucinations, all of which are subjectively based to some degree on dissociation. For example, the hypnotherapist may suggest, "It can seem to you as if you are a bodiless mind, just drifting in space and drifting in time." Elicited hypnotic phenomena promote the experience of dissociation, because dissociation is an integral part of every hypnotic phenomenon. (For detailed discussion of hypnotic phenomena see Edgette & Edgette, 1995.)

The dissociation instructions are added so that the patient can further experience dissociation in the form of something "just happening" and/or as being both "a part of and apart from" the experience.

*Responsiveness*

Subsequent to eliciting dissociation, the therapist further develops responsiveness. For example, in the style of Erickson, the clinician might suggest, "When next I say the word 'now,' you can take a deep breath *now*." In eliciting the patient's response to the unexpected suggestion, the therapist builds, perhaps in a stepwise manner, responses from the patient to the therapist's overt and implied directives. One of the major purposes of hypnosis is to establish a fertile climate of responsive cooperation.

*Resources*

Once the therapist elicits responses, especially to minimal cues, the process of "induction" is over. Eliciting resources is the purview of hypnotherapy. Because this chapter centers on "induction," a discussion of resource elicitation is beyond the present scope. In general, the therapist may use indirect suggestions, such as anecdotes and metaphors, to stimulate the patient's previously dormant resources. For example, patients with a specific phobia, such as a fear of flying, have many resources that allow them to be comfortable in situations that others would perceive as difficult. They may be great public speakers, for example. Those who overeat have many resources for controlling movements of their hands. In general, the job of the therapist is to help patients to access dormant resources experientially in such a way that patients can employ these resources to solve or cope with the problem for which they have sought treatment.

§

The primary purpose of induction is to set the stage for the therapy to follow. If the therapist intends to use indirect techniques—such as metaphors, anecdotes or symbols—to help the patient elicit the phenomenology of change, then the induction paves the way by indirectly eliciting the hypnotic phenomenology.

Three phenomenologies are involved in hypnotherapy: that of the problem, that of hypnosis, and that of the solution. In the assessment period of therapy, the clinician determines the patient-specific phenomenological components of the symptom. Consider a patient who presents with depression. Depression can be viewed as a phenomenological experience with components that include an internal focus of attention, negativity, an orientation to the past, inactivity, hopelessness, and a lack of goals.

The therapist establishes a new phenomenology, the phenomenology of hypnosis, which consists of the previously mentioned primary and secondary characteristics. It can be understood that if the patient can shift phenomenology once, it can be shifted again, in an even more positive direction.

In the therapy (resource-elicitation) period of hypnosis, the therapist works to help the patient to establish the phenomenology of the solution. For example, the phenomenology of happiness, in contradistinction to the phenomenology of "depression," consists of being more external, being positive, being active, being hopeful, and having constructive, future-oriented goals. In this conceptualization, hypnotic induction is a bridge between the land of the problem and the land of solutions. The patient comes into the therapy in "reverse," experiencing the phenomenology of the problem. Subsequently, the hypnotherapist puts props on the patient's stage so that the patient can move experientially into "neutral," the state of hypnosis. Then, the therapist helps the patient experientially to elicit "first gear," namely, aspects of the phenomenology of changing or coping adequately. The remaining "gears" accelerate patients into greater satisfaction and augment their ability to apply previously dormant resources to the conduct of their lives.

### References

Barber, T. X. (1969). *Hypnosis: A scientific approach.* New York: Brunner/Mazel.

Edgette, J. H., & Edgette, J. S. (1995). *The handbook of hypnotic phenomena in psychotherapy*. New York: Brunner/Mazel.

Erickson, M. H., Rossi, E. L., & Rossi, S. (1976). *Hypnotic realities: The induction of clinical hypnosis and forms of indirect suggestion*. New York: Irvington.

Geary, B. J. (1994). Seeding responsiveness to hypnotic processes. In J. Zeig (Ed.), *Ericksonian methods: The essence of the story* (pp. 295–314). New York: Brunner/ Mazel.

Zeig, J. K. (1988). An Ericksonian phenomenological approach to therapeutic hypnotic induction and symptom utilization. In J. K. Zeig & S. R. Lankton (Eds.), *Developing Ericksonian therapy: State of the art* (pp. 353–375). New York: Brunner/Mazel.

Zeig, J. K. (1990). Seeding. In J. K. Zeig & S. G. Gilligan (Eds.), *Brief therapy: Myths, methods, and metaphors* (pp. 221–246). New York: Brunner/Mazel.

# 3

# Social Influence, Expectancy Theory, and Ericksonian Hypnosis

*William J. Matthews*

It has been my experience that the average Ericksonian-oriented therapist, when asked to describe the defining characteristic of Milton Erickson's approach to therapy, would be likely to say, "Erickson had no limiting theory of psychotherapy or personality. He was interested in what worked." Rossi (Erickson & Rossi, 1980) makes this point in discussing Erickson's notion of the "limiting preconceptions of most schools of psychotherapy" (p. xv). Erickson (Erickson & Rossi, 1980) notes that in the field of psychotherapy, there has been an overemphasis on theory and rigidity of practice. This is particularly evident in psychoanalysis with its underlying psychodynamic orientation, which, although actually practiced by few therapists, continues to influence the field (e.g., notions of a repressed unconscious, defense mechanisms, stages of development). Erickson made these observations in the 1950s, at a time when these beliefs were probably even more pronounced than today.

## WHAT ACCOUNTS FOR CHANGES IN PSYCHOTHERAPY?

Lambert's (1986) classic study of psychotherapy provides empirical support for Erickson's earlier broad criticism. Lambert calculated the percentage of the variance that could account for client progress and concluded that 40% of change is attributable to spontaneous improvement (i.e., simple statistical regression, positive life events); 30% to nonspecific factors of the client–therapist interaction (i.e., trust, empathy, insight, warmth); 15% to placebo effect (i.e., hope, expectation of change); and, finally, 15% to the actual treatment. These data suggest that 85% of clients would improve with the help of a sympathetic friend, and 40% would improve doing nothing—simply as a function of everyday events. Lambert's study reflects the earlier work of Hans Strupp (Strupp & Hadley, 1979; Strupp, 1980, 1993) in which empirical support was found for the significance of the nonspecific factors mentioned previously and their effect on treatment outcome.

Based on the current research literature, Erickson's concern with the overemphasis on and rigidity of treatment was well placed. Erickson clearly understood the importance of a positive expectation for change, the value of rapport with the client, and the importance of the client's current life situation (Rossi in Erickson & Rossi, 1980). I would suggest that his willingness and ability to vary his treatment approach was in the service of increasing the expectancy of treatment by life event interactions.

Prior to discussing the importance of expectancy in psychotherapy outcome, it would be useful to present a brief discussion of the current empirical research on the principles underlying Ericksonian therapy. My intention here is to suggest that essential claims concerning Ericksonian notions of hypnosis, hypnotic susceptibility, and utilization strategies (e.g., indirect suggestion) lack empirical support and that perhaps the data and the rule of parsimony suggest that a social influence expectancy-based model would be a better frame in which to consider an Ericksonian approach.

## BASIC ASSUMPTIONS OF ERICKSONIAN HYPNOSIS

As I have discussed elsewhere (Matthews, Conti, & Starr, 1998), four basic notions underlie Ericksonian hypnosis: (1) hypnosis is an altered state of consciousness; and as such (2) there are markers of this altered state that distinguish it from the waking state; (3) hypnotizability of the subject/client is a function more of the hypnotist's skill (i.e., utilization strategies) than of the subject/client's ability; and (4) the use of indirect hypnotic suggestion is, at least in some instances, more effective in producing hypnotic responses than is direct suggestion.

## Hypnosis as a State

Milton Erickson was a strong proponent of the altered-state position (Haley, 1967; Erickson & Rossi, 1979, 1980), as have been a number of his followers (e.g., Dolan, 1991; Edgette & Edgette, 1995; Lankton & Lankton, 1983; Matthews, 1985; Gilligan, 1987). This altered state of consciousness is produced by some form of hypnotic induction in responsive persons. The state produced is distinguishable from other altered states, and although suggestibility is a characteristic of this altered state, it is not the only distinguishing characteristic (Kirsch & Lynn, 1995).

Sarbin and Slagle's 1979 review of the literature on physiological indicants of the hypnotic state considered a wide range of research on respiratory, cardiovascular, hemodynamic, vasomotor, genitourinary, gastrointestinal, endocrine, and cutaneous functions. These authors concluded that (1) there is simply no evidence that physiological changes in the aforementioned functions are attributable to a hypnotic trance state, and (2) such physiological changes can be influenced by stimulation conditions, symbolic processes, and imaginings (p. 300). Careful and systematic empirical research, at least as yet, has failed to yield any consistent replicable physiological indicants of a hypnotic state (Kirsch & Lynn, 1995; Sarbin & Slagle, 1979). However, as Kirsch and Lynn (1995) point out, there *could* be an identifiable indicator of state yet to be identified that makes the state hypothesis not falsifiable.

T. X. Barber (Barber, 1969, 1979; Barber & Ham, 1974) has been a prolific researcher in considering an alternative explanation for the hypnotic state. The data produced by Barber and his colleagues (i.e., Barber & Ham, 1974) have led them to conclude that hypnotic behaviors (e.g., production of blisters, wart removal, pain reduction) and phenomena (amnesia, age regression, age progression, visual and auditory hallucinations, arm catalepsy, etc.) are a function of the client/subject's motivations, attitudes, and expectations rather than a result of an altered state of consciousness.

Erickson (Erickson, Hershman, & Secter, 1961; Erickson & Rossi, 1979, 1980) was a strong proponent of literalism as a clear behavioral indicator of hypnotic trance. In two well-controlled studies on literalism (Green, Lynn, Weekes, et al., 1990; Lynn, Green, Weekes, et al., 1990), the data indicated that a great majority of the highly hypnotizable subjects were not literal in their responding. Lynn and colleagues also found no difference in literal responding between the hypnotized and nonhypnotized task-motivated subjects.

In the absence of clear distinguishable physiological changes or behaviors (e.g., literalism) that would define hypnosis as an altered state, state theorists focused on the subjective reports of clients/subjects (i.e., that subjects report *feeling* different in their experience of hypnosis than in the normal waking state). Kirsch, Mobayed, Council, and Kenny (1992) sought to ascertain the accuracy of this claim. Experts in the field of hypnosis were asked to rate the subjects' open-ended written expressions of their states of consciousness and responsiveness to suggestion. Subjects were in either a traditional hypnosis, relaxation, alert hypnosis, or imagination treatment condition. Kirsch and associates found that the experts' ratings failed to distinguish the traditional hypnotic induction from non-hypnotic relaxation training, that the subjective experience of hypnotic suggestions after imagination training is indistinguishable from that after hypnotic inductions, and that suggestibility is unrelated to state of consciousness as assessed by experts.

### Hypnotizability as a Trait or Skill of the Hypnotist

In the Ericksonian paradigm, essentially all individuals have the capacity for hypnotic responding. The essence of achieving this responding lies in the individualizing of the hypnotic technique.

Trait theorists (e.g., Brown & Fromm, 1986; Hilgard, 1965; Kihlstrom, 1985; Orne & Dinges, 1989; Spiegel & Spiegel, 1978) maintain that the ability to experience hypnosis exists primarily within the person, not in the hypnotist. As Kirsch and Lynn (1995), in their review of the trait debate, stated: "There is ample support for the hypothesis that hypnotic responsiveness is a traitlike, aptitudinal capacity of the person: Different measures of hypnotizability are moderately to highly intercorrelated, typically in excess of .60 and a test–test correlation of .71 has been reported for a retest interval of 25 years" (p. 849). E. R. Hilgard (1982) stated that "the main source of the belief held by many practicing clinicians that everyone is hypnotizable is a confusion between the success of their psychotherapy and the role of hypnosis in it" (p. 398).

### Indirect and Direct Suggestion

While Milton Erickson was no stranger to the use of direct suggestion in his hypnotic approach, he has perhaps become, rightly or wrongly, most celebrated for his extremely creative use of indirection (i.e., indirect suggestion, puns, metaphors, anecdotes, and the like) in the process of hypnosis and hypnotic induction. Erickson (Erickson & Rossi, 1980) suggested that indirect suggestion has utility in helping the client to access unique potential and earlier life experiences, as well as a way in which conscious resistance can be bypassed.

In their review of the available data, Lynn and colleagues (1990) conclude that "the best controlled studies provide no support for the superiority of indirect suggestions, and there are indications that direct suggestions are superior to indirect suggestions in terms of modifying subjects' experience of hypnosis. Nevertheless, the overriding conclusion is that differences between a wide variety of suggestions are either nonexistent or trivial in nature" (p. 138).

## ERICKSON: EXPECTANCY AND SOCIAL INFLUENCE

If there is no empirical support for the notion of a hypnotic state, if hypnotizability is perhaps more a function of the subject/client than of the hypnotist's utilization skills, and if there are no convincing empirical data that favor the superiority of indirect suggestion, then what do we have when we speak of Erickson and Ericksonian hypnotherapy? Matthews (Matthews, 1985; Matthews, Conti, & Starr, 1998) and Sherman and Lynn (1990) suggest that the clinical brilliance of Milton Erickson can be understood in a social psychological frame. Erickson's unique skill was his ability to increase client motivation, expectancy, and belief that therapeutic change could and would occur. We would suggest that hypnotic "trance," depth of "trance," and hypnotizability are constructs that ultimately convey less meaning than do expectancy and motivation. Sherman and Lynn (1990) suggest that Erickson's clinical mastery was attributable to his use of patient reactance: seeding, framing/reframing, increasing patient effort, and including the patient as an active participant within the context of social influence. Perhaps the most significant variable in this frame is that of expectancy.

### Expectancy

Kihlstrom (1985) stated: "Hypnosis may be defined as a social interaction in which one person, designated the subject, responds to suggestions offered by another person, designated the hypnotist, for experiences involving alterations in perception, memory, and voluntary action" (p. 385). Kihlstrom offers a parsimonious definition of hypnosis based on social learning theory that does not require the notion of state, but in its stead places importance on the interactional and meaning-making nature of the relationship between hypnotist and subject/client. In social learning theory, human behavior is a function of cognitive processes involving the acquisition of information. This information can be acquired by direct or vicarious experience. Expectancy and the reinforcement value are central concepts in social learning theory: What is the likelihood that an event will occur (expectancy) and what is the value placed on the event (reinforcement) in a specific context? (Compare Rotter, 1954.)

Kirsch (1990) has made a convincing argument, based on social learning theory, for the role of expectancy as a singularly powerful determinant of hypnotic behavior and psychotherapy in general. He has shown that correlations between expectancy and hypnotizability are higher than are correlations between imaginative involvement and hypnotizability. Goal-directed imagery, considered by Barber (1969) to be an especially important determinant of hypnotic behavior, has been shown to be mediated by expectancy (Vickery & Kirsch, 1985). Kirsch (1990) makes the point that a good hypnotic induction is defined by what the subject believes a good induction to be, a good "trance" experience is based on subject belief and expectations of what a hypnotic experience will be. Rather than an artifact of hypnosis, he concludes that "expectancy is an essential aspect of hypnosis, perhaps its most essential aspect" (p. 143).

Erickson was a master of social influence and expectancy manipulation. His pragmatic willingness and flexibility to achieve positive therapeutic goals are well documented. His goal in the context of therapy was to utilize the client's reactance or resistance such that client could develop a sense of personal mastery and associate or reassociate skills from one context to the desired context. As part of this process, Erickson provided the clinical atmosphere in which clients learned to modify beliefs, perceptions, and behaviors, (i.e., he sought to create the expectancy for change).

## Indirection

Many of Erickson's interventions were based on indirection and circumventing client reactance/resistance. It is important to make a distinction between indirect approaches and the specific use of indirect suggestions for particular hypnotic behavior. While the empirical data do not support the latter, there is some general support for the former (Sherman & Lynn, 1990). Social psychologists have long observed that in order for people to maintain a sense of personal mastery, they will often react to or challenge the perceived threat (a notion to which any clinician who has worked with adolescents can attest). To offset the possibility of reactance, social psychologists have used deception and unobtrusive measures in their research (Sherman & Lynn, 1990).

Clearly, Erickson understood this notion and used deception and disguise of specific goals in order to achieve the desired results (cf. Haley, 1967, 1973). Erickson realized that some clients, in order to maintain a sense of personal mastery, would challenge him by refusing to experience hypnosis. He typically assumed that ultimately the client wanted to have the hypnotic experience, and he was exceptionally skilled at exploiting the client's challenge by instructing the client to fail and/or by defining any client response as some form of success (Haley, 1967; Erickson & Rossi, 1980).

Recent developments in the cognitive sciences suggest limitations to clients' conscious self-reports of their cognitive processes, thereby necessitating the use of alternative methods to work with the tacit and analogical levels of human experiencing (Gonçalves & Craine, 1990). Metaphor, analogy, and/or stories can become useful tools to suggest the possibility of change at this tacit or unconscious level of cognitive representation. For Erickson, the value of such a manner of expression in therapy was the opportunity to redirect and restructure the client's view of self and his or her relationship to the presenting issue.

This notion of circumventing the client's reactance by indirection (i.e., with stories, anecdotes, metaphors) raises interesting questions with regard to how indirection may be perceived by the client. The fact that the therapist assumes that he or she is being indirect does not necessarily mean that the client perceives the intervention similarly. Matthews and Langdell (1989) conducted a clinical study using hypnosis and multiple embedded metaphors (Lankton & Lankton, 1983) with six clients from a university counseling center. All clients received eight therapy sessions (four sessions employing hypnosis and the multiple embedded metaphor protocol in concert with four sessions using a cognitive-behavioral approach).

In posttreatment interviews, five of the six clients essentially reported total recall for the metaphors each had received and recognized that the metaphors were related to their presenting issues. These clients also stated that their presenting problems (e.g., anxiety, moderate depression, study difficulties) had significantly improved. The sixth client, however, reported no memory for the metaphors he was told, and reported no clinical improvement. The five clients who reported a positive clinical improvement indicated that while they were aware of what the therapist was doing (i.e., the purpose of the stories), they liked and trusted the therapist and believed the therapist to be working in their interests. The sixth client, who reported total amnesia, did not like the process or feel comfortable with the therapist's approach. Whereas the Matthews and Langdell (1989) study has clear methodological and generalizability limitations, it is at least suggestive of the meaning that clients may attach to the process of indirection, which may differ significantly from that of the therapist.

### The Importance of Effort

Sherman and Lynn (1990) cite cognitive dissonance theory as support for the concept that the greater the effort exerted toward a goal, the greater is the worth attached to the goal. Erickson believed in the value of effort (Lankton & Lankton, 1983; Matthews, 1985). His homework assignments to carry objects, climb mountains, visit museums, and so on, were designed to increase the expenditure of client effort in achieving the desired therapeutic goals. The greater the effort expended by the client, the more likely it is that he or she will invest in the process.

### Seeding/Priming

Erickson was clearly interested in influencing clients' thoughts and their perception of events and frequently used the techniques of seeding or priming to begin to orient client thinking in the therapeutically desired direction. His case of reframing a husband's impotence as a compliment to his wife (Haley, 1973) is a dramatic example of influencing the client's perception and altering the meaning of the initial presenting problem. A number of studies (e.g., Higgins, Rhodes, & Jones, 1977; LaRue & Olejnik, 1980; Wilson & Capitman, 1982) provide empirical support for the effect of priming a subject with a particular concept or idea and its clear effect on subsequent behavior. There are numerous clinical examples of Erickson's seeding ideas of change or suggesting particular behaviors early in the course of therapy or a given session so that these might take place at a later time. Seeding ideas in this manner is directly related to the notion of expectancy discussed earlier (cf. Haley, 1967, 1973; Erickson & Rossi, 1980). Erickson would frequently ask clients to think about or imagine themselves engaging in some particular behavior. Sherman and Lynn (1990) state that "by guiding clients' imagery, and the kinds of outcomes they thought about and explained, Erickson presumably affected how these clients behaved when the relevant situation arose" (p. 41).

## The Client as Active Participant

In this process of guiding client imagery, Erickson, while clearly directing the therapeutic process, was also seeking to engage the client as an active participant. Sherman and Lynn (1990) note the ample psychological research supporting the concept that self-generated words and ideas have greater weight and meaning in memory than does information presented from an external source. In his use of metaphors, Erickson was giving the client an opportunity, and creating a context in which, to develop a new and different understanding of the presenting problem and its resolution from that held upon entering therapy. Matthews (1997) discusses Erickson in view of the relatively recent development of narrative therapy.

In describing the narrative paradigm, Lakoff (1987) stated that: (1) humans are seen as storytellers; (2) thoughts are essentially metaphorical and imaginative; (3) the manipulation of thoughts is an intentional pursuit of meaning; and (4) reality is seen as set of ill-structured problems that can be accessed through hermeneutic and narrative operations. Within this perspective, Erickson's clinical interventions can be seen as a form of narrative reconstruction using direct and indirect techniques (stories, metaphors, etc.) to assist the client in constructing a more useful life narrative.

## CONCLUSION

The empirical research reviewed in this chapter found little support for the traditionally held Ericksonian beliefs in hypnosis as a state with identifiable markers, the universality of hypnotic suggestibility, or the increased effectiveness of indirect as compared with direct hypnotic suggestion. Instead, we have argued that the effectiveness, creativity, and ingenuity of Milton Erickson can be understood in terms of his seemingly intuitive grasp of the importance of expectancy, belief, and motivation for both the client and the therapist. There is considerable empirically based support for this viewpoint. Matthews (1985) suggested a cybernetic or interactional frame in which to consider the work of Erickson, rather than a simple linear or causal frame. In moving away from a hierarchical model (i.e., therapist as expert, client as passive recipient), he suggested that the client informs and influences the therapist, as does the therapist the client.

It is the author's contention that the essence of Erickson's approach was to create an expectancy for change; to disrupt, distract, or otherwise occupy the limited conscious mind; and so to create a context (based on the nonspecific factors discussed earlier) for the client in which a change in his or her self narrative could occur. Within this perspective, hypnosis is used as a social interaction constructed by the therapist and client in which different multiple realities for the client can emerge. It becomes a form of communication in which clients are provided with a context in which to develop a more useful life narrative than that with which they entered therapy.

Finally, one might ask what purpose it serves to make so fine a distinction between hypnotic "trance" and expectancy if the end result is clinical success. Our task as scientist/practitioners is to be as precise as possible in our operational definitions and use of various constructs in our attempt to understand observed phenomena. The rule of parsimony requires the simplest explanations that fit the data. Not to obey this rule unnecessarily obfuscates and mystifies any attempt to understand the natural world.

## References

Barber, T. X. (1969). *Hypnosis: A scientific approach.* New York: Van Nostrand Reinhold.

Barber, T. X. (1979). Suggested ("hypnotic") behavior: The trance paradigm versus an alternative paradigm. In E. Fromm & R. Shor (Eds.), *Hypnosis: Developments in research and new perspectives.* New York: Aldine.

Barber, T. X., & Ham, M. (1974). *Hypnotic phenomena.* New Jersey: General Learning Press.

Brown, D. P., & Fromm, E. (1986). *Hypnotherapy and hypnoanalysis.* Hillsdale, NJ: Erlbaum.

Dolan, Y. (1991). *Resolving sexual abuse: Solution-focused therapy and hypnosis for adult survivors.* New York: Norton.

Edgette, J. H., & Edgette, J. S. (1995). *The handbook of hypnotic phenomena in psychotherapy.* New York: Brunner/Mazel.

Erickson, M. H., Hershman, S., & Secter, I. I. (1961). *The practical applications of medical dental hypnosis.* New York: Julian.

Erickson, M. H., & Rossi, E. (1979). *Hypnotherapy: An exploratory casebook.* New York: Irvington.

Erickson, M. H., & Rossi, E. L. (1980). *The collected papers of Milton H. Erickson, Vol. IV.* New York: Irvington.

Gilligan, S. G. (1987). *Therapeutic trances: The cooperation principle in Ericksonian hypnotherapy*. New York: Brunner/Mazel.

Gonçalves, O., & Craine, M. (1990). The use of metaphors in cognitive therapy. *Journal of Cognitive Psychotherapy, 4*, 135–150.

Green, J. P., Lynn, S. J., Weekes, J. R., Carlson, B. W., Brentar, J., Latham, L., & Kurzhals, R. (1990). Literalism as a marker of hypnotic "trance": Disconfirming evidence. *Journal of Abnormal Psychology, 99*, 16–21.

Haley, J. (1967). *Advanced techniques of hypnosis and therapy: Selected papers of Milton H. Erickson, M.D.* New York: Grune & Stratton.

Haley, J. (1973). *Uncommon therapy: The psychiatric technique of Milton H. Erickson.* New York: Norton.

Higgins, E. T., Rholes, W. S., & Jones, C. R. (1977). Category accessibility and impression formation. *Journal of Experimental Social Psychology, 13*, 141–154.

Hilgard, E. R. (1982). Hypnotic susceptibility and implications for measurement. *International Journal of Clinical and Experimental Hypnosis, 30*, 394–403.

Kihlstrom, J. F. (1985). Hypnosis. *Annual Review of Psychology, 36*, 385–418.

Kirsch, I. (1990). *Changing expectations: A key to effective psychotherapy.* Pacific Grove, CA: Brooks/Cole.

Kirsch, I., & Lynn, S. J. (1995). The altered state of hypnosis: Changes in the theoretical landscape. *American Psychologist, 50*, 846–858.

Kirsch, I, Mobayed, C., Council, J., & Kenny, D. (1992). Expert judgments of hypnosis from subjective state reports. *Journal of Abnormal Psychology, 101*(4), 657–662.

Lakoff, G. (1987). *Women, fire and dangerous things: What categories reveal about the mind.* Chicago: University of Chicago Press.

Lambert, M. J. (1986). Some implications of psychotherapy outcome research for eclectic psychotherapy. *International Journal of Eclectic Psychotherapy, 5*(1), 16–44.

Lankton, S. R., & Lankton, C. H. (1983). *The answer within: A clinical framework of Ericksonian hypnotherapy.* New York: Brunner/Mazel.

LaRue, A., & Olejnik, A. B. (1980). Cognitive "priming" of principled moral thought. *Personality and Social Psychology Bulletin, 6*, 413–416.

Lynn, S. J., Green, J. P., Weekes, J. R., Carlson, B. W., Brentar, J., Latham, L., & Kurzhals, R. (1990). Literalism and hypnosis: Hypnotic versus task-motivated subjects. *American Journal of Clinical Hypnosis, 33*(2), 113–119.

Matthews, W. (1985). A cybernetic model of Ericksonian hypnotherapy: One hand draws the other. In S. Lankton (Ed.), *Elements and dimensions of an Ericksonian approach.* New York: Brunner/Mazel.

Matthews, W. (1997). Constructing meaning and action in therapy: Confessions of an early pragmatist. *Journal of Systemic Therapies, 16*(2), 134–144.

Matthews, W., Conti, J., & Starr, L. (1998). Ericksonian hypnosis: A review of the empirical data. In W. Matthews & J. Edgette (Eds.), *Current thinking and research in brief therapy, Vol. II*. Philadelphia: Taylor & Francis.

Matthews, W., & Langdell, S. (1989). What do clients think about the metaphors they receive? *American Journal of Clinical Hypnosis, 31*(1), 242–251.

Orne, M. T., & Dinges, D. F. (1989). Hypnosis. In H. I. Kaplan & B. J. Sadock (Eds.), *Comprehensive textbook of psychiatry* (5th ed., pp. 1501–1516). Baltimore: Williams & Wilkens.

Rotter, J. B. (1954). *Social learning and clinical psychology*. Englewood Cliffs, NJ: Prentice-Hall.

Sarbin, T. R., & Slagle, R. W. (1979). Hypnosis and psychophysiological outcomes. In E. Fromm & R. Shor (Eds.), *Hypnosis: Developments in research and new perspectives*. New York: Aldine.

Sherman, S. J., & Lynn, S. J. (1990). Social-psychological principles in Milton Erickson's psychotherapy. *British Journal of Experimental and Clinical Hypnosis, 7*(1), 37–46.

Spiegel, H., & Spiegel, D. (1978). *Trance and treatment: Clinical uses of hypnosis*. New York: Basic Books.

Strupp, H. (1980). Success and failure in time-limited psychotherapy: A systematic comparison of two cases. *Archives of General Psychiatry, 37*, 595–603.

Strupp, H. (1993). The Vanderbilt psychotherapy studies: Synopsis. *Journal of Consulting and Clinical Psychology, 61*, 431–433.

Strupp, H., & Hadley, S. W. (1979). Specific versus non-specific factors in psychotherapy. *Archives of General Psychiatry, 36*, 1125–1136.

Vickery, A. R., & Kirsch, I. (1985, August). Expectancy and skill-training in the modification of hypnotizability. In S. J. Lynn (Chair), *Modifying hypnotizability*. Symposium at the meeting of the American Psychological Association, Los Angeles.

Wilson, T. D., & Capitman, J. A. (1982). Effects of script availability on social behavior. *Personality and Social Psychology Bulletin, 8*, 11–20.

# 4

# Utilization: A Seminal Contribution, a Family of Ideas, and a New Generation of Applications[1]

*Barry L. Duncan, Scott D. Miller, & Susanne T. Coleman*

Milton Erickson was unencumbered by the prevailing orthodoxy of his time. His creativity continues to reverberate profoundly in often unacknowledged ways. Perhaps the most important of Erickson's principles is utilization. Consider the following vignettes.

Erickson saw Kim, a teacher troubled by nude young men hovering just above her head. She told Erickson not to take her young men away, but rather stop their interference with her everyday life. He suggested that Kim leave the nude young men in a closet in his office where they would be secure and not interfere with her teaching. She checked on the young men at first, but gradually stopped. Much later, Kim moved to another city and worried about her "psychotic episodes." Erickson suggested that she put her psychotic episodes in a manila envelope and mail it to him. Occasionally, she would send Erickson a psychotic episode and meanwhile continued a productive life (Erickson, 1980).

---

[1] The authors wish to thank Jim Keim and Douglas Flemons for their invaluable input to this chapter.

Erickson saw Bob, who requested that his irresponsible, reckless, driving be corrected. Erickson asked what he could do to be helpful and Bob's answer was that Erickson could do nothing, that Bob would have to do it his own way. Erickson asked how soon he wished to make the changes and Bob said that by the next month he should be driving properly. Bob's statement that he would have to quit in his own way was repeated in various ways over two sessions. Two weeks later, Bob reported jubilantly that he had handled things in his own way. He had driven so recklessly that at one point he had to abandon his car just before it hurtled down a mountainside. Since that incident, he stated, he had been driving safely and within legal speed limits.

Consider these cases in the context of the following descriptions of utilization. "Exploring a patient's individuality to ascertain what life learnings, experiences, and mental skills are available to deal with the problem . . . (and) then utilizing these uniquely personal internal responses to achieve therapeutic goals" (Erickson & Rossi, 1979, p. 1).

"These methods are based on the utilization of the subject's own attitudes, thinking, feeling, and behavior, and aspects of the reality situation, variously employed, as the essential components of the trance induction procedure" (Erickson, 1980, p. 205).

"Utilization theory emphasizes that every individual's particular range of abilities and personality characteristics must be surveyed in order to determine which preferred modes of functioning can be evoked and utilized for therapeutic purposes" (Rossi, 1980, p. 147).

"The therapist's task should not be a proselytizing on the patient with his own beliefs and understandings. . . . What is needed is the development of a therapeutic situation permitting the patient to use his own thinking, his own understandings, his own emotions in the way that best fits him in his scheme of life" (Erickson, 1980, p. 223).

Erickson's brilliance transcended clever tasks or magical inductions and is best reflected in the principle of utilization. The utilization method encompasses an unwavering belief in the client's self-healing, his or her regenerative capabilities. Erickson counted on Kim's and Bob's inherent abilities to provide direction in attaining their desired goals. Such a belief fits 40 years of outcome data demonstrating the client to be the most important component of the change process, accounting for 40% of outcome variance (Assay & Lambert, 1999; Tallman & Bohart, 1999). Research makes it abundantly clear that the client is the star of the therapeutic drama.

Utilization requires an intense focus on clients' views of their concerns, their goals for therapy, and their ideas about change. Erickson understood the importance of not attempting to eliminate Kim's nude men or confronting Bob's desire to "do it his own way." This focus includes an uninhibited determination (considered reckless abandon by some) to work within and respect the client's world view. Erickson did not become mired in his own fears (e.g., that he might be "reinforcing Kim's delusions") or a priori treatment preferences (e.g., that he needed to do "something" with Bob). Erickson kept Kim's envelopes in case she showed up to look at them—and she did. This stance of putting the client's view first is also supported by outcome research. In total, client perceptions of the relationship account for 30% of positive outcome. Indeed, client ratings of the alliance are the best predictor of success (Bachelor & Horvath, 1999).

This chapter connects Erickson's principle of utilization to a community of both theoretical and empirical ideas, and suggests yet another application. Much has been written about the utilization of client resources and competencies by the therapist (e.g., Berg & Miller, 1992). Less often discussed is the utilization of the client's perceptions of the presenting complaint, and how therapy and the therapist may best address the client's goals and expectations of therapy—what we call the client's theory of change.

## UTILIZING THE CLIENT'S THEORY OF CHANGE: A COMMUNITY OF IDEAS

The notion that client perceptions of problem formation and resolution have important implications for therapy has a rich, although somewhat ignored, theoretical heritage. Many have noted the clinical wisdom in attending to the client's own formulations about change in therapy. As early as 1955, Hoch stated:

> There are some patients who would like to submit to a psychotherapeutic procedure whose theoretical foundations are in agreement with their own ideas about psychic functioning. ... We feel that it would be fruitful to explain patients' own ideas about psychotherapy and what they expect from it. (p. 322)

Later, Torrey (1972) asserted that sharing similar beliefs with clients about both the causes and treatment of mental disorders is a prerequisite to successful psychotherapy. Wile (1977), too, believed that clients enter therapy with their own theories about their problems, how they developed, and how they are to be solved. Wile stated that "many of the classic disputes which arise between clients and therapists can be attributed to differences in their theories of [etiology and] cure" (p. 437). Similarly, Brickman, Rabinowitz, Karuza, et al. (1982) hypothesized that "many of the problems characterizing relationships between help givers and help recipients arise form the fact that the two parties are applying models that are out of phase with one another" (p. 375).

Building on Erickson's tradition of utilization, the Mental Research Institute (MRI) (Watzlawick, Weakland, & Fisch, 1974) developed the concept of *position*, or the client's beliefs that specifically influence the presenting problem and the client's participation in therapy (Fisch, Weakland, & Segal, 1982). The MRI recommended rapid assessment of the client's position so that the therapist could tailor all intervention accordingly. Similarly, Frank and Frank (1991) suggested that "ideally therapists should select for each patient the therapy that accords, or can be brought to accord, with the patient's personal characteristics and view of the problem" (p. xv).

Held (1991) separates therapist and client beliefs into two categories. Formal theory, held by therapists, consists of predetermined explanatory schemes (e.g., fixated psychosexual development, triangulation) addressed across cases to solve problems. Informal theory, held by clients, involves their specific notions about the causes of their particular complaints. Held suggests that strategies may be selected from any model based on congruence with the client's informal theory. Duncan, Solovey, and Rusk (1992) clinically demonstrate such a selection process in their "client-directed" approach.

Duncan and Moynihan (1994) assert that utilizing the client's theory of change facilitates a favorable relationship, increases client participation, and, therefore, enhances positive outcome. Duncan, Hubble, and Miller (1997) view the client's theory of change as holding the keys to success regardless of the model used by the therapist, and especially with "impossible" cases. Similarly, Frank (1995) concludes: "I'm inclined to entertain the notion that the relative efficacy of most psychotherapeutic methods depends almost exclusively on how successfully the therapist is able to make the methods fit the patient's expectations" (p. 91).

Scholars representing a wide variety of clinical orientations tend to agree that the client's perceptions about a problem's etiology and resolution are likely to affect the process and outcome of therapy. Do these hypothesized impacts have empirical support?

## UTILIZATION-RELATED RESEARCH: A BRIEF SAMPLE

Attribution research has an important bearing on the theoretical issues raised above. Claiborn, Ward, and Strong (1981) placed clients in conditions that were either discrepant or congruent with the therapist's beliefs about problem causality. Clients in the congruent condition showed greater expectations for change, achieved more change, and rated higher levels of satisfaction than did those in the discrepant condition. Tracey (1988) investigated attributional congruence with regard to responsibility for the cause of the problem, and found that agreement between the therapist and client was significantly related to client satisfaction and client change, and inversely related to premature termination.

Two studies (Atkinson, Worthington, Dana, & Good, 1991; Worthington & Atkinson, 1996) found that clients' perceptions about the similarity of their causal beliefs to those of their therapists were related to ratings of therapist credibility and how satisfied the clients were with therapy. Similarly, Hayes and Wall (1998) found that treatment success depends on congruence between clients' and therapists' attributions concerning client responsibility for a problem. They suggest that attending carefully to clients' attributions and tailoring interventions accordingly enhances effectiveness.

Client expectancies and beliefs about the credibility of specific therapeutic procedures may be an important factor in predicting who will benefit from therapy. For example, Hester, Miller, Delaney, and Meyers (1990) compared traditional alcohol treatment with a learning-based approach. Clients who believed that alcohol problems were caused by a disease were much more likely to be sober at six-month follow-up if they had received the traditional alcoholic treatment. Clients who believed that alcohol problems were a bad habit were more likely to be successful if they had participated in the learning-based therapy. It was the congruence between client beliefs and expectations and therapeutic approach that proved crucial. Finally, Crane, Griffin, and Hill (1986) found that how well treatment seemed to "fit" clients' views of their problems accounted for 35% of outcome variance.

It seems to be a recurring finding that the degree of credibility of the intervention, or fit, or match with the client's theory of change is a variable worthy of attention. The alliance provides further support of the importance of utilizing the client's theory of change to effect a positive outcome.


## ALLIANCE

Contrast the position of utilizing the client's theory with the stance of applying the therapist's orientation across cases. For Erickson, theoretical loyalty could lead to oversimplifications about people, close off possibilities for change, and promote technical inflexibility: "Each person is an individual. Hence, psychotherapy should be formulated to meet the uniqueness of the individual's needs, rather than tailoring the person to fit the Procrustean bed of a hypothetical theory of human behavior" (Zeig & Gilligan, 1990, p. xix).

Rather than reformulating the client's complaint into the language of the therapist's orientation, the data suggest the opposite: that therapists elevate the client's perceptions above theory, and allow the client to direct therapeutic choices. Such a process all but guarantees the security of a strong alliance.

Gaston (1990) summarizes the alliance into four components: (1) the client's affective relationship with the therapist, (2) the client's capacity to work purposely in therapy, (3) the therapist's empathic understanding and involvement, and (4) client–therapist agreement as to the goals and tasks of therapy. Whereas items 1 and 3 reiterate the importance of the relationship, the client's participation in and agreement on goals and tasks refer to the congruence between the client's and the therapist's beliefs about *how people change in therapy* (Gaston, 1990).

Utilizing the client's theory, therefore, proactively builds a strong alliance by promoting therapist agreement with client beliefs about change, as well as about the goals and tasks of therapy. The therapist and client work jointly to construct interventions that fit the client's experience and interpretation of the problem. In this way, interventions represent an instance of the alliance in action.

## UTILIZING THE CLIENT'S THEORY: PRACTICAL GUIDELINES

Within the client is a uniquely personal theory of change waiting for discovery, a framework for intervention to be unfolded and utilized for a successful outcome. To learn the client's theory, therapists may be best served by viewing themselves as "aliens" seeking a pristine understanding of a close encounter with the clients' interpretations and cultural experiences. Clinicians must adopt clients' views on their terms, with a very strong bias in their favor.

After direct inquiries about the client's goals for treatment are made, questions regarding his or her ideas about intervention are asked. What the client wants from treatment and how those goals can be accomplished may be the most important pieces of information that can be obtained. Recall how Erickson asked Bob about his view of change and how he could be helpful to Bob.

Client responses to similar questions provide a snapshot of the client's theory and a route to a successful conclusion.

- What ideas do you have about what needs to happen for improvement to occur?
- Many times people have a pretty good hunch not only about what is causing a problem, but also about what will resolve it. Do you have a theory of how change is going to happen here?
- In what ways do you see me and this process as helpful to you in attaining your goals?

It is also of help simply to listen for or inquire about the client's usual method of or experience with change. The credibility of a procedure is enhanced when it is based on, paired with, or elicits a previously successful experience of the client. Recall how Erickson utilized Kim's previously helpful solution of containing the nude young men in the closet in his suggestion to put the psychotic episodes in an envelope.

- How does change usually happen in the client's life?
- What do the client and others do to initiate change?

Utilizing the client's theory occurs when a given therapeutic procedure fits or complements the client's preexisting beliefs about his or her problems and the change process. We, therefore, simply listen and then amplify the stories, experiences, and interpretations that clients offer about their problems, as well as their thoughts, feelings, and ideas about how those problems might be best addressed. The degree and intensity of our input vary and are driven by the client's expectations of our role. *The client's theory of change is an "emergent reality" that unfolds from a conversation structured by the therapist's curiosity about the client's ideas, attitudes, and speculations about change.* As the client's theory evolves, we implement the client's identified solutions or seek an approach that both fits the client's theory and provides possibilities for change.

## THE CASE OF TOM

For five years, Tom, an 18-year-old college student, had been becoming increasing distressed by thoughts about having sex with young boys.

**Session One**

C:     I am physically attracted to children, but I haven't acted on my thoughts. I'm a pedophile. I've done lots of reading about pedophiles. You can wean yourself out of your behavior if you're young and willing to do it. But just in case, I'm looking into chemical castration. But I know if I got help from an expert, my chances might improve. You know, a normal person's mind doesn't function like that, dreaming about children. It's programmed into my mind.

Tom shared his beliefs about his problem (he is a pedophile), how change will happen (wean himself out of it), and the role of the therapist (expert). Although the therapist did not believe Tom to be a pedophile, she did not challenge his view.

T:     Since you have given it much thought and research and you have your own diagnosis, have you given thought to how you would accomplish your goals?

C:     Yes. It will take time. All I want is to meet a woman who is very special to me. Someone who cares about me, someone with whom I feel comfortable and safe. But first I need to focus on the thoughts.

The client's theory of change is crystalizing. He will wean himself off his thoughts of children by meeting someone who will care about him. But first, Tom said, he needed to focus on the thoughts; therefore, he was assigned the task of embracing his thoughts and learning from them.

### Session Two

C:    I've learned there is something missing from my life. I need some-one besides my family to share my life, a relationship. But I really don't know where to start.

T:    So do you think that if you find a relationship, the thoughts of children will go away?

C:    Yes, I do—yes, I am convinced.

Tom's theory of change has unfolded. Finding a relationship is his chosen method of eliminating the thoughts. The therapist assigns another task that gives credibility to Tom's beliefs regarding the problem and its solution. Building on Tom's research skills and his success with therapeutic tasks, he is asked to observe relationships to identify the type that he would like to have.

### Session Three

C:    I looked into relationships, talked to people, and found some interesting books. I wanted to tell you that if the situation were to present itself, I wouldn't do anything with a child. Dreams are dreams and actions are actions. There has been positive change. I thought I was a pedophile. Now I know that I am a fantasizer. All I do is fantasize, and I could probably fantasize about anything.

Tom, without confrontation of his belief, shifts his view of himself as a pedophile. The therapist amplifies and empowers the change and Tom discusses his plan to talk to women. The therapist follows the client's lead.

### Session Four

C:    I gave a girl a kiss! I was talking to her and she put her cheek down and I gave her a kiss. It was fun and felt good. I know I'm interested in girls and I think things are changing, but how can I be sure?

T:      Have your thoughts decreased?

C:      I think so, but I'm not sure.

Tom shared his exciting news and his uncertainty about the extent of the change. The therapist again highlighted the change and reinforced the connection between finding a relationship and reducing the thoughts. To measure Tom's progress, he was asked to monitor and rate his thoughts.

### Session Five

C:      I completed the assignment and I found that my thoughts have substantially decreased. If I dream of a kid, I can now immediately transfer my thinking to a woman. I get turned on by my thoughts of women. I've reprogrammed my thinking. It feels great.

Tom had his own theory on how to resolve his problem, and honoring that theory created a space for him in which to employ his strengths. Throughout the therapy, the client's ideas directed the process; the therapist utilized Tom's theory of change to direct therapeutic actions. Follow-up revealed Tom's continued attraction to, and pursuit of, women.

### ERICKSON WAS ON TO SOMETHING

This brief historical review revealed a rich theoretical tapestry made up of different orientations woven together by their consistent agreement on the importance of matching the client's ideas about problem formation and resolution. We briefly sampled the attribution, expectancy, and alliance literatures and established that these disparate literatures are in concert in their empirical support for utilizing (matching, fitting, sharing attributions with, being credible to, etc.) the client's theory of change.

Historically, mental health discourse has relegated clients to playing nameless, faceless parts in therapeutic change. This attitude is changing. No longer interchangeable cardboard cutouts, identified only by diagnosis or problem type, clients emerge as *the* source of wisdom and the solution. They are the true heroes and heroines of the therapeutic drama.

Unfolding the client's map reveals not only the desired destination for the therapeutic journey, but also possible paths to get there. In that endeavor, our clients have shown us trails we never thought existed.

## Evolving Client-Directed, Outcome-Informed Discourse

While a client-directed discourse is familiar landscape to many, it remains uncharted as to how that discourse may legitimize our efforts to third-party payers. We believe that further utilization of the client's ideas and perceptions holds the key. The assessment and utilization of outcome information as defined by the client may be the best possibility for proving the value of our services to managed care.

Developing such an outcome-informed discourse need not be complicated or time-consuming. Therapists can simply choose from measures already in existence that are standardized, take only minutes to administer, and are accompanied by normative data for comparative purposes. Rather than repeating the failures of the past and attempting to determine "what approach works for which problem," these methods focus on whether or not a given encounter is working for an individual client at a given point in time. They focus on the factors that research has shown really do make a significant contribution to outcome: incorporation of client strengths and ideas and the development of a strong therapeutic alliance (Hubble, Duncan, & Miller, 1999). Using standardized measures would also eliminate "treatment plans" containing sensitive and potentially damaging personal information.

Information learned from these instruments is "fed back" throughout the therapy process itself (Duncan & Miller, in press). This radical departure from the traditional use of assessment instruments gives clients a new way in which to look at and comment on their own progress and their ongoing therapy. The process is simple: clients who are informed, and who inform, feel connected to their therapist and the therapy process; their participation is courted and utilized as a pivotal component of change itself (Duncan, Sparks, & Miller, in press).

The client has been woefully left out of the loop regarding outcome and service accountability. Using measures that acknowledge the client's experience of progress and satisfaction would allow clients to *really* direct their therapy. The client's voice would be formally utilized in all aspects of therapy, thereby establishing an entirely different discourse—not a pathology or treatment approach, but the discourse of the client.

### UTILIZING THE CLIENT'S THEORY OF CHANGE

- Think of oneself as an alien seeking a pristine understanding of the client and his or her culture of change.

- Explore client stories, experiences, and interpretations particularly relevant to the problem and its resolution.
- Ask about and listen for the client's goals for therapy and ideas about change.
- Ask about and listen for how change has previously happened, including previous attempts at change.
- Ensure that the therapy amplifies, fits, or complements the client's preexisting beliefs about the problem and the change process.

### References

Asay, T., & Lambert, M. (1999). The empirical case for the common factors in therapy. In M. Hubble, B. Duncan, & S. Miller (Eds.), *The heart and soul of change*. Washington, DC: APA Books.

Atkinson, D., Worthington, R., Dana, D., & Good, G. (1991). Etiology beliefs, preferences for counseling orientations, and counseling effectiveness. *Journal of Counseling Psychology, 38*, 258–264.

Bachelor, A., & Horvath, A. (1999). The therapeutic relationship. In M. Hubble, B. Duncan, & S. Miller (Eds.), *The heart and soul of change*. Washington, DC: APA Books.

Berg, I. K. & Miller, S. D. (1992). *Working with the problem drinker*. New York: Norton.

Brickman, P., Rabinowitz, V., Karuza, J., Coates, D., Cohn, E., & Kidder, L. (1982). Models of helping and coping. *American Psychologist, 37*, 368–384.

Claiborn, C., Ward, S., & Strong, S. (1981). Effects of congruence between counselor interpretations and client beliefs. *Journal of Counseling Psychology, 28*, 101–109.

Crane, R. D., Griffin, W., & Hill, R. D. (1986). Influence of therapist skills on client perceptions of marriage and family therapy outcome: Implications for supervision. *Journal of Marital and Family Therapy, 12*, 91–96.

Duncan, B., Hubble, M., & Miller, S. (1997). *Psychotherapy with "impossible" cases*. New York: Norton.

Duncan, B., & Miller, S. (in press). *The heroic client*. San Francisco: Jossey-Bass.

Duncan, B., & Moynihan, D. (1994). Applying outcome research: Intentional utilization of the client's frame of reference. *Psychotherapy, 31*(2), 294–301.

Duncan, B., Solovey, A., & Rusk, G. (1992). *Changing the rules: A client-directed approach*. New York: Guilford.

Duncan, B., Sparks, J., & Miller, S. (in press). Recasting the therapeutic drama: A client-directed, outcome-informed approach. In F. Datillio and L. Bevilacqua (Eds.), *Comparative treatment in couples relationships*. New York: Springer.

Erickson, M. (1980). *The nature of hypnosis and suggestion: The collected papers of Milton H. Erickson on hypnosis* (Vol. 1, E. L. Rossi, Ed.). New York: Irvington.

Erickson, M. H., & Rossi, E. L. (1979). *Hypnotherapy: An exploratory casebook*. New York: Irvington.

Fisch, R., Weakland, J., & Segal, L. (1982). *The tactics of change: Doing therapy briefly*. San Francisco: Jossey-Bass.

Frank, J. D. (1995). Psychotherapy as rhetoric: Some implications. *Clinical Psychology: Science and Practice, 2*, 90–93.

Frank, J. D., & Frank, J. B. (1991). *Persuasion and healing* (3rd ed.). Baltimore: John Hopkins University Press.

Gaston, L. (1990). The concept of the alliance and its role in psychotherapy. *Psychotherapy, 27*, 143–152.

Hayes, J., & Wall, T. (1998). What influences clinicians' responsibility attributions? The role of problem type, theoretical orientation, and client attribution. *Journal of Social and Clinical Psychology, 17*, 69–74.

Held, B. S. (1991). The process/content distinction in psychotherapy revisited. *Psychotherapy, 28*, 207–217.

Hester, R., Miller, W., Delaney, H., & Meyers, R. (1990, November). *Effectiveness of the community reinforcement approach*. Presented at the 24th annual meeting of the Association for the Advancement of Behavior Therapy. San Francisco.

Hoch, P. (1955). Aims and limitations of psychotherapy. *American Journal of Psychiatry, 112*, 321–327.

Miller, S., Duncan, B., & Hubble, M. (1997). *Escape from Babel*. New York: Norton.

Rossi, E. L. (1980). *Innovative hypnotherapy by Milton Erickson*. New York: Irvington.

Tallman, K., & Bohart, A. (1999). The client as a common factor. In M. Hubble, B. Duncan, & S. Miller (Eds.), *The heart and soul of change*. Washington, DC: APA Books.

Torrey, E. (1972). *The mind game*. New York: Emerson Hall.

Tracey, T. (1988). Relationship of responsibility attribution congruence to psychotherapy outcome. *Journal of Social and Clinical Psychology, 7*, 131–146.

Watzlawick, P., Weakland, J., & Fisch, R. (1974). *Change: Problem formation and problem resolution*. New York: Norton.

Wile, D. (1977). Ideological conflicts between clients and psychotherapists. *American Journal of Psychotherapy, 37*, 437–449.

Worthington, R., & Atkinson, D. (1996). Effects of perceived etiology attribution similarity on client ratings of counselor credibility. *Journal of Counseling Psychology*, *43*, 423–429.

Zeig, J. K., & Gilligan, S. G. (Eds.). (1990). *Brief therapy: Myths, methods, and metaphors.* New York: Brunner/Mazel.

## Suggested Readings

Dolan, Y. (1985). Ericksonian utilization and intervention techniques with chronically mentally ill clients. In J. Zeig (Ed.), *Ericksonian psychotherapy* (Vol. 2). New York: Brunner/Mazel

Duncan, B., Hubble, M., & Miller, S. (1998). Is the customer always right? Maybe not, but it's a good place to start. *Family Therapy Networker*, March/April, 81–90.

Duncan, B., Hubble, M., Miller, S., & Coleman, S. (1998). Escaping the lost world of impossibility: Honoring clients' language, motivations, and theories of change. In M. A. Hoyt (Ed.), *Handbook of the constructive therapies.* San Francisco: Jossey-Bass.

Gilligan, S. (1987). *Therapeutic trances.* New York: Brunner/Mazel.

Stern, C. (1985). There's no theory like no-theory: The Ericksonian approach in perspective. In J. Zeig (Ed.), *Ericksonian psychotherapy* (Vol. 1). New York: Brunner/Mazel.

Yapko, M. (1985). The Erickson hook. Values in Ericksonian approaches. In J. Zeig (Ed.), *Ericksonian psychotherapy* (Vol. 1). New York: Brunner/Mazel.

# 5

## Creating a Context for Hypnosis: Listening for a Resource Theme and Integrating It Into an Ericksonian Hypnosis Session

*Robert B. McNeilly*

---

When I first heard of hypnosis, I was interested. When I heard John Hartland speak in 1975 about his personal experiences with Erickson, I was intrigued. When I saw Lustig's (1975) videotape "The Artistry of Milton H. Erickson" in Philadelphia in 1976, I was smitten. When I read Haley's *Uncommon Therapy* (1973), I was mystified. When I met Erickson personally in 1977, I felt as if I'd come home. To hear him speak of respecting individuality, focusing on resources, and using what the client brings to therapy, and to see him put those ideas into action was enchanting. I was overwhelmed by the experience. It took me several years to get past being overwhelmed so that I could begin to use what I learned from him rather than try to emulate him. What follows is a reflection on how I have adapted what I learned and how that learning has evolved over the last 15 years.

Back then, I was plagued by questions: "What is Erickson doing?" "How does he know what to do, and when?" "How could I ever begin to do something like that?" "What should I be looking for?" "Now that I've observed something, how can I use it?"

What has emerged for me over the years is a growing appreciation for the experience that hypnosis can generate. I see the central importance of language and of listening for what the individual client wants. It is becoming increasingly apparent to me that effective therapy goes beyond any technique and necessarily includes creating a respectful, coherent therapeutic relationship.

One of the most important learnings for me is to listen to the client for "What's missing" rather than for "What's wrong." In this way, missing resources can emerge that serve as a direction or theme for the therapeutic process. This perspective provides some direction for dealing with concerns about where to begin, and what kinds of induction, metaphors, and suggestions will be most effective.

Key issues I have found most relevant are:

- How can we best listen for a resource?
- How can we identify a resource theme for a session?
- How can we integrate such a resource theme into a hypnosis session?

### Ericksonian Perspectives on Accessing Resources

In the foreword to *Change: Principles of Problem Formation and Problem Resolution* (Watzlawick, Weakland, & Fisch, 1973), Erickson wrote, "Psychotherapy is sought not primarily for enlightenment about the unchangeable past but because of dissatisfaction with the present and a desire to better the future." This alerts us to seek out resources that clients can use to effect such improvement.

### WHAT IS IT ABOUT HYPNOSIS?

### Hypnosis Generates Rapport

When we work hypnotically with someone, it is an intimate experience. It is an experience in which there is a sense of being with another person in a very special way. Hypnosis can generate rapport by setting a mood of respectful, trusting communication. So, when we ask the patient about the problem, the conversation can take place in a context of generating a respectful relationship.

## Hypnosis Allows New Observations

Erickson thought of problems as extensions of everyday experiences. He spoke about problems as if they were situations with which people had somehow become involved and didn't know how to get out. He normalized problems in order to reconnect them to experiences of everyday life.

A training nurse told me years ago that she wanted to lose some weight. She said the problem was the caramel custards they served at the nurses' home. At 11:30 a.m., the custards started "calling" her. She wanted me to hypnotize her so she would have some control. I introduced her to the idea that instead of my hypnotizing her, perhaps she could avoid being hypnotized by the custard. Since it was morning, I said, "Why don't you leave here and go to the hospital canteen and look those custards in the eye. See if you can hypnotize them to stay on the shelf before they hypnotize you into reaching out for them." She laughed. And she found that the custard was very responsive to her hypnosis! Instead of thinking of her issue about weight as being one of willpower, she looked at the parallels between her behavior and hypnotic behavior. This provided a way to interrupt unhelpful patterns.

## Hypnosis Generates Experience

Hypnosis provides an unusually predictable way of actually getting into an experience. Much therapeutic work can be accomplished by talking about an experience: "What was it like? When did it start? Why is it there?" While discussing an experience, there will be some recall of it. But hypnosis provides a way of intentionally getting into the physiology, the emotions, the processes of the experience itself.

## Hypnosis Facilitates Learning

People *learn* to have problems. People also can unlearn problems and learn new ways of behavior. In hypnosis, we expect alteration in perception, greater flexibility of experience. The past, present, and future can appear to merge and become interchangeable. Time can seem to speed up, slow down, or stand still. Shifts in memory occur. Sensations change. This fluidity of experience provides a basis for change and learning. And the idea of learning brings with it a mood of possibility for the future, a mood that is central to therapeutic change. Because hypnosis can generate experience, it can promote learning.

Hypnosis may not be the only way of working that generates rapport. Hypnosis may not be the only way of generating a set of observations. Hypnosis may not be the only way of directing an experience or fostering learning. But hypnosis is one way in which we can design our conversation and interactions to influence the likelihood of actually creating learning experiences.

## BEGINNING A SESSION

Asking "What do you like doing?" or "What is pleasing to you?" allows the clinician to listen for the individuality of each client. The answers to these questions provide a window to the client's life. Questions about likes inform us about clients' aspirations, their passions, their hopes for the future. We can listen for key words, phrases, and metaphors in their description of likes for use in working with the problem.

By beginning the session with a conversation about likes, the client is invited to respond as a person rather than as a case. We establish a mood, which fosters a therapeutic relationship of normality. From this perspective, problems can be viewed as circumstances in which resources that are functional elsewhere in the client's life are not being adequately utilized. Asking what the client likes can provide an opportunity for us to look for the missing resources that might be useful in the problem area.

### What's the Problem?

We can ask, "What's the problem?" Or we can ask presuppositional questions, such as, "If we could do something useful, what would that be?" "What would you like to work on today that would make some useful difference to you?" "At what would you like to succeed?" These questions assist in focusing on a solution from the beginning.

### What's Missing?

Instead of asking, "What's wrong that needs fixing?" we can ask our client, "What's missing?" We also might ask, "What's missing that would solve the problem?" These questions help to orient the conversation in the direction of looking for resources, of seeking solutions.

### Ways of Identifying a Resource Theme

We can ask, "How will you be different when we have finished here?" We can ask about how the client was before the problem began, wondering about resources that were used then. We can ask the client to go into hypnosis, imagine going into the future when the problem has been solved, and ask, "What's different?" The answer to these questions might include, "I'd feel calmer," "I'd be more confident," "I'd be having more fun." They provide a direction for induction, metaphors, and suggestions.

### INDUCTION OF HYPNOSIS

Once we have identified a resource theme for clients, they can be introduced in the induction. The induction can include an invitation to take their own time, to be unhurried, to notice only the experiences of increasing comfort.

### Metaphors

We can offer clients stories about other persons who were similarly troubled. Perhaps these others learned to take a break, to take some time out, to take a deep breath so they could get on with what needed to be done. By taking their own time, they were able to achieve more with less pressure.

In the induction, we could tell a story of someone, perhaps a young woman, who liked to walk in the country. This woman would forget about the time and just enjoy the experience. There was no need to count how many times her left foot touched the ground or how many times she breathed in or out or to remember the average gradient of the path. She was able to become absorbed in the experience of enjoying the walk so much that time went by and she finished her walk feeling satisfied and energized.

### On Completing Hypnosis

Instead of asking, "How was it?" we can ask, "What do you notice now that is different from when we began?" Anything useful can be ratified and amplified. If a client reports feeling calmer, and that is something the person wanted to accomplish, we can encourage it by saying, "That's good." We also can make observations about body changes by commenting, "You look more at ease than before," or "You look like you've had a rest," or whatever else may be useful to the process. By specifically eliciting signs of the presence of the resource theme, we can further the therapeutic process.

### Setting up Future Learning

Completing a session provides us with another opportunity to offer suggestions. We can suggest that the client might be interested in taking care to notice further evidence of improvement, noting the comments of others about the changes that have happened and personally enjoying the continuing improvements as the learning progresses in and out of awareness. The completion process provides yet another opportunity to speak to the resource theme, maintain the coherence and relevance of the session as a whole, and link the learning with the client's everyday life.

CLINICAL EXAMPLES

### Case 1

Eric, a 25-year-old university student, requested hypnosis for depression. He described it as a feeling of being overwhelmed and hopeless, as if everything were too much for him. He volunteered that he had memories of his father being verbally violent as Eric was growing up. What was missing for him was a feeling of peace, an ability to be more connected with his family, and the self-confidence to cope. He said he liked jazz (the saxophone in particular), walking in the country, and reading. I decided to work with a resource theme of feeling more peaceful and confident, with his music as a preferred area. At the initiation of induction, I suggested that he look around the room until he found something of his choosing. He could close his eyes when he was ready. He could imagine listening to his favorite music. He didn't need to listen to anything I said that wasn't interesting to him and he could feel confident in his ability to enjoy the music, since he knew it so well.

I reminded Eric that when he first learned to listen to music, all the instruments blurred together. He might have been overwhelmed by the complexity, but as he continued to listen, he learned to feel more confident about which instrument was which, what songs he liked best, what was pleasing to him. Then he could really connect with the music.

I told him about a client who contemplated giving up his career as a professional musician because he felt overwhelmed by the idea of performing. He created a novel solution by imagining that the music could play the instrument for him. All he needed to do was sit back and listen to the music that happened as a result.

I offered Eric a variety of suggestions as to how he might begin to feel more as he wanted to feel. I told him I wondered if it would happen slowly and gradually or intermittently at first, or in some other way. When he came out of hypnosis, he reported feeling peaceful. He said he felt more connected and believed that he could now cope. I congratulated him on demonstrating to himself how ready he was to learn. The following week, Eric told me that he had experienced only one down day, and that he was able to live through it without succumbing to his old feelings of doubt and despair. He had learned how to deal with his demon.

## Case 2

Simon, a 34-year-old lawyer, wanted help to overcome chronic anxiety. He was experiencing increasing stress at work brought on by demanding clients and senior partners. What he was missing was a feeling of greater self-confidence on his job. Outside the office, he liked golf and was a skilled player, and even had considered becoming a professional. I decided to work with a resource theme of being more confident and independent, more accepting of difficulties.

During the induction, I suggested that he could feel confident that his feet were resting on the floor and he would not fall out of the chair, and that he could feel this confidence independently of me or of anyone else. He could close his eyes with confidence when he was ready. I also suggested that he could go into hypnosis in his own way, to his own depth, and experience anything that he might find useful, independently of anything I might say.

I reminded him that learning to walk had involved learning to feel confident about the movement of his legs, the balance of his body. As an accomplished golfer, he knew a lot about standing and holding and swinging the club confidently. He could play with confidence while ignoring the onlookers and their expectations. He played his best when he attended to his own experience and adapted his game to the surroundings.

I told him about a champion swimmer who almost lost his heat because he was looking at the positions of the other swimmers. He won in the end by ignoring the competition and focusing on his own rhythm of swimming. He allowed the rhythm to take over and it brought him a gold medal.

I offered Simon a variety of other suggestions about feelings associated with being confident. And I wondered aloud who would be the first to notice his increasing self-confidence.

## CONCLUSION

When we ask a client about the client's problem, speculate about what's missing, and listen for a resource theme, we can integrate the client's report into the hypnotic session. In this way, the shape and content of the hypnotic experience are coherent with the resource theme. As a result, every aspect of the session has the possibility of being therapeutic. This process of observing and utilizing what clients bring in, emphasizing their resources and individuality, is a cornerstone of the Ericksonian approach. Effective therapy goes beyond any technique, and necessarily includes creating a respectful, contactful, coherent therapeutic relationship. In essence, it means promoting a resource theme and utilizing patients' behaviors in the process.

### References

American Society of Clinical Hypnosis. (1980). Taped lecture, 7/16/65.

Beahrs, J. (1977). Integrating Erickson's approach. *American Journal of Clinical Hypnosis, 20,* 55–68.

De Shazer, S. (1988). *Clues: Investigating solutions in brief therapy.* New York: Norton.

Dolan, Y. (1985). *A path with a heart.* New York: Brunner/Mazel.

Erickson, M. (1980) The First International Congress on Ericksonian Hypnosis and Psychotherapy. *The collected papers of Milton H. Erickson, Vol. II* (E. L. Rossi, Ed.). New York: Irvington.

Erickson, M. (1985). *Life reframing in hypnosis.* New York: Irvington.

Haley, J. (1973). *Uncommon therapy: The psychiatric techniques of Milton H. Erickson, M.D.* New York: Norton.

Haley, J. (1985). *Conversations with Milton H. Erickson, M.D.* New York: Norton.

Haley, J. & Richeport, M. (1993). *Milton H. Erickson, M.D.: Explorer in hypnosis and therapy.* Rockville, MD: Triangle.

Lustig, H. (1975). *The artistry of Milton H. Erickson, M.D.* (Videotape).

O'Hanlon, W., & Martin, M. (1992). *Solution-oriented hypnosis.* New York: Norton.

Watzlawick, P., Weakland, J., & Fisch, R. (1973). *Change: principles of problem formation and problem resolution.* New York: Norton.

Yapko, M. (1995). *Essentials of hypnosis.* New York: Brunner/Mazel.

Zeig, J. (1980). *A teaching seminar with Milton H. Erickson.* New York: Brunner/ Mazel.

Zeig, J. (1985). *Experiencing Erickson: An introduction to the man and his work.* New York: Brunner/Mazel.

### Suggested Readings

Echeverria, R. (1994). *Ontologia del lenguage.* Santiago: Dolmen.

Haley, J., & Richeport, M. (1993). *Milton H. Erickson, M.D. Explorer in hypnosis and therapy.* Rockville, MD: Triangle.

Lao-tzu. (1972). *Tao te ching.* New York: Vintage.

Maturana, H., & Varella, F. (1988). *The tree of knowledge: The biological roots of human understanding.* Boston: Shambhala.

McNeilly, R. (1997, February). Ericksonian hypnotherapy. *Psychotherapy in Australia, 3*(2).

McNeilly, R., & Brown J. (1994). *Healing with words.* Melbourne: Hill of Content.

Winograd, T., & Flores, F. (1986). *Understanding computers and cognition.* New York: Addison-Wesley.

# 6

# When to Use or Not to Use Hypnosis According to the Ericksonian Tradition

*Terry L. Argast, Richard E. Landis,*
*& Pennie Dexter Carrell*

In Ericksonian psychotherapy, the issue of when or when not to use hypnosis is often an extension of the decision of when or when not to use strategic communication. Betty Alice Erickson (1994) has pointed out that Milton H. Erickson, her father, often said he could not exactly distinguish the point at which hypnosis began and other forms of communication ended. Dr. Erickson emphasized in his writings and lectures that he did not use formal hypnosis with every patient who entered his office, any more than he used any other specific technique or tool. However, in observing him at work and reviewing his published accounts, some patterns of hypnotic utilization do emerge.

In this chapter, we will attempt to present what we feel are relevant issues, for both the novice and the seasoned clinician, regarding the appropriate use of hypnosis and hypnotic communication. In addressing the issue of when to use hypnosis in a clinical setting, we will contrast the more traditional view of hypnosis (where the therapist uses formal induction, deepening, and suggestions) with the Erickson approach, which can be less formal and more indirect.

For example, in an intervention with an adolescent girl who thought her feet were too big, Erickson employed a shock technique, "inadvertently" stepping on her foot and then telling her that her feet were too small to be seen by a man. This strategic communication brought about a change in the girl's behavior and social adjustment even though neither she nor her mother realized that Erickson had performed any intervention at all (Erickson, 1960). Another case example is of the young, unwed couple who came to Erickson to get his medical approval for an abortion their parents were pressuring the young woman to have. Erickson, recognizing that the couple truly did not want the abortion, told them that if they honestly wanted the woman to abort, then under no circumstances should they think of a name for the baby (Erickson, 1950/1980).

In neither of these cases was there a "formal induction" in a traditional sense; rather, in both cases, an altered state of consciousness was elicited by a pattern disruption and then a suggestion was given. These interventions actually fit a broader definition of hypnosis where indirect or strategic techniques are used paradoxically to create alterations in, or a depotentiation of, the conscious set. Conscious depotentiation tends to result in the acceptance of a given suggestion by the person's unconscious in the same way that might occur in a more formal state of hypnosis.

In exploring this idea of the "Erickson approach," we will address the issue of *when* a clinician should use hypnosis from the standpoint of *how* one uses the state of hypnosis and utilizes hypnotic principles in special circumstances.

When trained in traditional hypnotic approaches, the authors were routinely warned against using hypnosis with psychotic or depressed patients or with individuals who had character disorders. A review of the literature using traditional approaches continues to discourage the use of traditional hypnotic approaches with these disorders, and for good reason. Using traditional hypnotic techniques with certain disorders can be problematic and any clinician utilizing such approaches should be wary.

However, in our Ericksonian training we discovered that there is another way to approach these disorders, and to address the clinical concerns noted by more traditional hypnotists. Dr. Erickson knew of and respected the issues that could make hypnosis contraindicated for many patients. However, his emphasis on individualizing hypnotic techniques to meet the needs of each patient is in marked contrast to the standardized techniques commonly used in more traditional forms of hypnosis. Erickson viewed patients as so much more than their diagnoses, and it was this view of the uniqueness of the individual that provided a springboard for some very creative interventions. As Haley (1967) described of Erickson, "His therapeutic approach is characterized by the view that human problems are infinitely diverse while his therapeutic stance appears infinitely flexible" (p. 531).

It was this flexibility and Erickson's very broad understanding of communication that allowed him to induce hypnotic trances in people who were unresponsive to more traditional techniques. In fact, the Ericksonian tradition of hypnosis differs from the more traditional concept of hypnosis as a process in which an induction is recited by an operator and a susceptible subject goes into trance, uniformly responding to the suggestions. In the traditional model, the individual qualities of the operator and of the subject are seen as secondary to the innate power of the hypnotic trance. Thus, the model tends to lump all diagnostic classifications together as being either responsive or unresponsive to hypnotic interventions. Erickson emphasized how the individual differences in motivations, resources, expectations, and prior experiences of each operator and of each subject made an impact on whether or not someone would be responsive. Thus, in the Erickson approach, there is no one way of delivering, or of receiving, a hypnotic trance. Consequently, individuals are responsive or unresponsive based on the unique circumstances and the training and flexibility of the operator, not on their inability to go into a hypnotic trance.

Consistent with this view, Weizenhoffer (1989) stated that problems arise in hypnotic interventions as the result of the misuse of suggestion, rather than of the use of hypnosis itself. The literature is full of examples of situations where "clinical" suggestions were followed by the subject, but led to negative, and sometimes disastrous, results. Erickson would indicate that the negative outcome more likely had to do with the misalignment of suggestion to the individual needs of the patient.

Therefore, from an Ericksonian perspective, we offer the following elements as some of the more critical determinants for the use, or misuse, of clinical hypnosis.

The therapist must ask the following:

- What is my training?
- What are my experience and confidence?

- What are my consultative and supervisory resources?
- What are my motivations?

The therapist must assess the patient:

- What are the patient's motivations?
- What are the patient's underlying assumptions?
- How susceptible is the patient to decompensation?
- Are there possible medical conditions that must be considered?
- Is the patient under the influence of drugs or alcohol?
- Are there possible legal considerations?

Each of these questions will be addressed in turn.

## What the Therapist Must Ask
- *What is my training?*

The first criterion of when to use hypnosis is determined by the competence of the operator. In other words, the clinician using hypnosis needs to be adequately trained both in the technique of hypnosis and in its application to particular clinical issues. The operator must also have a thorough understanding of the psychopathology that is being treated in a particular patient. To use hypnosis indiscriminately outside of one's professional understanding is unethical. Therefore, it is very important to stay within one's area of competence.

Haley (1967) felt that Erickson had redefined and broadened our clinical understanding of the "unconscious" and its application to strategic communication and clinical hypnosis. Erickson utilized both direct and indirect techniques whenever clinically indicated. He felt that training in both approaches made the therapist more flexible and, therefore, more effective. Unfortunately, there is no universal definition of hypnosis that can distinguish all of its qualities from those of the naturalistic trance, which can result from the strategic use of indirect communication. This overlay of properties is perhaps attributable to the fact that the qualities of both naturalistic trance and hypnosis are found within the domain of altered states of consciousness.

## DEALING WITH COMPLICATIONS
## WHEN USING HYPNOSIS

One of the processes that make hypnosis so effective is that it deals directly with the unconscious in a way that can bypass normal conscious defense mechanisms. However, "what is a blessing can also be a curse" if one is not trained appropriately in dealing with unconscious processes and systems. In other words, when using a tool, such as hypnosis, that accesses the unconscious directly, certain complications can arise that are neither anticipated nor purposely elicited by the operator and that might not be as intense or arise as frequently in therapeutic approaches that emphasize conscious processes. Barber (1998) points out: "The first step in avoiding clinical complications is recognizing that they can occur" (p. 157). Adequate professional training can assist in preparing the clinician to deal with these unexpected complications, if and when they do develop. A solid therapeutic alliance between the patient and the therapist is especially important in keeping the negative effects of such complications to a minimum (Barber, 1998; Lynn, Martin, & Frauman, 1996).

### Intensification of the Transference

While transference is a substantial part of any ongoing therapy, it appears to be especially intensified when hypnosis is employed (Judd, Burrows, & Dennerstein, 1985). Barber (1998) emphasizes the suddenness with which these intense feelings can arise. The patient's normal defenses may be overwhelmed with the feelings or experiences elicited during the hypnotic procedure and thus the patient may have difficulty dealing with his or her own reaction. The feelings that are elicited usually involve intense erotic and sexual feelings or intense anger and resentment. These feelings are common in the psychotherapeutic relationship, but in the context of hypnosis, they are likely to be more immediate, frequent, and intense. Such a presentation, although often highly effective, may result in unexpected complications and create an interference with the therapeutic goal.

On the other hand, when properly handled, the transference can be used quite effectively to further the therapeutic goal. In fact, Erickson would often utilize the transference to develop a response potential when he gave a hypnotic suggestion. The result would often be that the patient would be "motivated" to perform some action just to prove Erickson "wrong": that action, of course, was actually the desired outcome. An example of this utilization of transference involves a case that Erickson treated in which a recently married woman was panicked about having sex with her husband, a reaction related to her moral and religious upbringing. In trance, Erickson told her that he would like her to consummate her marriage on a Friday, but she chose to consummate it on a Thursday. The anger over Erickson's "control" outweighed her anxiety about having sex (Erickson, 1954).

## Spontaneous Abreaction

Some people appear to experience emotional distress when going into trance (Cheek & LeCron, 1968; Frauman, Lynn, & Brantar, 1993). Even when doing very benign group inductions in our training workshops, we find that a small percentage of the participants will get "triggered" and may have a negative emotional response. This is also true in clinical situations, most often for those experiencing their first exposure to trance. For individuals having these negative reactions, the trance appears to be connected with dissociated material that occurred in the past. Thus, when the person begins to enter a trance state, often without any warning, the dissociated and usually emotionally charged material can surface and manifest as a spontaneous abreaction. Frequently, no suggestion from the therapist is necessary, but, of course, may be given unintentionally. In most cases, the spontaneous abreaction can be utilized in the service of the therapeutic goal and there is no negative outcome. However, sometimes the surprising nature of emotions or dissociated material can leave the patient apprehensive about future therapeutic work, especially if it involves trance. In our training workshops, we have learned that it is best to prepare individuals for this possibility and to instruct them to alert us, if it is not already obvious to us, so that the experience can be processed appropriately and any unnecessary negative fallout can be limited. This overlay of processes is again an example of how hypnotic trance and dissociated trance are both subsets of the broader category of altered states of consciousness.

## Unanticipated Awareness of Repressed Feelings, Thoughts, and Memories

Awareness of repressed material is almost always accelerated by the use of hypnosis (Judd, Burrows, & Dennerstein, 1985; Meares, 1960). Normally, but not always, the negative effects of recovering repressed information in hypnosis are dealt with by circumventing the normal defense mechanisms and creating a deep level of trance. However, sometimes the repressed information and/or feelings unexpectedly "leak" out into conscious awareness. When this conscious "knowing" occurs, it often leads to an intensification of the patient's symptomatology. Watkins (1987) states that it is important that the clinician using hypnosis always be prepared with a strategy to assist the patient with the conscious integration of the material. Erickson felt that there were always two patients with whom the hypnotist must deal: the conscious awareness of the individual and then the unconscious awareness. He indicated that hypnosis could be effective only if the clinician balanced the process of accessing unconscious information and, when appropriate, relating it to the conscious understandings. If the conscious mind was not prepared to deal with the information, it was important to "hide" it a bit longer. Erickson used many different techniques to balance the degree of processing the information, including stories, shock and confusion, amnesia, "slow leaks," and graduated awareness.

- *What are my experience and confidence?*

Experience is significantly different from just intellectually knowing about something. One can gain knowledge by reading and gathering second-hand information. However, there is no substitute for actual clinical experience. Each therapist will have more experience in one clinical domain than in another. Because of the potential power of hypnosis, it is wise initially to limit one's use of it to the areas in which one has had the most clinical experience. As the therapist expands into areas of lesser experience, it is necessary to increase the use of supervision and consultation.

Erickson (1978) emphasized practicing the elements of hypnotic trance work with one's colleagues. He felt that practicing hypnosis on a nonclinical population allowed the therapist time to develop the necessary skill and confidence for using hypnosis with patients. Clearly understanding that individuals are different, and that the same approach does not work with everyone, is a must for the successful hypnotist and/or therapist. To operate in this fashion, however, necessitates that the therapist maintain a stance of confident flexibility. Erickson was experimentally minded and was always exploring new ideas; some did not work, but many did. For example, in the case of the young bride who feared consummation because of her moral and religious beliefs (Erickson, 1954), the first intervention Erickson attempted failed, but his flexibility allowed him to utilize the failure and to develop a response potential for the intervention that was successful. Erickson felt that there was no substitute for practice and experimentation.

In the Erickson approach to hypnosis and psychotherapy, the therapist's skill in utilization is a primary determinant of with whom and when it is appropriate to use hypnosis. Zeig (1992) defines utilization as "the readiness of the therapist to respond strategically to any and all aspects of the patient or the environment" (p. 256). Zeig further observes that utilization is goal-directed. Therefore, one needs to have both confidence and experience in order effectively to utilize a patient's reactions to any intervention so that the outcome is in the service of the therapeutic goals. If one is lacking either the experience or the confidence in using hypnosis with a particular patient, regardless of the formal diagnosis, one should choose a different therapeutic intervention.

One of the things that Erickson emphasized about the success of hypnosis was the importance of the therapist's confidence level with regard to inducing a trance state. Of course, the same thing could be said of any therapist's belief in the effectiveness of a particular intervention. However, that variable is difficult to account for in controlled studies. Often the success or failure of any intervention is attributed to some dynamic inherent in the patient, such as suggestibility. Erickson firmly believed that the success or failure of an intervention was much more frequently a function of the level of training, experience, and conviction of the therapist. Certainly, we are all aware that nonverbal communication patterns often express at a manifest level those inner thoughts and feelings hidden at an unconscious level. At least, we may believe that ours, as therapists, are "hidden," but more often than not they can be picked up by patients.

Rossi and Ryan (1985) cite Erickson on this matter:

In the vast majority of cases, it is the competence you are willing to radiate that enables you to induce hypnosis. It is your willingness to know that you can do it. I carried on experiments with medical students wherein I told one group ... the subject was very poor ... and another group that the subject was an excellent subject. The first group failed, while the second group was successful. ... Now, if you can achieve such results experimentally, you can also achieve such results in your own practices. I think you ought to have confidence and trust in your own professional capacities. (pp. 125–126)

Ideally, the use of hypnosis is so integrated into one's clinical model that it reaches a level of sophistication where it can be used creatively and spontaneously within the bounds of the clinician's expertise and within the framework of the therapeutic goal (Parsons-Fein, 1998). Erickson (1952) said that there were certain techniques he would not touch with a "ten-foot pole," but that he could admire the results of the people who used them. Perhaps Erickson's warning would go something like this: Don't get wedded to your techniques, because you will be confronted with clients who won't respond to them. Why not have several techniques from which to choose that will be effective with a larger range of patients?

- *What are my consultative and supervisory resources?*

One of the primary concerns is that hypnosis be used ethically and safely. As the clinician enhances his or her knowledge in treating certain problems in general, it is important to have clinical consultation and/or supervision in the specific applications of hypnosis. In addition to regular consultative procedures, special collaboration is necessary when the patient is presenting with physical symptoms. Yapko (1984) warns: "When working on a physical symptom, unless you are a physician you should have a medical referral and medical clearance to work with the problem. Practicing medicine (psychology, nutrition, etc.) without a license or without adequate knowledge and backup is nothing short of irresponsible" (p. 312).

For many clinicians, private practice can be very isolating. The authors have been meeting on a regular basis since 1978 to share clinical experiences and ask questions of each other. We have found that meeting for training and case review is significantly different from the solitary experience of keeping current with the literature. These meetings were a big factor in our decision to develop a professional society where informal supervision, consultation, and shared information about hypnosis and its clinical application could be made readily available to professionals.

- *What are my motivations?*

As in all therapeutic situations, while using hypnosis there is a danger of the therapist's abuse of power. In his conversations with Rossi and Ryan (1985), Erickson stated,

> When you are working hypnotically with a patient, your orientation should center around the patient and the patient's needs. Whenever you try to maximize your own ego through a patient you start losing ground. That is why we are so much opposed to the teaching of stage hypnosis techniques, because stage hypnotists are oriented about themselves as operators, not about their subjects. In medical and dental hypnosis, you need to orient everything about the patient. It is the patient who is the important person. (p. 179)

When the therapist's personal motivations are not clear, it can pave the way for contratherapeutic countertransferences, which can be heightened through the use of hypnosis. Judd, Burrows, and Dennerstein (1985) state: "When hypnosis is used destructively, it is often the result of countertransference factors" (p. 4). Cheek and LeCron (1968) go so far as to say that the dangers in hypnosis result from the personality difficulties of the hypnotist. "Patients will protect themselves from harm when the therapist shows respect for their ability to do so" (p. 3).

The therapist's motivations need to respect the patient's integrity and be in the service of the patient's personal welfare and therapeutic goals. When a therapist's personal motivations conflict with a patient's needs, the effectiveness of treatment is compromised. Erickson (Rossi & Ryan, 1988) presented a clear example of this situation:

> Whenever you try to use hypnosis for a purely selfish purpose, you lose. I can think of the doctor who was very pleased with his son, Johnny, who was a prized hypnotic subject. Johnny was 12 years old. Then Johnny brought his report card home and there was one D, plenty of C's, and one B. Papa put Johnny into a trance and explained to him that he had to get some B's and A's. Then Papa discovered that Johnny wouldn't go into a trance for him ever again, because, you see, Papa tried to use hypnosis to make Johnny do Papa's bidding. That is wrong, it is unfair; it is unjust. It is a violation of Johnny; it is a violation of Johnny's unconscious. (p. 122)

Orne (1972) has identified several "red flags" that can alert the therapist to possible unresolved power fantasies that may be influencing the therapist's use of hypnosis:

- Is hypnosis used indiscriminately with all patients?
- Is there more concern for the inductions than for the applications?
- Is the induction experienced as a battle of wills?
- Is there an overconcern about the patient's possibly deceiving the therapist or faking hypnosis?
- Is there greater positive anticipation in hypnotizing attractive as compared with less attractive patients?

If the answer to any of the above is Yes, Orne suggests that the therapist review his or her own motivations. We would add that the therapist should get supervision, consultation, and perhaps refrain from using hypnosis until the motivational problem is remedied.

## Assessing the Patient
- *What are the patient's motivations?*

Erickson received many referrals from other professionals where either other forms of treatment had not been effective or therapists had unsuccessfully attempted to use hypnosis. While this type of referral might not afford the most desirable time to use hypnosis, it is usually a time when the patient is desperate and motivation is high. A positive outcome of hypnosis is actually much more limited when the primary motivation is curiosity, as is frequently the case with many well-defended graduate psychology students who have to undergo a required number of hours of their own therapy!

Erickson would frequently assess the level of a patient's motivation by assigning some task to the patient. He would then determine what therapeutic approaches he could use based on the patient's level of compliance in performing the task. For example, one of Erickson's favorite tasks was to ask a potential patient coming in to stop smoking to climb Squaw Peak, a 2,600-foot mountain on the outskirts of Phoenix. If the person followed through with the task, then the motivation for treatment was judged to be higher than if there were no, or little, compliance. When motivation for change was judged to be low, Erickson would use this information to determine what therapeutic intervention he could best employ. Erickson said that if the patient was compliant, that also increased the patient's motivation for future compliance in therapy (Rosen, 1982).

- *What are the patient's underlying assumptions?*

Sometimes patient expectations are unrealistically high, as can be the case with the therapist as well. Idealistic expectations are frequently a two-edged sword. The patient may be very motivated, but may become discouraged if the results do not live up to the initial expectation. Weitzenhoffer (1989) emphasized that it is important to know the patient's history in order to determine whether a prior hypnotic experience could influence the patient's expectations. Furthermore, Weitzenhoffer suggests that this history can be helpful in determining any misconceptions about hypnosis. Erickson was very attentive to these personal attitudes of the patient when employing hypnotic suggestions. To remedy this "discouragement dynamic" in the patient, one technique that Erickson frequently used was to suggest that the symptomatic change would be gradual and slow. In this way, if the symptom did not disappear right away, or reemerged at some point, the patient would not lose faith in the power of the hypnotic intervention.

Erickson felt that it oversimplified the complexity of the problem and limited the uniqueness of the patient to expect a standardized intervention to be effective with every individual. He believed it was critical to understand the basic underlying assumptions that supported the patient's presenting problems, and that it was often much more useful to focus the hypnotic interventions on these underlying assumptions, than to attack the presenting symptoms directly. For example, in approaching sexual issues, Erickson (Rossi & Ryan, 1985) stated:

> I wouldn't try any direct suggestion. In fact, I wouldn't use hypnosis to correct the impotence or the frigidity, because both impotence and frigidity are rather deeply involved problems employing faulty attitudes toward the body, faulty orientations toward the body, and a lot of confused understanding on the subject of sex and emotion in general. Therefore, I would use the hypnosis for the purpose of providing a different psychological orientation. (p. 125)

- *How susceptible is the patient to decompensation?*

In all forms of therapy, decompensation of the patient can be unexpected and can take many forms, including psychosis, suicide attempts, and acting out sexual or aggressive impulses. When using hypnosis in particular, on rare occasions the elicitation of intense feelings can result in the person's normal ego-defense system being overwhelmed. When this situation does occur, the patient may act out in a manner that seemingly would be unusual for that patient. When the authors met with Dr. Erickson for training, he instructed us that hypnosis should never be used with a patient where its employment might lead to a decompensation, *regardless of the patient's diagnostic classification.*

The therapist's assessment of the patient's psychological makeup is often the best way to determine when to use hypnosis and when to avoid it. Watkins (1987) emphasized that the ego strength of the patient was a major criterion for determining how much information a patient could safely integrate without its precipitating a psychological crisis. The authors believe that if hypnosis is going to be used with someone with limited psychological resources, the focus would best be oriented toward ego-building goals, rather than attacking the patient's symptoms or defenses directly.

We would like to emphasize at this point that the most common criterion as whether or not to use hypnosis is: Does using hypnosis run the reasonable risk of leading to a decompensation in the patient? However, while this is a good rule of thumb, it is not infallible. It is impossible always to determine beforehand who will respond negatively or positively to the use of hypnosis. For this reason, Erickson cautioned healthcare providers who had limited training and experience with clinical situations about utilizing hypnosis. When asked about contraindications to its use in dentistry, Erickson (Rossi & Ryan, 1985) replied:

When I consider how difficult it is for me to recognize a potential psychotic patient when he first comes into my office, I am at a loss to suggest to dentists—who do not have psychiatric training—those personality disturbances that contraindicate hypnosis. I am very much at a loss, because it is only in the very obvious cases that immediate recognition is possible. I have seen some awfully nice, sweet people in my office. I studied them, I thought them over, and I missed the goal entirely—because all of a sudden they developed an acute psychosis. And yet when I first saw these patients there was no real evidence of psychosis that I could detect. So my general tendency, no matter who enters my office, is to look at the person and wonder just how soon he or she will be committed—until I can answer that question for myself as accurately as possible. In general, when [extreme conditions are] perfectly obvious, avoid hypnosis; but otherwise, you are going to miss the mark just as many times as I do. (pp. 124–125)

- *Are there possible medical conditions that must be considered?*

Hypnosis is used as an adjunctive intervention in the treatment of many physical illnesses. The dangers with using it in such situations may result, not from the hypnosis per se, but from a failure to appreciate the effects that hypnosis can have on the physical condition being treated (Judd, Burrows, & Dennerstein, 1985). Erickson had the advantage of a medical education and his knowledge enabled him to treat physical conditions with which most therapists would not be equipped to deal.

Hypnosis should not be attempted with a person with a physical problem without consulting a physician. The literature gives many examples of hypnotic suggestions being successfully carried out, but with a negative outcome (Judd, Burrows, & Dennerstein, 1985; Watkins, 1987; Weitzenhoffer, 1989). The danger arises when a therapist, no matter how well meaning, uses hypnosis without the appropriate knowledge of, or concern for, the physical nature of the illness. For example, using hypnosis for the symptom removal of pain can have serious consequences if masking the pain prevents the patient from recognizing problems that may require medical treatment.

- *Is the patient under the influence of drugs or alcohol?*

When asked what he thought about using medication as an aid in doing hypnosis, Erickson (Rossi & Ryan, 1985) replied:

Personally, I don't like the use of medication. I have tried everything. The only drug I think is at all good is about an ounce of $C_2H_5OH$ (ethyl alcohol—whiskey) about half an hour in advance. Sometimes by the operator, sometimes by the patient! All kidding aside, I don't think much of drugs as an aid. If the patient insists on drugs, the best to use is a placebo. If you use a drug, you are then dealing with a patient plus drug effects. Therefore, use a placebo whenever possible. (p. 117)

It is important to understand that many drugs, including alcohol, are in the same classification as hypnosis, in that they can result in an altered state of consciousness. However, the distinction can be made, and one to which Erickson alludes in the above quote, that hypnosis is a special type of altered state, in that its emergence and benefits depend on the interaction between the hypnotist and the subject. When an individual is being influenced by a substance, it becomes difficult to know whether or not the rapport is with the hypnotist or with the intoxification by the drug.

- *Are there possible legal considerations?*

There are many legal and ethical pitfalls to be considered when applying hypnosis in a forensic setting. In such a setting, the primary purpose of using hypnosis is usually to enhance the memories of victims and witnesses. A word of warning: Because of the mercurial nature of what is, and what is not, admissible in court, if hypnosis is employed during therapy sessions, that fact could be used by the opposing attorney to bring into question the accuracy of a patient's testimony.

## THE ERICKSON TOUCH

The following are examples of how Dr. Erickson used hypnosis with patients who were traditionally placed in the "contraindicated for hypnosis" category. Note that the function of the hypnosis in these cases was not to attack the symptoms directly, but to create an amicable environment that would facilitate the use of other forms of therapeutic intervention, or to modify underlying assumptions that maintained the unwanted symptomatic pattern.

### Depression and Hypnosis

Traditionally, hypnosis is thought to be contraindicated for people with depression, especially if they are suicidal (Meares, 1960; Judd, Burrows, & Dennerstein, 1985; Crasilneck & Hall, 1975; Hartland, 1971). One reason given in the literature for avoiding hypnosis with these cases is that, owing to the patient's emotional instability, any unanticipated reaction to the trance could be fatal. Another reason given is that due to the intensification of the transference, as well as to the tendency for emotions to be heightened in hypnosis, the patient can be overwhelmed by the emergence of intense feelings. In severe depression, the person's normal defense mechanisms may not be fully operative, and thus the use of a technique (in this case, hypnosis) that might intensify negative emotions could lead to impulsive acting out, suicidal or otherwise. One final issue that we will mention here is that using hypnosis for symptom removal in severely depressed individuals—or any diagnostic category, for that matter—may uncover additional underlying symptomology. The risk in this situation involves the possibility that decompensation or impulsive acting out will become an issue for the patient, where it was not present in the original presentation.

Dr. Erickson's criterion for whether to use hypnosis with depressed or suicidal patients appears to be consistent with what he outlined as important considerations for determining the appropriateness of using hypnosis with any other patient. Erickson felt it was more important to look at the symptoms and to assess the individual strengths of the patient than to make a determination based on a global diagnosis of depression or suicidality. His tendency was not to attack the suicidality or depression directly, but rather to address the underlying assumption of the patient that suicide was the only option and an inevitable conclusion.

An excellent example of how Erickson used hypnosis to address underlying assumptions is the case of Dottie (Haley, 1985). At the age of 21, Dottie broke her back and her fiancé left her. She had no sense of feeling from the waist down, suffered complete paralysis, and bladder and bowel incontinence, and was wheelchair bound. She came to Dr. Erickson at age 31, undecided about suicide. Erickson generated a formal trance with amnesia for the trance experience. He then attacked the two main beliefs that made suicide a serious option for Dottie. The first belief was that no one could find her attractive because of her loss of bladder and bowel control; the second was that the paralysis had left her sexless.

To address the first belief of nonattractiveness, Dr. Erickson described some of the more unusual standards of beauty in the world, such as the duck-billed women of Africa and the enormous fat-buttocked Hottentot women, whom some men find attractive. Then he said, "I stated that men have a variety of tastes. What made her think that, because she was incontinent with feces and urine, there wasn't some nice guy in the world who would find her attractive if she were she?" (p. 24). In the hypnotic state, this generated an attitude of expectation that would allow a man to approach her. Curiosity and possibilities were seeded.

The second belief was attacked by using displacement of symptoms. While displacement of symptoms is usually associated with negative sensations, it can be associated with positive sensations in the same way that the existence of phantom-limb pain demands the possibility of phantom-limb pleasure. Continuing Dottie's trance state, Dr. Erickson listed the physical and hormonal connections that make up sexual response. He linked the external genitalia to the vagina, to the uterus, to the ovary, to the adrenal gland, to the hormone system, to the breast, to the thyroid, to the pituitary. In discussing this case, he said, "I was quite certain that the paralysis, the lack of sensation, hadn't interfered with the adrenals. They weren't paralyzed. The kidneys weren't paralyzed, even though they were connected with the adrenals. The adrenals and the kidneys were connected with the bladder. Her own wetting of herself proved that her kidneys weren't paralyzed. While she had lost the external genitalia, still the internal genitalia were connected" (p. 25).

As therapy progressed, Dottie's two "fixed" beliefs changed dramatically. Interestingly enough, Dr. Erickson reported that Dottie had no memory of the hypnosis when he talked with her ten years later. By that time, Dottie had married a pathologist who was doing research on urine and feces, and they had two children. Dottie told Dr. Erickson that she had sexual relations with her husband three to five times a week and had "excellent orgasms," which she experienced throughout her upper body.

### Psychosis and Hypnosis

Although there is some disagreement, it is generally accepted that hypnosis should be avoided with people who are psychotic. However, Erickson did use hypnosis with this diagnosis, again addressing the patient's symptoms and resources in making the determination as to whether or not to use it. The three main reasons given in the literature for not using hypnosis with psychotic patients are:

1.  Psychotics are not good hypnotic subjects in that they have difficulty responding to normal hypnotic inductions (Weitzenhoffer, 1989).
2.  If a psychotic individual could be hypnotized, he or she would not be responsive to hypnotic-based intervention (Weitzenhoffer, 1989).

3.  The psychotic patient has diminished psychological defenses. Because hypnosis is thought to increase psychotic symptoms, there is the fear that decompensation will result (Meares, 1960).

For these reasons, Brenman and Gill (1946) specified that hypnosis is to be especially avoided for psychotic patients who are paranoid. Wolberg (1948) warned that the transference with schizophrenic patients has to be handled carefully when using hypnosis. Furthermore, he warned against giving posthypnotic suggestions in an attempt to induce behavior, which, in the past, was ego-dystonic for the patient. Meares (1960) indicated that using hypnosis with psychotic individuals could lead to a situation in which the therapist would be incorporated into the negative delusional system or become a part of the patient's hallucinations. In the opinion of the authors, these concerns can become issues in all therapeutic modalities, but certainly can be intensified with hypnosis.

There are also traditional concerns that the use of hypnosis with fragile patients can precipitate a psychotic break. However, according to a review of the literature, these concerns are not supported. Abrams (1964) found that most of the reports of psychotic breaks with the use of hypnosis were based on anecdotal material. Heron (1953) and Conn (1972) were skeptical that hypnosis per se was the primary reason for these reports. Cheek & LeCron (1968) asserted that it is the inappropriate use of hypnosis, not the hypnosis itself, that might cause a person to become psychotic: "A skilled therapist might even use hypnosis with such a patient to prevent a psychotic break. In itself, being hypnotized never caused anyone to become psychotic" (pp. 69–70).

In reviewing Dr. Erickson's written articles and listening to his audiotaped lectures, no reference to his use of formal hypnosis with floridly psychotic patients could be found. Likewise, Erickson never referred to such use of hypnosis in any of our conversations with him while in training. In fact, from what we can ascertain, he strongly recommended against using hypnosis with psychotic patients who might decompensate. However, there are records of his using hypnosis with patients who were in less than florid states of psychosis. In each of these instances where Erickson used trance with psychotic or prepsychotic patients, he wrote about the special circumstances that were unique to each patient rather than the common elements of the diagnosis. In examining such cases, the exaggerated elements of the psychotic presentation provide some clear examples of how the Erickson approach respects the potentially delicate nature of some mental conditions.

One example of Dr. Erickson's use of hypnosis with a psychotic individual is discussed in his article on resistance (Erickson, 1964). In this case, a 24-year-old woman was diagnosed as a paranoid schizophrenic, but was not florid at the time of her first session. The young woman had persecutory, auditory, and visual hallucinations and was very antagonistic toward her parents and siblings. A college student with superior intelligence, she had made a mockery of previous, psychodynamically oriented therapists who had tried to treat her. Dr. Erickson said that her pattern was to make the therapist either very self-conscious, defensive, or angry at her, and then treatment would end. She knew that Dr. Erickson used hypnosis, and so offered him an antagonistic challenge by saying, "I have a family that thinks you can hypnotize me into sanity, as they call it" (p. 27).

In dealing with this young woman, Dr. Erickson used a confusion method to provide a safe avenue for her hostility. He did this by accepting her attacks on both his profession and himself. Then he creatively utilized her patterns of attack to get her to listen to a prewritten induction, which included an ideodynamic ratification of his ability to "speak" with her unconscious mind, and the potential of his ability to help her with her problem. Erickson stated that the purpose of using hypnosis during the first session was to gain cooperation and rapport, not necessarily to make any significant clinical changes. As a result of using the hypnosis, Erickson reported that the woman was "... now a most eager, cooperative, and thoroughly responsive patient, making excellent progress" (p. 28).

In actuality, Erickson recognized that the young woman was motivated to fight and ridicule what she anticipated he represented. Because he agreed with her and utilized her attack patterns, he became an "us" rather than a "one of them." Therefore, she gave up her adversarial position and joined Dr. Erickson in a more appropriate therapeutic alliance. Erickson placed the therapeutic emphasis on the woman's intelligence, motivational energy, and history as a student, not on the diagnosis. As Zeig (1997) says, "Thinking of schizophrenia as a 'degenerative brain disease' does not promote interventions." Let us emphasize again that Dr. Erickson always saw the uniqueness of the person, and then responded accordingly.

In another article, Erickson (1954) reported treating a clinically psychotic woman who was catatonic. The woman's husband was a petty criminal, voyeur, and sexual exhibitionist. Shortly after her husband was arrested and sentenced, the woman hallucinated roses floating in Erickson's office. Dr. Erickson states: "She knew that the psychiatrist was a hypnotist and, on entering the office, she had gone into a trance" (p. 217). Thus, a formal induction was not necessary. Dr. Erickson recognized that the woman had spontaneously gone into a trance, so he utilized it in the service of the therapy. He had the woman manipulate the roses by first having her let them float into a vase, change color, and then change into a rose bush. This hypnotic guidance caused a spontaneous age regression, where the patient talked about a little girl who watched her father cut roses. Subsequent sessions involved the woman's spontaneously going into trance and reprocessing elements of her life. By the time she had reprocessed her college experiences, she was no longer clinically psychotic. In this case, Dr. Erickson utilized the patient's natural and spontaneous trance states. The patient determined the appropriateness of hypnosis as a phenomenon, while Erickson determined the appropriateness of hypnosis as a tool with this particular patient.

Erickson (1977) describes another case in which he used hypnosis with a possible psychotic diagnosis. He states, "I think you would call her psychotic, although she had sufficient insight so that you could have some doubts about it. She wasn't quite certain whether she was having dreams or whether her experiences were real" (p. 31). "I was very much afraid that ... [she] ... was going to develop schizophrenia" (p. 30). He described her spontaneous age-regressed symptoms, which were a function of a fixation on early traumas. Using only the most minimal suggestions, Dr. Erickson was able to get her to hallucinate 13 crystal balls. He then had her use the hallucinated crystals to view previously isolated information about age-related events in her life. Then he had her hallucinate a 14th crystal ball that held a positive event that was to happen two months in the future. The use of hypnosis involved making it safe for the patient to observe each isolated traumatic experience and then assisting her conscious mind to integrate the pretrauma child with the 14th-crystal future event. He used this patient's natural strength of insight to dictate the nature of the hypnotic intervention.

These are examples from Dr. Erickson's writings of cases in which he did use hypnosis with psychotic patients. However, according to our research, at no time did he attempt direct and systematic hypnotic techniques when the patient was in a florid state of psychosis. Again, it would appear that when he worked with psychotic patients, whether or not he used hypnosis, he would utilize the symptom and the personal strengths presented in the service of the patient. If the patient hallucinated roses, then the manipulation of the hallucinated roses would redirect the patient into a therapeutic direction where an intervention could take place. If a psychotic patient came into his office and spontaneously went into a trance state, Erickson would utilize and redirect the spontaneous state into a therapeutic trance of rapport without any need for a formal induction. If one were to draw a conclusion from his examples, it would be that at no time did he attempt to alter or challenge a psychotic symptom directly using hypnosis. In contrast to the "attack" approach, Erickson used hypnosis in the above case gently to enhance or utilize a personal strength within the patient to decrease the inner chaos that might have been created by the psychosis. In employing hypnosis in this manner, Erickson's "artificial" enhancement of the personal strength alleviated the psychotic symptoms and reinforced the patient's ego structure.

### Symptom Removal and Hypnosis

In some situations, symptom removal is contraindicated regardless of the diagnosis or the therapeutic technique. For instance, whenever a particular symptom still performs a function to maintain an internal psychological equilibrium, caution is advised when using hypnosis, or any other method, to alter the symptom. Gardner and Olness (1981) warned that, in the treatment of children, symptom removal should be avoided if the symptom is providing a type of "secondary gain" for the child. Hilgard, Hilgard, and Newman (1961) specified that, in some cases, symptom removal as a process in and of itself may result in a severe breakdown. Weitzenhoffer (1989) stated, "I have a simple rule for symptom removal: If a symptom is refractory to treatment or repeatedly reappears after removal, it is best to let the symptom alone until further therapy of a different type has been done" (vol. 2, p. 25).

The caution about symptom removal for the sake of symptom removal is consistent with Dr. Erickson's views. According to the Ericksonian perspective, if a symptom is respected, rather then attacked, the dangers commonly associated with direct symptom removal can be avoided. For example, Cheek and LeCron (1968) advise giving the suggestion in a permissive manner (e.g., "Is it all right for you to lose this symptom?" p. 68) in order to maintain the safety and integrity of any critical functions that the symptom may represent.

Another strategy Erickson would use to create therapeutic relief was to shape the symptom so that it did not create as much of a problem for the patient. An example is the case of a truck driver who had a terrible stuttering problem (Erickson, 1962). Erickson realized that the man's stuttering was associated with pent-up anger. He discovered that the patient was angry with his employer, because he did not keep the trucks in top running condition, and he associated the stuttering with the man's hatred of his noisy truck. He had the man do all of his stuttering in the truck when he was alone. Erickson suggested to him that no one liked his "damn stuttering. It's just a bunch of noise." Because the man didn't like the "damn noise" of his truck, Erickson suggested that he keep his "noisy stuttering" in his "noisy truck." In this case, Erickson felt that the stuttering was a symptom of the man's anger and that he really needed an outlet for the anger, but did not need to stutter all the time.

In conclusion, according to the Ericksonian perspective, when to use hypnosis and when not to use it is not a categorical decision. Each clinical situation must be evaluated on its own merits. The crucial elements in the evaluation are more limited by the qualities of the therapist than by those of the patient. It is unrealistic to think that a therapist can use hypnosis to deal with every problem. Erickson could not work with every patient. Some patients he did not like; some did not like him; and some did not comply with treatment. It is just a little refreshing to know that someone as skilled as Dr. Erickson had failures. However, he was able to succeed in many cases where others could not, and his innate wisdom of human nature and his magnificent skill at applying his knowledge to often very complex manifestations of psychopathology continue to baffle the therapeutic community. Perhaps Erickson's success can best be exemplified in his own words. Haley (1967) recounts the story Erickson used when discussing the therapeutic principles of his work with patients:

> Each case is unique. Another difficulty in generalizing about Erickson is that inevitably there seems to be an exception to whatever one says. He will go to considerable trouble to emphasize that fact about his work. Once, many years ago, a research investigator was engaging in long conversations with Erickson to obtain generalizations about his therapeutic "method" and Erickson was doing his best to educate him. At a certain point, Erickson interrupted the discussion and took the young man outside the house to the front

lawn. He pointed up the street and asked what he saw. Puzzled, the young man replied that he saw a street. Erickson asked if he saw anything else. When he continued to be puzzled, Erickson pointed to the trees which lined the street. "Do you notice anything about those trees?" he asked. After a period of study, the young man said they all were leaning in an easterly direction. "That's right," said Erickson, pleased. "All except one. That second one from the end is leaning in a westerly direction. There's always an exception." (pp. 548–549)

Some therapists have the personality, training, experience, and skill to be effective with patients with whom other therapists cannot work at all, and vice versa. This individuality of the patient–therapist relationship outweighs the effectiveness of any technique, including hypnosis. It is important to remember that a clinical tool is only as effective as the person using it. Just like the saying, "If you're a hammer, everything looks like a nail," it is necessary for the successful clinician to remain flexible and to be able to recognize when, and when not, to use whatever tools there are in the therapeutic armentarium. This was Erickson's gift.

Hypnosis is an extremely valuable tool that needs to be used carefully and selectively. Although it is a complex technique, it can be employed in a variety of ways: from putting individuals into a trance, to taking them out of a preexisting trance; from giving suggestions to remember to giving suggestions to forget; from creating a state of vigilance to creating a state of relaxation. Once the therapist realizes the endless ways in which hypnosis can be utilized, the emphasis is on *how* hypnosis will be used, not on *if* it will be used.

Finally, in approaching any patient, the therapist must ask:

- Do I have adequate clinical training to understand and to anticipate the probable responses from this specific patient?
- Do I have an adequate foundation in my hypnotic training to use hypnosis as an adjunctive tool in the treatment of this particular patient?
- Do I have sufficient understanding about my patient's unique strengths, concerns, and motivations to utilize them within the context of hypnosis toward a therapeutic outcome?
- Do I have the flexibility and experience to employ the responses

of this specific patient in the service of the therapeutic goal?

• Do I have sufficient supervision available with which to confer as I expand the boundaries of my skills and experience in the use of hypnosis as a therapeutic tool?

If the answer is No to any of these questions, then the use of hypnosis is contraindicated.

We end with a quote from Milton Erickson (Haley, 1985), where he defines hypnotic psychotherapy and what makes it effective:

... By such an indirect suggestion, the patient is enabled to go through those difficult inner processes of disorganizing, reorganizing, reassociating, and projecting of inner real experience to meet the requirements of the suggestion, and thus [the suggestion] becomes a part of his experiential life instead of a simple superficial response ... not until he goes through the inner process of reassociating and reorganizing his experiential life can effective results occur ... hypnotic psychotherapy is a learning process for the patient, a procedure of reeducation. Effective results in hypnotic psychotherapy, or hypnotherapy, derive only from the patient's activities. The therapist merely stimulates the patient into activity, often not knowing what the activity may be, and then guides the patient and exercises clinical judgment in determining the amount of work to be done to achieve the desired results. How to guide and to judge constitute the therapist's problem, while the patient's task is that of learning through his own efforts to understand his experiential life in a new way. Such reeducation is, of course, necessarily in terms of the patient's life experiences, his understandings, memories, attitudes, and ideas; it cannot be in terms of the therapist's ideas and opinions. (pp. 28–29)

### References

Abrams, S. (1964). The use of hypnotic techniques with psychotics. *American Journal of Psychotherapy, 18*, 79–94.

Asaad, G. (1994). *Understanding mental disorders due to medical conditions or substance abuse.* New York: Brunner/Mazel.

Barber, J. (1998). When hypnosis causes trouble. *International Journal of Clinical and Experimental Hypnosis, 46*, 157–170.

Brenman, M., & Gill, M. M. (1946). Some recent observations on the use of hypnosis in psychotherapy. *Bulletin of the Menninger Clinic, 10,* 104.

Cheek, D. B., & LeCron, L. M. (1968). *Clinical hypnotherapy.* New York: Grune & Stratton.

Conn, J. H. (1972). Is hypnosis really dangerous? *International Journal of Clinical and Experimental Hypnosis, 20,* 61–79.

Crasilneck, H. B., & Hall, J. B. (1975). *Clinical hypnosis.* New York: Grune & Stratton.

Erickson, B. A. (1994). Ericksonian therapy demystified: A straightforward approach. *Hypnos, 20,* 68–78.

Erickson, M. H. (1950/1980) The abortion issue: Facilitating unconscious dynamics permitting real choice. In E. L. Rossi (Ed.), *The collected papers of Milton Erickson on hypnosis* (vol. 4, pp. 370–373). New York: Irvington.

Erickson, M. H. (1952). *The 1952 lectures at U.C.L.A.* (audiotaped lectures). Phoenix, AZ: Milton H. Erickson Foundation.

Erickson, M. H. (1954). Special techniques of brief hypnotherapy. *Journal of Clinical and Experimental Hypnosis, 2,* 109–129.

Erickson, M. H. (1960). *The Chicago lectures.* (audiotaped lectures). Phoenix, AZ: Milton H. Erickson Foundation.

Erickson, M. H. (1960/1980). Explorations in hypnosis research. In E. L. Rossi (Ed.), *The collected papers of Milton Erickson on hypnosis* (vol. 2, pp. 313–336). New York: Irvington.

Erickson, M. H. (1964). An hypnotic technique for resistant patients: The patient, the technique, and its rationale and field experiments. *American Journal of Clinical Hypnosis, 7,* 8–32.

Erickson, M. H. (1977). Hypnotic approaches to therapy. *American Journal of Clinical Hypnosis, 20,* 20–35.

Erickson, M. H. (1978) *Now you wanted a trance demonstrated* (video teaching tape). Laguna Niguel, CA: Southern California Society for Ericksonian Psychotherapy and Hypnosis.

Erickson, M. H., & Rosen, H. (1954). The hypnotic and hypnotherapeutic investigation and determination of symptom-function. *Journal of Clinical and Experimental Hypnosis, 2,* 201–219.

Erickson, M. H., & Rossi, E. L. (1979). *Hypnotherapy.* New York: Irvington.

Frauman, D. C., Lynn, S. J., & Brantar, J. P. (1993). Prevention and therapeutic management of "negative effects" in hypnotherapy. In J. W. Rhue, S. J. Lynn, & I. Kirsch (Eds.), *Handbook of clinical hypnosis* (pp. 95–120). Washington, DC: American Psychological Association.

Gardner, G. G., & Olness, K. (1981). *Hypnosis and hypnotherapy with children.* Orlando, FL: Grune & Stratton.

Haley, J. (1967). Commentary on the writings of Milton H. Erickson, M.D. In J. Haley (Ed.), *Advanced techniques of hypnosis and therapy: Selected papers of Milton H. Erickson, M.D.* (pp. 530–549). New York: Grune & Stratton.

Haley, J. (1973). *Uncommon therapy.* New York: Norton.

Haley, J. (Ed.). (1985). *Conversation with Milton H. Erickson, M.D. Changing individuals, Vol. 1.* New York: Triangle (Norton).

Hartland, J. (1971). *Medical and dental hypnosis and its clinical applications* (2nd ed.). London: Bailliere Tindal.

Hartland, J. (1974). An alleged case of criminal assault upon a married woman under hypnosis. *American Journal of Clinical Hypnosis, 16,* 188–198.

Heron, W. T. (1953). *Clinical applications of suggestion and hypnosis.* Springfield, IL: Charles C. Thomas.

Hilgard, J. R., Hilgard, E. R., & Newman, M. (1961). Sequelae of hypnotic induction with special reference to earlier chemical anesthesia. *Journal of Nervous and Mental Disease, 133,* 461–475.

Judd, F. K., Burrows, G. D., & Dennerstein, L. (1985). The dangers of hypnosis: A review. *Australian Journal of Clinical and Experimental Hypnosis, 13,* 1–15.

Lynn, S. J., Martin, D. J., & Frauman, D. C. (1996). Does hypnosis pose special risks for negative effects? A master class commentary. *International Journal of Clinical and Experimental Hypnosis, 44,* 7–19.

Meares, A. (1960). *A system of medical hypnosis.* Philadelphia: Saunders.

Orne, M. T. (1972). Can a hypnotized subject be compelled to carry out otherwise unacceptable behavior? *International Journal of Clinical and Experimental Hypnosis, 20,* 101–117.

Parsons-Fein, J. (1998). Reply to Lazarus's article. *Hypnos, 25,* 213–216.

Rosen, S. (1982). The value and philosophy of Milton H. Erickson. In J. K. Zeig (Ed.), *Ericksonian approaches to hypnosis and psychotherapy* (pp. 462–476). New York: Brunner/Mazel.

Rossi, E. L., & Ryan, M. O. (1985). *The seminars, workshops and lectures of Milton H. Erickson, Vol. 1: Life reframing in hypnosis.* New York: Irvington.

Spiegel, H., & Spiegel, D. (1978). *Trance and treatment.* New York: Basic Books.

Watkins, J. G. (1987). *Hypnotherapeutic techniques, Vol. 1.* New York: Irvington.

Weitzenhoffer, A. M. (1989). *The practice of hypnotism, Vols. 1–2.* New York: Wiley.

Wolberg, L. R. (1948). *Medical hypnosis, Vol. I: The principles of hypnotherapy.* New York: Grune & Stratton.

Yapko, M. (1984). *Trancework.* New York: Irvington.

Zeig, J. K. (1992). The virtues of our faults: A key concept of Ericksonian psychotherapy. In J. K. Zeig (Ed.), *The evolution of psychotherapy: The second conference*
(pp. 252–269). New York: Brunner/Mazel,

Zeig, J. K. (1994). *Ericksonian methods. The essence of the story.* New York: Brun-
ner/Mazel.

Zeig, J. K. (1997, September 19). *Entering delusions.* Milton H. Erickson Forum, Internet communication.

### Suggested Readings

Barber, J. (1998). When hypnosis causes trouble. *International Journal of Clinical and
Experimental Hypnosis, 46,* 157–170.

Erickson, M. H., & Rossi, E. L. (1979). *Hypnotherapy.* New York: Irvington.

Haley, J. (Ed.). (1985). *Conversation with Milton H. Erickson, M.D. Changing individuals, Vol. 1.* New York: Triangle (Norton).

Rossi, E. L. (Ed.). (1980). *The collected papers of Milton Erickson on hypnosis, Vols. 1–4.*
New York: Irvington.

# 7

# Transference/Countertransference

*Eric Greenleaf*

I knew a great deal is said about this transference relationship, and while I like to have my patients like me, and like me immensely, I want them to like me in such a fashion that I, as a therapist, can be pleased.
— Milton Erickson (Haley, 1985, vol. 2, p. 68)

## UTILIZATION AND IMAGINATION

The relational forms encouraged by a hypnotic psychotherapy lead in different directions from those engaged in by the several "dynamic" psychotherapies. In the latter, the concepts of *resistance* and *transference* predominate, whereas the former are guided by notions of *utilization* and *imagination*.

Freud, we know, derived the concepts of resistance and transference from his hypnotic experiences. He observed that Bernheim would restore memories of experiences from the trance state by pressing firmly with his hands on the patients' foreheads after they awakened from trance. The physical and emotional pressure required for this gave Freud (1935, pp. 50–51) his metaphor for resistance:

When the subject awoke from the state of somnambulism he seemed to have lost all memory of what had happened while he was in that state. But Bernheim maintained that the memory was present all the same; and if he insisted on the subject remembering, if he asseverated that the subject knew it all and only had to say it, and if at the same time he laid his hand on the subject's forehead, then the forgotten memories used in fact to return, hesitatingly at first, but eventually in a flood and with complete clarity.

Freud's lively image of Bernheim's insisting that patients remember, and accompanying his words with pressure on a patient's forehead, gives us some sense of the experiences that generated the concept of resistance as an analogy to such physical events as hydraulic pressure. And the rhetorical element in this hypnosis, the relational aspect expressed in ordinary language, reminds us that across the room from every resistant patient we may encounter a stubborn therapist.

Freud's observations of the social interactions in therapy were lost in the later development of psychoanalysis as a theory of intrapsychic conflict and accommodation. In modern narrative therapies (White & Epston, 1990), "resistance" is once again used to denote an interpersonal refusal to allow influences from another, and is encouraged as a means of recovery, rather than disparaged as an impediment to desired change.

The entire strategy of *utilization* derives from the highly original work of Milton Erickson. This concept, like Freud's resistance, was developed in hypnotic work with difficult patients (Erickson, 1980, vol. 4, p. 178):

Ordinarily trance induction is based upon securing from the patients some form of initial acceptance and cooperation with the operator. In techniques of utilization the usual procedure is reversed to an initial acceptance of the patients' presenting behaviors and a ready cooperation by the operator, however seemingly adverse the presenting behaviors may appear to be in the clinical situation.

This explanation, like a plain wool coat with a gorgeous silk lining, covers some charming and spectacular therapy. Erickson (Haley, 1993), confronted with a man who thought himself to be Christ, opined that the man must have experience as a carpenter and helped him develop work in that field and a life with other people. Met at an initial session by a man who cursed Erickson, psychiatry, and much else, Erickson said, "I'm sure you can say that and even more," opening the conversation between them to therapy.

We have been taught that "acceptance" of emotion in therapy is communicated to patients by saying, in effect, "I understand that you feel such and such to be so." Differences between the therapist's formulation and the patient's are often ascribed to patient resistance. Utilization approaches to communication take the patient's formulation as a given and extend it to action that helps to meet the goals of the patient: "You are [Christ] a skilled carpenter, therefore, take on meaningful work," or, "You have a lot to say [about me of a rude, negative sort] so you can say even more." As Rossi noted of Erickson (Erickson & Rossi, 1979, p. 234):

> The most common reason the senior author gave for both his successes and failures was the degree to which he was able to evoke and utilize the particular patient's motivation and repertory of experiential learning. The most remarkable hypnotic effects could be evoked because of the nature of the transference relationship and the importance of these hypnotic responses for the patient's much desired therapeutic outcome.

In current usage in many therapies, transference has come to mean a patterned response to the therapist that imitates the pattern of the patient's childhood relationships with parents. Freud's own use of the term is much broader (Freud, 1935, p. 80):

> Transference ... decides the success of all medical influence, and in fact delineates the whole of each person's relations to his human environment. We can easily recognize it as the same dynamic factor that the hypnotists have named "suggestibility" which is the agent of hypnotic rapport and whose incalculable behavior led to such difficulties with the cathartic method. When there is no indication to a transference of emotion ... then there is also no possibility of influencing the patient by psychological means.

The difficulties Freud refers to in this treatment of human relations are those that gave rise to the "grave doubts" about hypnotism with which generations of therapists are familiar. The origins of both doubt and transference are found in this narrative from Freud's *An Autobio-graphical Study* (1935, pp. 45–50):

> One day I had an experience which showed me in the crudest light what I had long suspected. One of my most acquiescent patients, with whom hypnotism had enabled me to bring about the most marvellous results, and whom I was engaged in relieving of her suffering by tracing back her attacks of pain to their origins, as she woke up on one occasion, threw her arms round my neck. The unexpected entrance of a servant relieved us from a painful discussion, but from that time onwards there was a tacit understanding between us that the hypnotic treatment should be discontinued ... I felt that I had now grasped the nature of the mysterious element that was at work behind hypnotism. In order to exclude it ... or to isolate it ... it was necessary to abandon hypnotism.

It's striking that Freud allowed "tacit understanding" to replace "analysis of the transference" and that the drama of this event was used to clothe Freud's scarecrow conception of hypnosis and of the unconscious mind. Dynamic therapists came to adopt versions of this point of view, as exemplified by Hill (Erickson & Hill, 1994, p. 216), who confuses Erickson's lack of interpretation of the transference relationship with an absense of utilization of it:

> Analysts have found that the transference is a vital part of the therapeutic process and that the intrapsychic conflict would not continue its disturbing existence were it not for current difficulties in personal relationships according to a pattern of transference and provoked by the individual's relationship to his environment. The hypnotist evidently holds the view that the intrapsychic conflict exists as an entity complete in itself although modifiable by extra-psychic influences. The transference of the hypnotic subject to the hypnotist is ignored or at least not utilized as a therapeutic instrument by the hypnotist. Psychoanalytic technique explores precisely the transference as the essential focus of therapy.

Therapists employing hypnotic therapy in ways other than hypnoanalysis also wrestled with the narrow notion of transference. Cheek and

LeCron (1968, pp. 44, 69) are good examples of authors caught between terms from different approaches:

> Rapport is not only related to hypnosis but is a factor in all good physician-patient relationships. Rapport seems to become stronger when one is under hypnosis ... [it] can be said to be empathy on the part of the subject with a strong desire to please the operator. It is closely related to what Freud called transference. ... As to transference, in brief therapy it is seldom of any importance and usually is disregarded or does not even develop. Ordinarily it can be handled easily through hypnosis.

Rossi (Erickson, 1980, vol. 3, pp. 250–251), trained as a Jungian analyst, tries on that theory's view of hypnotherapeutic relationship for size:

> In actual practice ... the analyst mediates the transcendent function of the patient, i.e., helps him to bring consciousness and unconsciousness together and so arrive at a new attitude. In this function of the analyst lies one of the many important meanings of the transference. The patient clings by means of the transference to the person who seems to promise him a renewal of attitude. ...

Restoring Freud's original, broad use of the term "transference," with its homology to hypnotic rapport and suggestibility, we can proceed to develop the modern sense of hypnotic psychotherapy as a focused and collaborative relational enterprise whose meanings are constructed through imaginative acts during a continuing conversation.

The analysts held that analysands "imagined" the nature of their relationship to the analyst. Rossi (Erickson & Rossi, 1981, p. 156) said, "In every analytic treatment there arises, without the physician's agency, an intense emotional relationship between the patient and the analyst which is not to be accounted for by the actual situation." Ericksonian therapists, taking responsibility for their influence on the relationship and guided by the principle of utilization, seek ways to use the imagined relationship as the actual situation to aid their patients in meeting their own goals.

Erickson's "February Man" monograph (Erickson & Rossi, 1979) is one striking example of the uses of imagination in forming therapeutic relatedness. Here Erickson utilizes the patient's feelings towards him—her rapport with him, her liking of him, her dependence on him—to help her meet her goals in therapy. He does this by informing her that she can revisit troubling times in her life with him as company. The widely quoted induction of this companionship is familiar to most Ericksonian therapists (Erickson & Rossi, 1979):

> And I want you to choose some time in the past when you were a very, very little girl. And my voice will go with you. And my voice will change into that of your parents, your neighbors, your friends, your schoolmates, your playmates, your teachers. And I want you to find yourself sitting in the schoolroom, a little girl feeling happy about something, something that happened a long time ago, that you forgot a long time ago.

Erickson's approach to or attitude toward patients is clear in this: The patient has an experience of free choice and can seek a positive outcome according to her goals. Her imagination can include Erickson, her past, and strong emotions in a safe and interesting relationship.

To replace the analytic concept of "working through the transference," with its implication of interpretation and conscious understanding, Erickson chooses to utilize transferential feelings unconsciously, in pursuit of desired changes. Freud (1935, p. 80) was clear on the distinction:

> It is perfectly true that psychoanalysis, like other psychotherapeutic methods, employs the instrument of suggestion (or transference). But the difference is this: that in analysis it is not allowed to play the decisive part in determining the therapeutic results. ... The transference is made conscious to the patient by the analyst and it is resolved by convincing him that in his transference-attitude he is *re-experiencing* emotional relations which had their origin during the repressed period of his childhood.

Erickson, utilizing these relationships, rather than convincing his patient of their interpreted meaning, describes his approach to Rossi, again using "February Man" as an example (Erickson & Rossi, 1979, p. 97):

MHE: When I ask, "How do you think you will like me three or four years from now?," I've got a good rapport with her. She answers with, "It will be *nice*." I come back with, "I think it will be nice to meet you then." I've depotentiated a little girlish crush.

ELR: To diminish the transference?

MHE: Um-hum.

ELR: You do these things in such a literal, concrete way!

MHE: And so very easily!

J. O. Behrs, in *Understanding Erickson's Approach* (Zeig, 1982, p. 79), discusses aspects of this difference between Erickson and the range of dynamic therapists:

> The implication that, even in borderline patients, intact hidden observers may be present and may perceive the therapist accurately, no matter how intense the transference may be overtly, suggests a possibly major revision in psychoanalytic method without significantly violating its theory. Talking directly to the hidden aspects, or "communicating with the unconscious," as Erickson defined the hypnotic modality, might serve the same function as working through the transference but more expeditiously.

Another modern understanding of this difference is expressed by an experienced psychologist and hypnotherapist (Stott, 1998), who has herself experienced both dynamic and Ericksonian therapies as a patient:

> I remembered that I had been trying to explain to my analytically oriented friend how it could be acceptable for me to attend a seminar that my psychotherapist was presenting. "It's not a problem to see him in these two roles," I explained. "In fact, the two contribute to one another. I think it is not problematic because the transference in our work together is so different from what I've experienced in the past. "What do you mean?" she said.
>
> My response: When Eric and I work together, there is an area between us where we meet and work. We both come there out of our own lives, bringing with us what we need to do the work. I am usually there as myself, but with a willing vulnerability to be open and direct, and as disclosing as possible, sometimes with a curiosity to understand something, and sometimes with just a need

to be understood, knowing that as Eric understands me I will come to understand myself.

There's the third place in the room: there's him and there's me and there's the place we work together. If there were a transference, it would be to the relationship. But I don't think you can really call it transference. It allows the work to develop, it enables it and it's quite freeing. It allows for basic processes to occur in a very supportive, nurturing, holding environment.

You don't go through all that stuff about boundaries. You effectively strengthen ego functioning as opposed to the traditional transference of attachment-individuation. It is more direct, but an entirely different experience.

He seems to come as himself; his personal life is somewhat visible (although the details are unknown) but largely irrelevant except as it lends understanding to something I'm trying to understand. It is present in a pleasant way; it imparts a kindness and a keen interest in people, but is nonintrusive in the work. Thus the "transference" is much less personal than in a more traditional framework. He never feels like my father to me, for example, even though there are times when I take from him the kindness and gentleness or the wisdom or the challenge that one would wish to receive from a father.

It is as though the interpersonal aspects of the therapy are all channeled through this working space between us, and in that way become personal yet impersonal and have to do with our work in that room, not who Eric is when he is presenting a seminar. Much as one can learn to dance from a talented dance instructor, experience the dance, learn to whirl and soar on the dance floor, by experiencing the instructor without ever needing to know him or her, it's that way with therapy. Thus seeing him in a seminar setting has very little bearing on the work we do together in the office. They are just two different ways of experiencing the same person.

## THE PERSON OF THE THERAPIST

Freud's patients came to his home office, read his books, knew his colleagues. Erickson's patients came to his home office, read his books, met his family. In distinction to the idea that the therapist can be a "blank screen" for a patient's projections, Ericksonian therapists hope to use their persons—voice, posture, humor, presence, social circumstance—to influence the other person's recovery and growth. We assume strong emotional responses, positive and negative, as a correlate of any real human relationship.

The "negative countertransference" was used by Erickson to train his medical students in developing a therapeutic attitude toward and feelings for their patients. He describes his approach to the therapist's emotions using the analytic language his students understood. His description comes from a 1965 workshop on using hypnosis in pain control (Erickson, 1983, vol. 1, pp. 271–272):

> Now here is an important question: In your endeavor to analyze and control the attitudes of patients, how do you subdue your own countertransference so that anxiety is therefore not aroused?
>
> I have often taken my medical students through cancer clinics because I think they ought to see terminal cases of cancer; I think they ought to see all the ulcerations and all the very difficult things that result from neglectful cases. This was in the County Hospital ... and my medical students were rather repulsed by the appearance of the patients' wounds and by their generally depressing condition.
>
> After my students were thoroughly repulsed and had manifested thoroughly their adverse reactions, I pointed out: "You are reacting adversely to these patients. Why? Aren't they the patients that are affording you a medical education? How do you expect to make your living except by meeting your patients, by respecting and liking them—by thoroughly liking them. ... Don't you think you ought to be grateful to those patients?"
>
> I also would take medical students through the back wards of the psychiatric section and do the same thing with them. You simply ought not to have any other attitude toward patients but one of sympathy and liking and respect.

In his own experience as a therapist, Erickson tolerated all manner of emotions toward patients, as he did in his students, but with the same emphasis on providing the patient with "sympathy, liking, and respect."

His response to his own emotional adjustments is both characteristic and charming (Haley, 1985, vol. 1, p. 89):

> I had an experience of countertransference the other night. This woman irritates the life out of me. Horribly so. The previous patient had come in a bathing suit and got the chair of the seat all wet. So I got a towel and draped it over the seat of the chair. Then the patient that irritates me so much came in, sat down on the towel, and irritated me very much. I suddenly realized, with a great deal of amusement, that after she left I had taken hold of the corner of that towel and very carefully, gingerly, picked it up and put it in the laundry. [*Laughter*] That really amused me. My own more or less phobic response to the towel—which took up all my anger. I think I must have looked funny taking that towel out to the laundry.

### THE THERAPIST AS STAND-IN

Even the most brilliant results were liable to be suddenly wiped away if my personal relationship with the patient became disturbed, proving that the personal emotional relation between doctor and patient was after all stronger than the whole cathartic process and escaped every effort at control.

— Sigmond Freud (1935, p. 48)

The stand-in is a member of the theatrical troupe or film cast who takes the place of the major characters, says their lines, and allows the other players to block their scenes and take their cues in the absence of the star. At the actual performance, the stand-in waits in the wings while the main actors take the stage. In active therapies, such as psychodrama, with its metaphorical space of theater, a stand-in's role can be central to rehearsals of the action.

Traditional therapies might benefit from this way of thinking of relationship. Rather than taking umbrage at being considered stand-ins for parents, friends, or lovers, therapists may enjoy and encourage this use of their abilities. They may say, "Let me talk to you like a mother (or a 'Dutch uncle,' friend or brother)." They may even say, "If I were a different sort of therapist, I might say ..."

An example of the stand-in approach to troubles and of the idea of imagination replacing that of transference is found in "Conjoint Therapy with an Imagined Co-therapist" (Greenleaf, 1985). I was consulted by Melody, a happily married woman who, although orgasmic with her husband and experiencing a wide range of sexual activity and emotion, suffered a feeling of sexual restraint. Her inhibition, although shameful and secret to her, was manifest in a fearful reluctance to undergo routine gynecological examinations. She also experienced nausea and dizziness when attempting to use tampons. In addition, and more unsettling still to Melody, herself a psychotherapist, she had contracted a series of "crushes" on a succession of therapists she consulted, the first one some three months following her marriage, the others over the course of the next 15 years.

Melody's therapy with me continued through the resolution of her inhibition, lasting over a year. We met for an hour each week and dealt in turn with themes in her life that seemed to offer a way to the relief of her distress. Meanwhile, Melody's "crush" on her therapist grew and flourished. As Melody said, "I need to keep doing this until I exhaust myself and let go of it."

Melody was encouraged repeatedly to express all her sexual feelings by words and in letters and to enjoy these feelings as the natural expression of her strong, womanly emotions. As she said, "It happens a little bit with the writing, but the experience of relief is much stronger after I actually have put these letters and dreams in your box."

Now, the experience of having an attractive, intelligent woman of honest conviction declare sexual passion week after week is a heady one, no matter how trivialized, demonized, or interpreted in the therapeutic literature. My box was piled high with letters. I thought I could use some help, and so suggested that Melody solicit a woman's view of her intense emotions. To save the expense involved, she was to consult, in her imagination, with a woman therapist of her choosing. She chose the distinguished and innovative family therapist Mara Selvini Palazzoli. Then, at home, she held the first of four long conversations with Mara.

In the first talk, Mara gave Melody a blue and red cloth blanket, telling her:

It belonged to your grandmother many years ago. She gave it up, put it away, far away, so that it was lost even in memory, when her first love died. This was the mantle of her womanhood. Under

its warm protection she would surrender fully to him—but more
important, she would yield to the mysteries of her own nature.

Mara told her, too, that Melody's husband would be as enriched as she
was by her "secret treasure."

The second conversation had Melody ask Mara for understanding of
"this dream about the small girl-child and the male torso with the large
penis." Placing Melody and the three-year-old girl on the magic blue blanket, Mara transported them to the hill that is the dream's most frightening place. She said, "No harm will come to either of you. I will help you
discover what to do." Melody and the child were naked. "Suddenly I was
aware that a shadow had fallen over us. Mara called to me, 'Melody, open
your eyes and look now.'"

It was a tall, dark, handsome stranger. Mara took the child away with
her, then returned to Melody. Mara coaxed Melody to speak with him, sit
with him, touch him, make love with him. Melody and the man are car-
essed. "Suddenly, I felt afraid. At that moment, Mara's singing came to
me with the breeze—she was comforting the child, and I, too, felt
soothed." Melody and the stranger made love until both were satisfied.
The child returned and Mara told Melody, "Your body holds all the
meaning you need."

Mara brought together the themes of the frightened little girl, the
alluring stranger, and a grown woman's sexual knowledge. And she placed
these in the context of the patient's history—her imitation of a grandpar-
ent's inhibited love. For their third conversation, I asked Melody to speak
with Mara about her strong, sexual feelings toward me.

In this conversation, Mara led Melody to describe her sexual imaginings and emotions. Then Mara suggested that she imagine being in the
office with me. Melody asked that Mara accompany her in this imagining
and warned her, "If you get me into hot water, I'm leaving!" She was encouraged to express her natural feelings in words—they turned out to be
words of warmth and affection—and was told, "It's the holding back that
creates difficulty. Long ago you learned to suppress these natural and very
right feelings."

The fourth conversation with Mara concerned ways in which Melody
might schedule her time and care for herself in the world, at work, among
her friends. Of the conversations with Mara, Melody said:

They seem to be supporting this important shift from my regarding you as the one to be revered and idolized to simply one who is my equal. I'm not speaking here of the content of the conversations; but rather of the structure itself. In addition, Mara's femaleness . . . in some way is allowing me to reown my own wisdom and power, rather than project them onto some male figure (you, most recently). I feel happy. Yes! I feel happy! I think I am finally falling in love with myself.

The resolution of issues of emotion was not accompanied by sexual disinhibition, although it did produce real changes in Melody's sense of herself, changes noted with approval by her friends and husband. Even into the next year, Melody insisted on bringing forth the remaining aspects of her family drama for experiencing, talking about, dreaming with, and understanding:

I dreamed that as I was looking into the deepest part of the water, which was at the beginning, a man who was alternately my husband and my father came up behind me as I was looking.

In February, Melody tearfully "confessed" that she had yet to overcome her sexual inhibition, and in March she asked to discontinue therapy, then changed her mind and continued until her successful completion of the experiences she had set for herself as the task of therapy. Her ability to endure gynecological examination comfortably was affirmed early that year, the disinhibition of her sexual fear in April, and the ability to insert a tampon without nausea and dizziness was hers by September.

These goals and investigations had to be accomplished, as Erickson always insisted, "In your own way; in your own good time; in the right way; at the right time." So, the acknowledgment of sexual passion as a natural emotion, the expression of sexual activity toward the right partner, respect for the emotions brought forward in psychotherapy and between therapist and patient, and trust in one's own wisdom, power, and love—all of these themes of emotion must coexist and be expressed. As Melody put it: "The charm would be to feel what I feel neither more nor less than what is actually so in the moment, and to find a way to stay in contact with you at the same time."

To illustrate the work further, and to give the reader its flavor, I include a transcript of the session in which Melody and I met and employed the aid of Mara as an imagined co-therapist. Here, "G" is Eric Greenleaf and "P" is Melody Palmer:

G:    I thought we might have a joint session today.

P:    With?

G:    Mara.

P:    I thought about that the other day. (*Laughs.*) And?

G:    I had the idea that she and I could show you something about this dilemma that you're in. All right. Just suppose you just sit back and close your eyes. (*Pause*) Now, I don't know when you started going to "blue movies," but if you started going to blue movies a long time ago, you probably remember that the male characters in those movies often wore masks. If you didn't start going that long ago, take my word for it. (*P. laughs.*)

    Now, in the letters you wrote to me you told me some interesting things. And, one of the interesting things you told me was that it's different to have sexual feelings in a daydream than it is to have a variety of feelings right here, talking with me, and that the contrast is intriguing to you—isn't bedeviling you. So, I thought, Mara and I would sit with you, and let you see a blue movie of your daydream, and then, at some point, when you are satisfied with the erotic content of this daydream, the male character in it will peel off his mask, and then you could see, and then he will peel off his mask again—as many masks as he has. And so, Mara will turn on the film. You can watch to your heart's content. Just have to watch the screen—you'll see it. She'll sit to one side of you and I'll sit to the other, and you can just watch, and when you finish watching the movie, open your eyes and tell me what you saw.

P:    And this male is supposed to have a mask?

G:    Well, you know, he'll probably look like your therapist, to begin with. At least, that's the mask he's always had in the past.

P:    How true. (*Laughs.*) Oh, God.

G:    Now, while you watch the movie, I'm not going to watch you. I'm going to go out to get coffee. Do you want coffee? Do you want tea? Do you want milk?

P:    You're supposed to say, "Coffee, tea or me?" (*Laughs.*) All right.

Tea, with one sugar.

*(Ten minutes pass while P sits by herself. G leaves to get coffee and tea. Then he returns.)*

P:     You came in just at the good part. Now, what about this "mask" business? Am I supposed to know who he is?

G:     Not necessarily. He might look like a complete stranger. If you have any questions, ask Mara what she knows about this odd event, that this complete stranger has such strong sexual attraction for you.

P:     So strange. I have this little, vague image of this older man. I imagined there'd be more masks, but it's the same. I'm sort of surprised though that even ... like when I saw this older man who's a stranger *I didn't feel horrified.*

G:     I wonder if you'd ask Mara if she's felt in her life strong, powerful sexual attraction for strangers, or if she knows that in other women? Just listen as she tells you about it.

P:     She has a very positive view on this subject (*Laughs.*). She says that it's an experience many people have and it's not something to be afraid of or ashamed of, but something you should be glad for. Sometimes it's easy to have your head up in a cloud perhaps, and these feelings can be reminders of something more rooted.

G:     Something more lifelike. Is her stranger an older stranger?

P:     She doesn't have only one. Well, she's older. (*Laughs.*) She has older and younger ones. Likes variety. (*Laughs.*)

G:     Yes, she does. (*Pause.*) And you can just open your eyes. Well, how did you enjoy it?

P:     What do you say I do when I do that? When I get into my thing, what am I doing? When I get into these fantasies it's like I give over conscious function to you. You being the teacher or being in charge. And then, that lets me imagine myself to get more and more intensely into sexual feelings. But actually, I'm doing the whole thing. I'm just using you in a sort of convenient way.

G:     Ah! That's me—a sexual convenience!

P:     (*Laughs.*) But here that's appropriate.

G:     I think that's exactly so.

Following this exchange, Melody was treated to a long, complicated lecture on the various psychoanalytic and Jungian analytic interpretations of the "stranger" in sexuality and of the utility of denial as a gradual way of allowing information to enter consciousness. The concept of the archetypes of the collective unconscious was invoked to encourage a rearrangement of emotions and actions better suited to Melody's individual needs and sensibilities than the arrangement bequeathed her by her family.

Then, in the last minutes of the hour, we spoke about relationship:

G:     So, what makes people special is the experience of doing something unique together. You know the story "The Little Prince"? You know what the fox says to the Little Prince when he's leaving? He says, "There are millions of little boys in the world, and millions of foxes. But what is it that makes you special to me? You're special to me because you've 'tamed' me," says the fox to the boy. "So, wherever I go I will see the color of your hair in the waving wheat and the color of your eyes in the blue sky." He didn't think he was the blondest boy in the world or the fox the reddest fox in the world, but it was special for them because of the relationship between them, although the world is full of foxes and boys.

It is important, when doing psychotherapy, to respect the emotions brought forth and the reality of the relationships formed during the work. Even Freud said, "Psychoanalysis is in essence a cure through love" (Bettelheim, 1983, p. v). Everyone has recognized, though, that these relationships and emotions are embedded in a complex context, now thought of in terms of narratives, structures, or families, or conceived of as complexes or introjects.

When interacting with others, we are all aware of the "voice of conscience," and some of us, too, of "voices" or "visions," the haunting presence of our dealings with others, or of the aspects of our "unconscious minds," carried by persons both in dreams and in waking life. Wise counsel from friends, family, and therapists also provides us with authority for our conduct. We may remember the voice of a friend, or, indeed, of Milton Erickson, during periods of doubt or struggle.

That said, it is a hallmark of effective therapy that people come more and more to depend on their own wisdom and emotions in living life and to feel equal with all other humans they may meet along their way. As Melody said to me that August:

> You will perhaps enjoy hearing what my friend said to me this morning as we were standing on the porch at work: "Melody, you have been looking so sexy lately. Are you going through a little sexual revolution or something?" I said, "Yes!"

## SUMMARY AND CONCLUSIONS

Alongside differences in approach to resistance and transference, some of the other important differences between older dynamic therapies and the modern strategic and narrative forms of Ericksonian psychotherapy should be kept in mind. To summarize: (1) The therapist in the dynamic model is meant to be emotionally neutral and reflective in tone while oriented toward the patient's past. Modern therapists are urged to be emotionally positive, humorous, and expectant, active in tone and future oriented. (2) The patient in a dynamic therapy is held responsible for change, and yet is enjoined to understand rather than to act. Modern therapists hold themselves responsible for change and encourage the patient to act, although the responsibility is often thought to be collective and the actions may be imaginative acts, or small changes in simple patterns of action. (3) Dynamic therapies entertain the concept of resistance and hold that the goal of therapy is to make the unconscious conscious. Modern therapies employ utilization of the unconscious alongside consciousness. (4) The method of dynamic psychotherapy is interpretation, an analytic tool with which to conceptualize the past differently. The modern method is storytelling, a didactic tool with which to imagine different futures. (5) Insight is held to yield change in dynamic models of therapy, whereas in many modern ones change is held to yield foresight

The practices of hypnotherapy involve a focus of attention on the entirety of the person before us: posture and physiology, language, figures of speech, patterns of action, culture, and personal style. Although it is true that hypnotherapists learn to give directives and to tell stories, they also practice a mutually focused relationship of ease and intensity, which contrasts with both the stereotyped authoritarian hypnotist and the stereotyped neutral analyst. Hypnotherapeutic practices encourage surprising and imaginative possibilities in social roles, as well as in emotions, images, and actions.

---

**Ideas About Thinking About Ericksonian Principles**

- Enjoy Erickson's maxim (Erickson, 1980, vol. 1, p. 146): "The need to appreciate the subject as a person possessing individuality which must be respected cannot be overemphasized."
- Think of communicating and of relationship, not of the intrapsychic.
- Utilize the therapy relationship to help patients realize their goals.
- Use the imagined relationships that are available as tools in therapy.
- Discuss anything openly with people while remaining un(self)-conscious.

---

## References

Bettelheim, B. (1983). *Freud and man's soul.* New York: Knopf.

Cheek, D. B. and LeCron, L. M. (1968). *Clinical hypnotherapy.* New York: Grune & Stratton.

Erickson, M. H. (1980). In E. L. Rossi (Ed.), *Collected papers of Milton H. Erickson on hypnosis* (4 vols.). New York: Irvington.

Erickson, M. H. (1983). E. L. Rossi, M. O. Ryan, & F. A. Sharp (Eds.), *Healing in hypnosis: The seminars, workshops and lectures of Milton H. Erickson* (4 vols.). New York: Irvington.

Erickson, M. H. & Hill, L. B. (1944/1980). Unconscious mental activity in hypnosis: psychoanalytic implications. In E. L. Rossi (Ed.), *Collected papers of Milton H. Erickson on hypnosis* (vol. 3, pp. 207–220). New York: Irvington.

Erickson, M. H. & Rossi, E. L. (1979). *Hypnotherapy: An exploratory casebook.* New York: Irvington.

Erickson, M. H. & Rossi, E. L. (1981). *Experiencing hypnosis: Therapeutic approaches to altered states.* New York: Irvington.

Erickson, M. H. and Rossi, E. L. (1989). *The February man: Evolving consciousness and identity in hypnotherapy.* New York: Brunner/Mazel.

Freud, S. (1935). *An autobiographical study.* New York: Norton.

Greenleaf, E. (1985). Conjoint hypnotherapy with an imagined co-therapist. In J. K. Zeig (Ed.), *Ericksonian psychotherapy, Vol. III: Clinical applications* (pp. 507–514). New York: Brunner/Mazel.

Haley, J. (Ed.). (1985). *Conversations with Milton H. Erickson, M.D.* New York: Triangle Press.

Haley, J. (1993). *Jay Haley on Milton H. Erickson.* New York: Brunner/Mazel.

Rosen, S. (Ed.). (1982). *My voice will go with you: The teaching tales of Milton H. Erickson.* New York: Norton.

Stott, F. (1998). *Note on transference in dynamic and Ericksonian therapies* (unpublished).

White, M. & Epston, D. (1990). *Narrative means to therapeutic ends.* New York: Norton.

Zeig, J. K. (Ed.). (1982). *Ericksonian approaches to hypnosis and psychotherapy.* New York: Brunner/Mazel.

## Suggested Readings

Erickson, M. H. & Rossi, E. L. (1989). *The February man: Evolving consciousness and identity in hypnotherapy.* New York: Brunner/Mazel.

Haley, J. (1993). *Jay Haley on Milton H. Erickson.* New York: Brunner/Mazel.

Rosen, S. (Ed.). (1982). *My voice will go with you: The teaching tales of Milton H. Erickson.* New York: Norton.

# 8

# Storytelling

*Betty Alice Erickson*

Milton H. Erickson, M.D., became legendary for therapeutic story-telling. Telling stories is now a recognized psychotherapeutic tool, principally because of the way Erickson used them. Those who came to work and study with him recognized the charm and power of the stories he told his patients and used in his teaching. Students began not only to write about the technique, but also to use stories in their own teaching and practice of therapy.

Erickson told stories for fun and also for specific reasons. He learned the attractions, the purposes and the power of stories early in his life. As a very young man, he told stories to fishermen he met while canoeing on the Mississippi and Wisconsin rivers, as he worked to recover from effects of infantile paralysis. He later took great pleasure in recounting how he had earned meals by telling stories. More important, he learned a great deal about people and storytelling.

In the 1940s, he was a frequent contributor to a newspaper column of vignettes about average people during World War II. He told his children bedtime stories throughout their lives. He told stories to virtually all his patients and all his students. And then he told stories about the stories he had told.

Most of the time, his stories had multiple purposes. First and fore-most, they were engaging and entertaining for both Erickson and the listener. They also provided examples of understanding and behaving, as well as offering people the opportunity to learn in multilevel, nonthreatening, and pleasing ways.

Over the years, Erickson perfected his skill of weaving deep messages into his stories. Each listener was then able to hear and understand on the level most appropriate and useful at that time. Erickson trusted that the listener would remember the salient message within and understand on a deeper level when the need for that understanding arose. Each story he told was an opportunity to teach, to give information, and to direct thinking. It was usually wrapped in metaphors with both obvious and more hidden meanings. Listening to a story developed a trance or a trancelike state, and the listener could incorporate important and profound lessons without conscious awareness or understanding of the changes in internal experience and learning.

Erickson was content to tell stories that would give useful information. He believed that giving was the supreme gift. He relied on his belief that the listener's unconscious would use knowledge in ways most suitable and helpful to that person. He didn't need to ask for validation that the message was used, or even received.

His son Lance was born with a heart murmur and the risk of a shortened life span. When Lance was a youngster, Erickson would often point out a huge white oak tree that stood in front of their home. Lance still remembers how Erickson talked about that wonderful tree, which was hundreds of years old. Trees live a long time, he told his son. They live a long time and grow tall and strong. They are something to admire. It's nice, Erickson emphasized, to know that there are old things and that things can live a long time.

As Lance grew up, he always looked for the oldest tree around. To this day, he remains, in his words, a huge admirer of old trees and enjoys just looking at them. He now recognizes the message contained in the stories his father told him. Even though he had a heart defect, there was no reason he couldn't live a long life.

It would be impossible to prove that the stories about trees, which Erickson told exclusively to Lance, helped increase his life span. It is also impossible to prove that the stories alleviated worries or concerns Lance may have had about his heart defect. From Erickson's point of view, he was giving information that could only help, and he relied on the wisdom of the unconscious to use that information.

He told bedtime stories to all of his children. The central character in the stories he told most often was a larger-than-life frog named White Tummy, who was learning the same life lessons and values that Erickson wanted his children to learn. As Erickson continued using and telling stories, he learned an increasingly trance-inducing way of introducing the message, often using the story itself as a metaphor for the message within: "Once upon a time there was a frog who lived on a lily pad in the middle of a pond. And he had a green back and a white tummy and that was his name—White Tummy. White Tummy liked to sit on his lily pad in the middle of the pond, with the warm sun shining down on him and the cool water beneath him, and wait for flies to buzz past him. Big flies, little flies, red flies, green flies, blue flies, yellow flies, and once in a while, his very favorite kind of fly, a great, big, fat, juicy, purple fly would fly by. One day, while White Tummy was sitting there, in the warm sun, waiting, waiting ..." The story would continue and weave Erickson's point into the magical adventures. We children would hear the parenting messages on multiple levels while we enjoyed the story.

Whether Erickson did psychotherapy, worked with hypnosis, or merely taught, he communicated in a succinct, relevant way. The divisions among psychotherapy, hypnosis, and teaching were often deliberately blurred. A carefully constructed story allowed that blurring of distinct lines and helped communicate with the conscious and unconscious resources that each person has.

Erickson did not write about the way he used stories in his therapy. He did not attempt to teach others how to use storytelling in therapy. What he did was to demonstrate it in virtually every session, in almost every trance induction, whenever he worked with students and as he talked with people on a social or casual basis. Some stories were very carefully crafted for specific purposes, and others were told because he liked a good story. He believed in the power of stories. The way he lived, his work with his students and with his patients, and the memories of everyone who interacted with him all stand as a monument to the importance he placed on storytelling as communication, as a gift of love, and as therapy.

## HOW THE EXPERTS VIEW ERICKSON

Virtually every student of Erickson's work has spent much energy analyzing and trying to understand the ways in which Erickson would create stories that would carry within a multiplicity of relevant meanings. Jeffrey Zeig (1980), in *A Teaching Seminar with Milton H. Erickson*, devotes an entire chapter to the therapeutic use of anecdotes (pp. 3–27). He includes a careful overview of the efficacy of this method, as well as an analysis of several short stories from the transcript of the seminar. In other books, and in his teaching, Zeig has continued to describe and discuss Erickson's storytelling. In *Experiencing Erickson*, Zeig (1985b) includes a transcript of some of the teaching he received directly from Erickson; storytelling makes up a good part of this instruction. There is also an account of long-term therapy with schizophrenics in which stories played a significant role (pp. 20–27).

Others have also focused on the power of stories. In *My Voice Will Go With You: The Teaching Tales of Milton H. Erickson, M.D.*, editor Sydney Rosen, M.D. (1982) categorizes some of Erickson's stories. Rosen analyzes the goals of the stories and discusses specific word choices and sequencing. Even the title of the book comes from a trance induction that Erickson often used: "And my voice will go with you. And my voice will change into that of your parents, your neighbors, your friends, your schoolmates, your playmates, your teachers. . . . feeling happy about something, something that happened a long time ago, that you forgot a long time ago."

Ernest Rossi worked with Erickson to publish a transcript of work that hypnotically explored the childhood of a chronically depressed woman. Replete with stories, part of the therapy involved Erickson's use of a mythical character, the February Man, to help the patient reconstruct her psychological past (Erickson & Rossi, 1989).

Jay Haley, legendary himself as a master therapist and communicator, first became intrigued with Erickson's style of communicating in the early 1950s. He and John Weakland spent many hours studying with Erickson, and Haley's (1985) three volumes of *Conversations with Milton H. Erickson, M.D.* contain verbatim transcripts of much of their work, including many stories from Erickson. Haley (1986) also used these stories in *Uncommon Therapy: The Psychiatric Techniques of Milton H. Erickson, M.D.* In this seminal volume of brief and strategic therapy in which Haley discusses how therapy was accomplished, the use of stories, analogies, and metaphors is reflected on at length. Haley, in his own work, has developed storytelling to the status of an art.

Virtually all of the people who worked directly with Erickson and who are now regarded as eminent Ericksonian-based therapists found the use of stories intriguing and a potent tool for therapy. Stephen and Carol Lankton, Joseph Barber, Stephen Gilligan, Bernhard Trenkle, and the late Kay Thompson are only a few who have written and taught extensively worldwide, emphasizing the impact that stories can have. The books containing presentations of the last several International Conferences on Ericksonian Hypnosis and Psychotherapy provide a wealth of varying perspectives on storytelling and the uses of metaphors and anecdotes (Zeig, 1995a, 1992; Zeig & Gilligan, 1990; Zeig & Lankton, 1988).

## APPLYING THE TECHNIQUES

Storytelling is one of the most powerful tools of psychotherapy. The concentration required to focus on a story has value in itself. A naturalistic trance tends to develop. In a trance, communication to the unconscious is possible. All the phenomena of a trance take place in quick and conversational ways.

We are all accustomed to learning from stories. When a story is told in the therapy room, the client is expecting to learn something. There is an openness, an implicit willingness to receive new information. New information is a basic tenet of therapy. When a client uses the learning from a story to make internal changes, the responsibility for and pleasure received from making the change belong to the listener. The therapist has merely told a story; the client has used it in the most productive way.

Stories can afford wisdom on multiple levels. The listener can understand relevant information for that particular life moment. Later, that same story can be remembered and becomes useful on a deeper level when the listener is able or ready to hear and understand more.

Stories also illustrate boundaries of ordinary and normal behaviors and options. They provide reassurances and redefine a situation, as well as illustrating the commonalties of human experiences.

And they are fun. The story and the sense of that story are easy to remember because they are tagged with pleasure. A poignant story provides a deep and easily remembered connection that calls forth an emotional response.

A therapeutic story is constructed by listening to what is told in the therapy room. This listening must be done on a meta-level. The therapist, frequently focusing in a personal naturalistic trance, hears what is said and takes a facet of it, a portion of the problem, and creates a story that deals with that theme, that keystone of the issue. Once that piece of the problem has been expanded, has changed, and can be seen from a different perspective, the understanding of the larger issue is changed. One tiny shift or alteration can snowball into much larger modifications and the problem becomes different.

## To Illustrate

One story I tell illustrates many of these points. Like most stories, this one has details that can be added or deleted to change the focus. Years ago, my family lived in a very small town where, because of my husband's occupation, I was recognized by many. We had a wonderful cat named Goat. Goat came when we whistled. She followed my son on his paper route. We spoiled and adored her. One day, Goat died tragically. Grief-stricken, we buried her in our backyard as neighbors stood sadly by.

Two days later, I was in the town's only grocery store and I saw a package of mahi-mahi. That fish had been Goat's favorite food. Every time I saw it, I bought some for her. I picked up the package and burst into sobs.

As I stood there, flooded with tears and memories, I became aware of the silence in the store. Glancing around, I saw employees and customers had gathered there, staring at me, obviously trying to figure out why I was standing in a grocery store, sobbing aloud, with a package of frozen fish clutched to my heart.

I remember thinking that an explanation, any explanation, could only make things worse. So I put the fish back in the case, wiped my eyes, and continued shopping. No one spoke to me or even came near me during that entire shopping trip.

Listeners engage with this story for many reasons. Even if one has never owned or loved a pet, one can surely understand and accept the grief felt when a beloved pet dies. The parameters of normal grief are illustrated, as well as the acceptance of an unexpected wave of pain that causes surprising behavior. On a deeper level, I am saying clearly that pain passes, and even though something is painful, it can be remembered later without that pain. There can be a shift from discomfort or guilt over lasting grief and sadness, a change to understanding that sadness passes, and recognition that expressions of pain are not necessarily logical. And the story itself is wrapped with a smile.

Another illustration is one that a client taught me. That explanation alone piques interest as well as carrying the message that we all learn from each other. My client was a lovely lady who sought out men who were unavailable. She had been married to an emotionally distant man and every man to whom she was attracted after her divorce was also unavailable. Either he was already married, planned to move across the country, was an alcoholic, or was unavailable in some other clear and unmistakable way. She wanted desperately to change this situation. She knew, as was clear to me, that this behavior had ties to the fact her father had abandoned the family when she was eight.

Nothing worked. Finally, I asked her to write an essay on the word "unavailable." She was a high-school English teacher and I thought this assignment might be helpful.

The next week, she returned. "I now know what 'unavailable' means," she announced.

"I went home," she said, "and got out my daughter's crayons. I sat at the kitchen table and drew pictures." In a naturalistic trance, she was clearly recreating the experience as she talked, as well as reliving a part of her emotional life that took place when she was eight. "I drew picture after picture and none of them were right. I would crumpled up each sheet of paper and throw it on the floor and then take another sheet and draw some more. Finally, I had my picture of 'unavailable.'

"I drew a picture of myself when I was eight. In the picture, I have a little skirt on and my hair is in pigtails. I am standing in front of a McDonald's with its big golden arches. Coming out of my mouth is a balloon, like in the cartoons, with words in it. I am asking, 'Do you have spaghetti?' There is another balloon coming out of McDonald's. It says, 'Spaghetti is unavailable here.'

"Suddenly I understood. No matter how much I want it, no matter what I pay, no matter how hard I ask, no matter how good I am, spaghetti is unavailable at McDonald's. It's nothing personal. McDonald's is not doing it to hurt me. It is just not there. It is not available there. It doesn't exist there.

"I put my head on the table and I cried and cried and cried. Then I put the picture on my refrigerator. My daughter came in and asked about it. I told her that the picture was meant to show what unavailable is—spaghetti is unavailable at McDonald's. She looked at me as though I were crazy and said, 'Everybody knows that. If you want something, you don't go where they don't have it.'"

This example gives clear unmistakable information in a way that cannot be misunderstood. The telling of the story, including the fact that the client went into a naturalistic trance as she told me about what she had done, is an invitation to the listener to go into a trance as well. The verbal picture of the little girl with pigtails standing in front of the golden arches of McDonald's adds to the invitation, as does imagining an eight-year-old drawing pictures with crayons in order to understand something. The trance allows the listener to hear the hard fact that no matter how much you want something, no matter what you do, if it is unavailable, you can't have it. Further, the unavailability has nothing to do with you. It is impersonal.

In a trance, this information can be heard on a very deep level. The internal experience of wanting and wishing and yearning for something can be changed into a new internal experience, into an acceptance that what you want simply doesn't exist. Blame or self-responsibility cannot exist simultaneously with this new internal learning.

The central cores of yearning for change in another and of believing that somehow "if only" one could be different, one could get whatever it is that is needed are both addressed in this story. The story itself models learning. It delivers its message wrapped not only in a trance, but in the world of an eight-year-old, coloring pictures to figure out what is happening in her life. The listener can learn, one step removed from the pain of that little girl. Last, but far from least, the story is tagged unforgettably with the juxtaposition of the high-school English teacher having to draw pictures with her daughter's crayons in order to understand and the humor of the daughter's instant recognition of the central truth.

## CONCLUSION

Storytelling has become recognized as a powerful psychotherapeutic tool that gives a client the ability to understand on multiple levels. These understandings can then create new internal experiences that can alter that client's perceptions and then help the client to choose behaviors that are more productive. Options become available to that client. Because the changes are built on the person's own internal experiences, self-responsibility is a part of the cluster of different perceptions and behaviors. The therapy contained within a story is direct and indirect at the same time. It is truly therapy, one step removed.

Although stories have been told since humans first sat around fires and talked about their past, their future, and their dreams, Milton H. Erickson is generally recognized as the father of psychotherapeutic storytelling. His legacy is contained in the stories about him and his work and in the stories told by other therapists, those Ericksonian in orientation, as well as those who have built other frameworks that include using metaphors and stories as a help to their clients.

---

**Points to Remember**

- Storytelling can create trances to facilitate communication with the unconscious.
- Storytelling creates a new internal experience upon which all behaviors are built.
- Storytelling can provide options and alternatives for the client.
- Storytelling is a direct way of approaching a problem indirectly.
- Storytelling promotes independence as clients tailor the information to suit their current needs.

---

### References

Erickson, M. H., & Rossi, E. L. (1989). *The February man: Evolving consciousness and identity in hypnotherapy*. New York: Norton.

Haley, J. (Ed.). (1985). *Conversations with Milton H. Erickson, M.D.*, Vol. I, II, & III. New York: Triangle Press.

Haley, J. (Ed.). (1986). *Uncommon therapy: The psychiatric techniques of Milton H. Erickson, M.D.* New York: Norton.

Rosen, S. (Ed.). (1982). *My voice will go with you: The teaching tales of Milton H. Erickson, M.D.* New York: Norton.

Zeig, J. (Ed.). (1980). *A teaching seminar with Milton H. Erickson*. New York: Brunner/Mazel.

Zeig, J. (Ed.). (1985a). *Ericksonian psychotherapy, Vols. I & II*. New York: Brunner/Mazel.

Zeig, J. (Ed.). (1985b). *Experiencing Erickson: An introduction to the man and his work*. New York: Brunner/Mazel.

Zeig, J. (Ed.). (1992). *Ericksonian methods: The essence of the story*. New York: Brunner/Mazel.

Zeig. J., & Gilligan, S. (Eds.). (1990). *Brief therapy: Myths, methods and metaphors.* New York: Brunner/Mazel.

Zeig, J., & Lankton, S. (Eds.). (1988). *Developing Ericksonian therapy: State of the art.* New York: Brunner/Mazel.

## Suggested Readings

Close, H. (1988). *Metaphor in psychotherapy: Clinical applications of stories and allegories.* San Luis Obispo, CA: Impact.

Erickson, M. H. (1980). *The collected papers of Milton H. Erickson on hypnosis* (Vols. I–IV). (E. L. Rossi, Ed.). New York: Irvington.

Erickson, M. H., & Rossi, E. L. (1979). *Hypnotherapy: An exploratory casebook.* New York: Irvington.

Gilligan, S. (1987). *Therapeutic trances: The cooperation principle in Ericksonian hypnotherapy.* New York: Brunner/Mazel.

Gordon, D., & Meyers-Anderson, M. (1981). *Phoenix: Therapeutic patterns of Milton H. Erickson.* Cupertino, CA: Meta Publications.

Haley, J. (Ed.). (1967). *Advanced techniques of hypnosis and therapy: Selected papers of Milton H. Erickson, M.D.* New York: Grune & Stratton.

Havens, R. A. (Ed.). (1996). *The wisdom of Milton H. Erickson.* (Vols. 1–2). New York: Irvington.

Lankton, S., & Lankton, C. (1986). *The answer within: A clinical framework of Ericksonian hypnotherapy.* New York: Brunner/Mazel.

Lankton, S., & Lankton, C. (1986). *Enchantment and intervention in family therapy training in Ericksonian approaches.* New York: Brunner/Mazel.

Rossi, E., & Ryan, M. (Eds.). (1985). *Life reframing in hypnosis: The seminars, workshops and lectures of Milton H. Erickson.* 1985. New York: Irvington.

Rossi, E., & Ryan, M. (Eds.). (1992). *Creative choice in hypnosis: The seminars, workshops and lectures of Milton H. Erickson.* 1992. New York: Irvington.

Rossi, E. L., Ryan, M. O., & Sharp, F. A. (Eds.). (1983). *Healing in hypnosis.* New York: Irvington.

9

# Psychobiological Principles of Creative Ericksonian Psychotherapy

*Ernest L. Rossi*

An overview of the 200-year history of therapeutic hypnosis reveals a continuing effort to formulate an adequate theory and practice of the psychobiological principles of healing. We continue this tradition by organizing current research to formulate a general model of the creative process of mindbody communication and healing. Our main thesis is that we can resolve many of the mysteries and paradoxes of Milton H. Erickson's approaches to psychotherapy only by a deeper investigation into their fundamental psychobiological mechanisms. In this chapter, the dynamics of psychotherapeutic communication and healing from the cognitive-behaviorial to the cellular-genetic level is outlined in four stages: (1) the neuroendocrine loop between the subjective experiences of the mind and the limbic-hypothalamic-pituitary system; (2) the psychosomatic network of messenger molecules and their receptors; (3) the immediate early gene protein cascade; and (4) state-dependent memory, learning, and behavior. Recent research in neuroscience and psychoneuroimmunology is outlined for its contributions to an understanding of how psychotherapy and the placebo response could facilitate healing at the cellular-genetic level. A series of principles is proposed as a guide for the theory, research, and clinical practice of the art and science of Ericksonian approaches to healing in the new millennium.

ERICKSON'S POSITION: THE ACTIVITY–PASSIVITY PARADOX
OF HISTORICAL HYPNOSIS

The relatively primitive state of our understanding of psychophysiology during the first century of research in hypnosis meant that its effects
could be conceptualized only as some sort of reflex or pathology. Bernheim (1886/1957), the leader of the Nancy school of suggestive therapeutics in France, for example, described hypnosis as the "exaltation of the
ideomotor reflex excitability, which effects the unconscious transformation of the thought into movement, unknown to the will ... The mechanism of suggestion, in general, may then be summed up in the following
formula: increase of the reflex ideomotor, ideo-sensitivity, and ideo-excita-
bility." The idea that hypnosis involved an *increase in "sensitivity" and
"excitability"* was in striking contrast to the view of the Salpêtrière school
in Paris led by Charcot who maintained, to the contrary, that hypnosis
was a pathological condition of *passivity* that progressed from *lethargy* and
catalepsy to somnambulism. This paradox in our fundamental understanding of the nature of hypnosis—*Is hypnosis heightened activity or passivity?*—
continued into the next generation of leading researchers. The Russian
physiologist Ivan Pavlov, for example, believed hypnosis to be a state of
*cerebral inhibition*, a kind of "partial sleep," whereas the American learning theorist Clark Hull maintained the opposite view, seeing hypnosis as
a state of *arousal* characterized by *hypersuggestibility* as follows:

> We seem forced to the view *that hypnosis is not sleep* ... Thus the
> extreme *lethargic* state is not hypnosis, but true sleep: *only the alert
> stage is hypnotic*. Lastly, evidence has been presented which indi-
> cates not only that conditioned reflexes may be set up during hyp-
> nosis, but that this may perhaps be accomplished with even greater
> ease than in the waking state. This probably disproves Pavlov's hy-
> pothesis that hypnosis is a state of *partial sleep* in the sense of a
> partial irradiation of *inhibition*. (Hull, 1933/1986, p. 221)

Milton Erickson, who was a student of Clark Hull, developed new
methods of hypnotherapy that could utilize either the *passive*, relaxed, and
sleeplike tendencies of his patients ("You don't even have to listen to my
voice"; Erickson, 1976) or their more *active*, compulsive, and even "acting
out" behavior, such as pacing around the therapy office in an agitated
manner (Erickson, 1958/1980). The approach to hypnotherapy Erickson

chose to use in any particular case was always a function of the patient's ongoing mood, attitudes, and behavior in the therapy session. Erickson's utilization of both the active and passive components of the patient's on-going behavior is the most recent expression of what we may call the "activity–passivity paradox of hypnosis." Erickson described many of his apparently paradoxical approaches to hypnotherapy that made use of the full range of the patient's ongoing behavior as the "naturalistic" or the "utilization" approach (Erickson, 1959/1980).

## THE POSITION OF ERICKSONIAN THERAPISTS: RESOLVING PARADOX

The first modern effort to integrate Milton Erickson's utilization of both activity and passivity in hypnosis with the psychophysiology of healing was undertaken by his early student and colleague, Bernard Gorton. The main focus of Gorton's two papers on "The Physiology of Hypnosis" (1957, 1958) was on how the autonomic nervous system (ANS) with its two main branches, the sympathetic system (arousal) and the parasympathetic system (relaxation), may be the major avenue through which therapeutic suggestion achieves its psychophysiological effects. These two review papers documented how hypnosis could be used to optimize peak performance associated with an arousal of the sympathetic branch of the autonomic system, as well as relaxation associated with the parasympathetic branch. As such, Gorton's review was a challenge to the then dominating but erroneous view of behaviorism that hypnosis was nothing more than relaxation. More recent research supports the essential view that there is "a positive correlation between hypnotic susceptibility and autonomic responsiveness during hypnosis..." (DeBenedittis, Cigada, & Gosi-Greguss, 1994, p. 140) and that the nature of the "physiological responsiveness [arousal or relaxation] is dependent on the type of suggestions during hypnosis..." (Sturgis & Coe, 1990, p. 205).

It has been proposed that this view of how hypnosis, together with a variety of other psychosocial processes, might modulate the activating, sympathetic branch as well as the passive, parasympathetic branch of the ANS could resolve centuries of debate about the fundamental nature of hypnosis (Rossi, 1986/1993, 1996). As is typical of many great debates in science, both sides expressed parts of a larger truth. It has been proposed that "high-phase hypnosis" might be used to facilitate performance in the outer world (e.g., hypnotherapeutic suggestions for improved work and sports) by engaging the activating sympathetic branch of the ANS, while "low-phase hypnosis" might be used to facilitate stress reduction and healing by engaging the parasympathetic branch of the ANS (Rossi, 1996). Even today, however, the implications of this basic psychobiological capacity of hypnotic suggestion to influence the active as well as the passive branches of the ANS is not well understood by researchers, who report the "paradoxical" nature of their results. In one of the all-too-rare efforts to measure molecular variables during therapeutic hypnosis, for example, Weinstein and Au (1991) reported that norepinephrine levels were significantly higher in the hypnotized group of patients undergoing angioplasty than in the control group. They report that this was "unexpected and seemed *paradoxical* (p. 29) ... One would expect that if hypnosis does cause relaxation, then those patients who were hypnotized would have a lower arterial catecholamine level than their controls. This was not the case. Just the opposite occurred and is hard to explain" (p. 35). But this so-called paradox is hard to explain only if one assumes, as these authors do, that hypnosis is essentially a state of relaxation. On the contrary, we propose that hypnosis is something vastly more than a state of relaxation. The activity–passivity paradox of hypnosis may be resolved by recognizing that the psychobiological basis of creative work in general, and of Ericksonian hypnotherapeutic work in particular, may utilize both the active and passive phases of the natural rhythms of the autonomic and related systems on all levels, from the cognitive-behavioral to the cellular-genetic (Rossi, 1996).

## THE PSYCHOBIOLOGICAL MODEL OF HEALING: THE DOMAIN OF HYPNOTHERAPY

Selye (1976) introduced a dynamical conception of the role of the autonomic, endocrine, and immune systems in response to trauma, emotional stress, and other challenges to adaptation that is consistent with a new model of the psychobiological domain of creative and hypnotherapeutic work (Rossi, 1996). The psychobiological model of therapeutic suggestion is consistent with a generation of research in experimental hypnosis that firmly established, contrary to popular belief, that there is no transcendence of normal abilities in hypnosis (Wagstaff, 1986). Current researchers, however, openly acknowledge that they have no adequate theory to explain the source and parameters of hypnotic performance. One prominent researcher, for example, summarized the current situation as follows: "As [hypnotic] susceptibility is normally assessed, a high scorer is one who produces the behavior, the reason for its production remains unknown ... the claim was frequently made that cognitive processes are involved in the production of 'hypnotic' effects. However, the exact nature of these processes generally remained obscure" (Naish, 1986, pp. 165–166). The psychobiological model of hypnotherapeutic work proposes that what seems to be an extension of the normal parameters of mindbody performance skills via hypnosis is actually the optimization of the individual's normal range of abilities in response to the general process of adaptation to challenge and stress.

The limitations of traditional theories of therapeutic suggestion have been discussed by a number of highly respected researchers, who emphasize that, whatever hypnosis may be, its domain cannot be limited to the behavioral or psychosocial level (Kirsch & Lynn, 1995). The more general psychobiological model of hypnotherapy proposed here expands the domain of suggestion beyond the cognitive-behavioral level to include all systems of mindbody communication and healing at the molecular level that are responsive to psychosocial cues. It has been proposed that the hormonal or messenger molecule-receptor dynamics of the neuroendocrine, neuropeptide, autonomic, and immune systems mediate stress, emotions, memory, learning, personality, behavior, and symptoms in a "psychosomatic network" (Pert, Ruff, Spencer, & Rossi, 1989; Pert, Ruff, Weber, & Herkenham, 1985). This leads to our first basic principle concerning the psychobiological domain of healing, creative work, and Ericksonian psychotherapy.

*Principle I: The psychobiological domain of creative work in general, and of Ericksonian hypnotherapy in particular, consists of the entire cybernetic loop of information transduction between the psychosocial environment, the central nervous system (CNS), and the psychosomatic network of the autonomic, neuroendocrine, and immune systems at the organ, tissue, and cellular-genetic-molecular levels.*

Let us explore what is currently known about the psychobiological mechanisms of creative work and hypnosis at each level and the types of research that are now needed for further progress in a systematic approach to mindbody medicine.

## Level 1: The CNS and the Mind–Brain

The experience of dissociation, automaticity, or involuntariness so characteristic of hypnotic experience has been reformulated as the theory of dissociated control (Woody & Farvolden, 1998). This theory emphasizes the contrast between explicit memory and a sense of conscious control over cognition and behavior versus implicit memory and the sense of automaticity or involuntariness of cognition and behavior. The active processes of high-phase hypnosis are thought to engage the explicit or voluntary conscious controls (associated with the prefrontal cortex) whereas passive processes of low-phase hypnosis engage the implicit memory systems (associated with the basal ganglia and related subsystems) of involuntary or automatic experience (Rossi, 1996). It is currently believed (Spiegel, 1998) that highly susceptible hypnotic subjects are able to engage the more automatic, unconscious, or implicit memory systems more closely associated with the subcortex, illustrated as the generalized limbic-hypothalamic-pituitary system at the first level, the amygdala and hippocampus, associated with emotions, memory, and learning.

Papez (1937) originally traced the anatomical pathways by which an emotional experience of the brain was transduced into the physiological responses of the body in a circuit of brain structures that are now generally recognized as the limbic-hypothalamic-pituitary system. The Scharrers (1940) documented how secretory cells within the hypothalamus could mediate molecular information transduction between the brain and body. Cells within the hypothalamus transduce the electrochemical impulses of neurons of the cerebral cortex that encode the phenomenological experience of "mind" and emotions into the hormonal or "primary messenger molecules" of the endocrine system. These primary messenger molecules are then communicated to the body through the blood stream in a cybernetic loop of information transduction called the neuroendocrine system.

The adaptive and complex cybernetic loop of communication of the neuroendocrine and neuropeptide systems modulates the action of neurons and cells at all levels, from the basic afferent pathways of sensation and perception in neurons of the brain to the intracellular dynamics of gene transcription and translation throughout the body. This leads to the neuropeptide hypothesis of hypnotherapy and emotional catharsis (Rossi, 1990), which relates the fundamental dynamics of high- and low-phase hypnotherapy to a major source of mindbody communication and regulation at the limbic-hypothalamic-pituitary level.

*Principle II: The high (arousal) and low (relaxation) phases of hypno-
therapy are mediated by the transduction of psychosocial experience
into neuropeptide cascade, beginning with the corticotrophin-releasing
factor (CRF) and proopiomelanocortin (POMC), leading to the release
of corticotrophin (ACTH) and beta-endorphin, which coordinate the
chronobiological processes of mindbody communication and healing at
all levels, from the cognitive-behavioral to the cellular-genetic.*

The experimental database for the neuropeptide hypothesis of hypnotherapy and catharsis comes from research in psychoendocrinology (Brush
& Levine, 1989; De Wied, 1990), chronobiology (Lloyd & Rossi, 1992),
and hypnosis (Rossi, 1986/1993, 1990, 1996). The current consensus in
neuroscience is that the CRF is the psychobiological coordinator on the
molecular level of the generalized arousal/stress response. Whereas neurons releasing CRF are found throughout the brain, their largest concentration is in the paraventricular nucleus of the hypothalamus, where they
receive inputs from the forebrain and limbic system encoding stress from
the cognitive-behavioral level that integrates nociceptive information from
the somatosensory cortex and related sources (Rainville, Duncan, Price, et
al., 1997). CRF is secreted via the fenestrated capillaries of the hypophy-
seal-portal venus plexus to signal the anterior pituitary to induce POMC
that is cleaved into about a dozen messenger molecules, including ACTH
and beta-endorphin, that have varying effects on the psychobiology of
arousal, memory, learning, and relaxation (Brush & Levine, 1989). ACTH
and beta-endorphin are now known to modulate a variety of mindbody
rhythms on the organ, tissue, and cellular-genetic levels. One of the most
prominent of these mindbody rhythms is the 90-120-minute basic rest activity cycle (BRAC) associated with rapid eye movement sleep (REM
sleep) and the periodicity of most hormonal systems of mindbody regulation (Lloyd & Rossi, 1992). Available evidence indicates that this typical,
but readily adaptable, 90–120-minute ultradian cycle of psychobiological
arousal, work, and performance is initiated by the ACTH-cortisol phase
of the BRAC and then brought to a natural conclusion by the action of
the beta-endorphin phase of the BRAC that initiates a signaling cascade at
the cellular-genetic-protein level to facilitate an "ultradian healing response" (Rossi & Nimmons, 1991). Iranmanesh, Veldhuis, Johnson, &
Lizarralde (1989, p. 1019), for example, report that "cortisol was considered to lead beta-endorphin by 20 or 30 minutes. We conclude that beta-

endorphin is released physiologically in a pulsate manner with circadian and ultradian rhythmicity and a close temporal coupling to cortisol." Because cortisol is a final common path of the informational CRF-POMC-ACTH-cortisol cascade, this research is consistent with the neuropeptide hypothesis that proposes that high-phase hypnosis is associated with cortisol activity while low-phase hypnosis is associated with beta-endorphin activity. Research is now required to monitor continuously the release of ACTH, cortisol, beta-endorphin, and related messenger molecules during creative work, hypnotherapy, and the cathartic approaches to psychotherapy, as described previously (Rossi, 1990; Rossi & Cheek, 1988). This leads to an integration of research on the chronobiology of adaptation, stress, and hypnotherapy.

*Principle III: Psychobiological stress engendered by chronic interference with the quasi-periodic circadian and ultradian rhythms by traumatic and/or excessive work loads is a major etiology for mindbody problems that may be ameliorated by Ericksonian hypnotherapy.*

Well-replicated research on the normal psychobiological dynamics of the major systems of mindbody regulation and healing is currently evolving out of time parameter research on many levels, ranging from the molecular biology of the cell cycle to the neuroendocrinal and behavioral levels (Lloyd & Rossi, 1992, 1993). It now appears that many of the highly adaptive processes of mindbody regulation that manifest a natural quasi-periodic circadian/ultradian periodicity are modifiable by hypnosis (Rossi, 1982, 1986/1993). "Quasi-periodic" is a term from modern chaos theory that means that these natural rhythms are not strictly regular in their periodicity like an accurate clock; rather, they are adaptive rhythms that continually shift in the process of creative adaptation to a changing outer environment (Lloyd & Rossi, 1992; Rossi, 1996). This implies the next principle of Ericksonian hypnotherapy.

*Principle IV: What has been traditionally called "hypnotherapeutic suggestion" may be, from a chronobiological perspective, the Ericksonian accessing and utilization of the natural periodicity of ultradian and circadian processes on all levels, from the cognitive-behavioral to the molecular, that respond to psychosocial cues.*

Within this framework, many of the classical phenomena of hypnosis may be conceptualized as extreme manifestations and/or perseverations of time-dependent psychobiological processes that are responsive to psychosocial cues. That is, what the hypnotherapist calls "therapeutic suggestion" is what the chronobiologist calls "the entrainment of biological processes by psychosocial cues." Research consistent with the significance of chronobiological parameters in a general psychobiological model of hypnotherapy has been reported by a number of investigators in the past decade. It was initially assessed by Aldrich and Bernstein (1987), who found that "time of day" was a statistically significant factor in hypnotic susceptibility. They reported a bimodal distribution of scores on the Harvard Group Scale of Hypnotic Susceptibility in college students with a sharp major peak at 12 noon and a secondary, broader plateau at around 5 to 6 P.M. Further research found a very prominent circadian rhythm with a peak between noon and 1 P.M. in self-hypnosis, as well as an ultradian periodicity of about 90 to 180 minutes throughout the day, which appears to coincide approximately with Kleitman's 90–120-minute BRAC (Kleitman, 1969; Kleitman & Rossi, 1992). The BRAC has an approximately 20-minute peak level of performance associated with a peak in cortisol that may be utilized in high-phase hypnosis that alternates with a 20-minute rest or ultradian healing period associated with a peak in beta-endorphin, when most people feel a need to take a break that may be utilized in low-phase hypnosis (Rossi & Nimmons, 1991; Rossi, 1996). It is interesting, and probably not coincidental, that most research assessing the therapeutic value of meditation and many other forms of alternative medicine, such as acupuncture, biofeedback, imagery, music, and therapeutic touch, also use a core 20-minute therapeutic period. This core therapeutic period may be condensed or extended, depending on practical exigencies, but it is rarely extended beyond Kleitman's typical 90–120-minute BRAC. Similar chronobiological parameters were found to be associated with hypnosis (Brown, 1991a, 1991b; Lippincott, 1992; Osowiec, 1992; Sommer, 1993; Wallace, 1993) and imagery (Wallace & Kokoszka, 1995). Two studies noted that a strictly periodic chronobiological model (Mann & Sanders, 1995; Saito & Kano, 1992) does *not* fit the data; these two studies are consistent with the quasi-periodic model, however (Rossi, 1996).

*Level 2: Stress, Immediate-Early Genes, Psychoneuroimmunology*

Studies of the modulation of the immune system by hypnosis imply that hypnosis may modulate the process of mindbody communication at level 2. Early studies by Black (1963) and others demonstrated that highly hypnotizable subjects could suppress the Mantoux reaction. Smith and McDaniel (1983) replicated Black's results with a cognitive-behavioral paradigm to demonstrate the role of cognitive expectation rather than hypnosis per se. A more recent study reported by Brewerton (1992) used hypnotic suggestion to suppress local blood vessel dilation following the Mantoux test. No fluid came to the site and there was no local swelling of the tissues as is typical of allergic reactions. Skin biopsies, however, revealed that the usual number of immune system cells arrived at the site of the injection. Hypnosis had suppressed that part of the Mantoux inflammatory response by blood vessel constriction but there was no clear evidence that the immune system itself was modulated. A long line of clinical observations implies that the modulation of blood flow is a major psychobiological mechanism of hypnosis (Barber, 1984; Rossi, 1986/1993). This view is entirely consistent with our neuropeptide hypothesis of the effects of high- and low-phase hypnosis on the sympathetic and parasympathetic branches of the ANS that can modulate blood flow throughout the brain and body.

Olness, Culbert, and Uden (1989) originally reported that 6- to 10-year-old children can use self-hypnosis voluntarily to modulate blood flow and salivary immunoglobulin A (IgA) after viewing a 15-minute videotape, "The Toymaker's Magic Microscope," which illustrated some of the basics about the immune system. Because the children also listened to a general relaxation audiotape while their peripheral temperature was monitored during the suggestion period, we can infer that their modulation of salivary IgA was associated with low-phase hypnosis. Consistent with these findings, Turner, Dewerth, and Fine (1993) found evidence of the modulation of the immune system by low-phase hypnosis by using a form of restricted environmental simulation therapy (REST) to induce a heightened secretion of salivary IgA. A study by Ruzyla-Smith, Barabasz, Barabasz, and Warner (1995), by contrast, used a more active high-phase hypnosis with instructions to: "Imagine your white blood cells attacking and destroying germ cells in your body." This form of high-phase hypnosis led to enhanced immune system functioning as measured by the activated response of B-cells and helper T-cells to mitogens. Suppressor cells of the immune systems were not modulated by this form of suggestion. These types of studies, however, are all very limited in the inferences that can be drawn about the actual cellular-genetic mechanisms of the immune system and hypnosis.

A more revealing demonstration of how psychosocial stress can modulate the actual mechanisms of gene expression in the immune system is a series of papers by Ronald Glaser and his colleagues (Glaser, Kennedy, Lafuse, et al., 1990). Their research traces the effects of psychological stress (experienced by medical students during academic examinations) in turning off the transcription of the interleukin-2 receptor gene and interleukin-2 mRNA production. Since interleukin-2 is a messenger molecule of the immune system, its down-regulation by psychological stress is the first demonstration of how the immune system's optimal functioning can be impaired by psychosocial cues at the cellular-genetic level. This molecular-genetic essence of the effect of emotional stress in psychoimmunology is now known to be mediated by immediate-early genes. Further evidence of how the immune system's functioning can be impaired at the cellular-genetic level was provided when Glaser and colleagues (1993) found that academic stress experienced by medical students led to the down-regulation of the two immediate-early genes (also called proto-oncogenes) c-myc and c-myb in peripheral blood leukocytes. The immediate-early gene c-myc is part of an informational loop at the cellular level that activates growth-promoting genes that are involved with breast cancer, as well as stomach and lung cancers and leukemia. Glaser's team also found a significant decrease in the level of mRNA leading to the formation of proteins for the glucocorticoid receptor and gamma interferon in the emotionally stressed medical students. These findings led the researchers to state: "The decrease in mRNA content of c-myc and c-myb, the glucocorticoid receptor, and gamma interferon in peripheral blood leukocytes obtained from subjects during examinations is consistent with data from previous studies using the same models that have demonstrated a down-regulation of T-lymphocyte activation and proliferation in response to mitogens" (Glaser, Lafuse, Bonneau, et al., 1993, p. 525). The current research frontier in psychoneuroimmunology is to document the reverse. Could hypnotherapy now be used to optimize the immune system by reducing emotional stress and thereby facilitating the expression of the interleukin-2 receptor gene, interleukin-2, and other proteins involved in the mind-gene loop of mind-body communication and healing? This would be the first demonstration that hypnotherapy could modulate gene expression.

*Level 3: Proteins, Time, Trauma, and Healing*

The time required to make new proteins in response to stress and trauma provides an important window into level 3 in the informational dynamics of alternative medicine in general, as well as in hypnotherapy. Todorov's (1990) research on how cells maintain their stability in response to environmental demands reveals three major "blocks" or stages of gene transcription and translation in response to physical trauma and stress. Immediate-early genes are turned on first to initiate the formation of M (metabolism) proteins *within an hour* to produce proteins required for energy dynamics. The next R (ribosomal) proteins are turned on to facilitate a heightened state of mRNA translation processes of healing *within a few hours*. The third stage produces the N (nuclear) proteins, such as DNA polymerases and histones required for deeper healing in a slower process requiring *12 hours to a day or more*.

A new research frontier of the psychobiology of creative work and hypnosis is to demonstrate how these stages of physical stress at the genetic-protein level will also be found in response to severe psychological trauma and stress. These time responses to trauma and stress are but one example of the quasi-periodic parameters for a complete cycle of mind-body healing. It has been proposed that these quasi-periodic rhythms are characteristic of the time parameters of information transduction on all levels of psychobiological communication and healing that may be facilitated with hypnotherapy (Rossi, 1986/1993; Rossi & Nimmons, 1991). Ewin (1986), a surgeon and specialist with emergency burn patients, has documented, for example, how hypnotherapeutic suggestions for cooling administered within two hours of a severe burn can reduce inflammation and facilitate healing to a much greater degree than they will after two hours. This is the same time frame for the formation of "stress proteins," whose overproduction can complicate the healing process in these patients (Pardue, Feramisco, & Lindquist, 1989). Research is now needed to determine whether hypnosis achieves this therapeutic effect by reducing the expression of stress proteins within the first two hours of experiencing a burn.

*Level 4: State-Dependent Memory, Learning, and Behavior (SDMLB)*

On level 4, messenger molecules that have their origin in the processing of larger protein "mother molecules," such as POMC discussed above, may be stored within cells as a kind of molecular memory. Messenger molecules from the peripheral cells of the body, such as epinephrine and norepinephrine from the adrenals, may then be released into the bloodstream, where they can complete the complex cybernetic loop of information transduction to the brain's neural networks. The current view is that such localized neuronal networks of the brain are modulated by signaling systems from the synapse to the nucleus of the neuron (Routtenberg & Meberg, 1998) as well as by a complex field of informational substances that can reach the limbic-hypothalamic-pituitary system and certain areas of the cerebral cortex. The extracellular fluid (ECF) of the brain makes up about 20% of the brain's volume. It has been theorized that informational substances can diffuse as much as 15 mm in the extracellular fluid to any site of the brain.

There is ample intercellular space for the dynamic interplay of many kinds of informational substances to diffuse from release points throughout the body to receptors within the neuronal networks of the cerebral cortex and other loci of the brain that encode the phenomenological experiences of mind and behavior. In the simplest case, a 15 mm$^2$ neuronal network containing at least 10,000 neurons could be turned on or off by the presence or absence of specific informational substances that modulate the phenomenology of mind in psychological time. That is, the activity of neuronal networks and the psychological experience they encode would be "state-dependent" (also called "state-specific") aspects of mind and behavior (SDMLB); an experience of mind, such as a thought or emotion, is dependent on the presence or absence of a specific complex of informational substances. There are potentially hundreds of informational substances communing with their corresponding families of receptors on the brain neurons. This means that the state-dependent neuronal networks are ever-changing dynamic structures, as they would certainly have to be in order to function as the psychophysiological basis for the phenomenology of mind, emotions, and behavior.

Recent research indicates that most forms of learning (Pavlovian, Skinnerian, imprinting, sensitization, etc.) are now known to involve messenger molecules or informational substances involved in the construction and reconstruction of memory (Izquierdo, Netto, Dalmaz, et al., 1988). Insofar as these classical forms of learning use informational substances, they *ipso facto* have a state-dependent component (McGaugh, 1989). Of central significance is the fact that when subjects are given memory and/or learning tasks while under the influence of stress hormones, such as ACTH or epinephrine (as well as psychoactive drugs that mimic natural hormonal messenger molecules), there is a varying degree of amnesia when the stress hormone or drug has been metabolized out of the system. That is, when memory is encoded under conditions of high emotional arousal, shock, surprise, stress, or trauma, it tends to become state-dependent or state-bound to that psychobiological condition. This state-dependent (or state-specific) memory becomes dissociated or "lost" after the person apparently recovers when the stress hormones or drugs are metabolized out of the system. Reactivating stress in another context, however, has a tendency to reestablish the original psychobiological stress-encoding condition and the cognitions, emotions, and behaviors associated with it with varying degrees of memory. It is important to recognize how SDMLB completes the information transduction loop of mindbody communication so that the psychosomatic network entrained by hypnotherapy becomes a two-way street.

*Principle V: The state-dependent pathways of mindbody communication and healing encoded by the messenger molecule receptor systems of the CNS, the autonomic system and the psychosomatic network, are two-way streets. Just as the messenger molecules' receptor system can modulate cognitive-emotional experience, so can the accessing and focusing of cognitive-emotional experience with creative Ericksonian hypnotherapeutic work modulate the messenger molecule system to facilitate healing.*

This is a proposed mechanism of how the molecules of the body can modulate mental experience, as well as how mental experience can modulate the molecules of the body (Rossi, 1986/1993, 1996). On the most reductive level, it can be understood as a simple extension of the reversibility of most stochastic life processes at the molecular level. This is the basis for emphasizing the view that SDMLB is a common denominator that bridges the mindbody gap: the so-called Cartesian dichotomy between mind and body. What is most interesting about research in this area is that it enables us to study the parameters of "reversible amnesia," which have been important criteria in understanding the phenomenology of psychoanalysis and therapeutic hypnosis (Rossi, 1996). Just as most experiments in state-dependent memory and learning demonstrate that this "reversible amnesia" is only partial (that is, there is usually some memory/learning available even in the dissociated condition after the stress hormones return to normal levels), so most of the hypnotic literature documents that hypnotic amnesia is usually fragile and partial in character. Since the earliest days of psychoanalysis, it has been noted that a sudden fright, shock, trauma, or stress could evoke "hypnoidal states" that were somehow related to amnesia and dissociated and neurotic behavior. A full amnesia that is completely reversible, however, is relatively rare in state-dependent memory/learning experiments, or in psychoanalysis and therapeutic hypnosis. In the historical literature on hypnosis and psychoanalysis, this same fragile and partial character of reversible amnesia may have been responsible for many of the paradoxes of memory.

These relationships between the psychosomatic network of messenger molecule receptor systems, stress, and SDMLB encoded mindbody problems suggest a new research frontier for the psychobiological investigation of classical psychoanalytic concepts, such as repression, dissociation, and emotional complexes, as well as hypnotherapy. A new paradigm for such research was provided recently by Cahill, Prins, Weber, & McGaugh (1994), who compared the effects of the beta-adrenergic receptor antagonist propranolol hydrochloride on the long-term memory for an emotionally arousing and emotionally neutral short story. Their results supported the hypothesis that the enhanced memory associated with emotional experiences involves activation of the messenger molecules of the beta-adrenergic or fight-or-flight channel of mindbody communication. Their research model could be extended to many forms of alternative medicine and hypnotherapy.

One theoretical objection to the idea that the psychosomatic network entrained by hypnotherapy is a two-way street is that the brain has long been regarded as a privileged organ that has a "blood–brain barrier" that normally protects the brain from toxic substances that may be circulating throughout the rest of the body. This suggests that many stress hormones and messenger molecules from the body could be blocked from entering the brain by the blood–brain barrier. Recent research, however, has demonstrated that during highly stressful emotional conditions, the blood–brain barrier is lowered, so that many messenger molecules and other substances can enter the brain. During the Gulf War, Israeli soldiers took pyridostigmine to protect themselves against chemical and biological weapons that might be launched by Iraq. This was considered a safe procedure because under the normal, unstressed living conditions in which pyridostigmine was tested, it was found that it did not cross the blood–brain barrier. To their dismay, however, researchers later found that during the stress of real battle conditions, pyridostigmine did cross the blood–brain barrier in 25% of the soldiers who, consequencely, experienced distressful mental symptoms. Further research then demonstrated that many other toxic substances, such as blue ink, that are normally blocked by the blood–brain barrier can enter the brains of animals under stressful conditions (Soreq & Friedman, 1997).

If we are willing to grant that information is encoded within the neuronal networks of the brain via protein-modulated changes in the activity-dependent Hebbian synaptic connections (that is, synaptic neural connections that grow stronger with activity), then we could say that meaning is to be found in the complex dynamic field of messenger molecules that continually contextualize the information of the neuronal networks into new state-dependent patterns of meaning. Freeman (1995), for example, has pointed out how oxytocin is a hormonal informational substance released during childbirth and lactation that encodes memory and learning, as well as unlearning (forgetting), in a state-dependent manner that would provide a survival advantage during evolution. Oxytocin, in concert with a complex of other messenger molecules in the extracellular fluid of the brain, makes up the ever-changing state-dependent field of meaning that is expressed in the phenomenological experience of "mind," consciousness, and intentional behavior during childbirth.

### SUMMARIZING ERICKSONIAN APPROACHES TO HEALING

An overview of Erickson's psychobiological approaches to healing and hypnosis can be found in his practical clinical demonstrations (Erickson, 1958/1980, 1959/1980). However varied his many approaches may seem, they fall into two distinct psychobiological categories: (1) the seemingly passive or low-phase approaches that appear to be similar to the traditional hypnotic methods of relaxation, comfort, and sometimes sleep; and (2) the more active and dynamic approaches of high-phase hypnosis that evoke emotional arousal and intense inner work. I once asked Erickson which state was more useful for healing: the seemingly passive, low-phase state when he had patients focus on a spot and listen quietly, or the more active, high-phase state of emotional arousal (evidenced by sweating, warmth, catharsis, etc.) that was often evoked with Erickson's method of hand levitation. Erickson responded with one of the most important psychotherapeutic principles of his work.

*Principle VI: To deal effectively with any problem, the patient must be actively experiencing it during the psychotherapeutic session. The therapist's basic task is to access and engage the patient's state-dependent experience of the problem and then to evoke and utilize the patient's own inner resources to deal with the problem in the patient's own way.*

Let us now review examples of how Erickson used both traditional, passive, low-phase (relaxation) hypnosis and active, high-phase hypnosis (emotional arousal) in his typically creative manner.

CLINICAL EXAMPLES

### Case One: State-Dependent Memory, Psychological Enrichment, and Personality Maturation

Many hypnotherapists report interesting case histories of how they accidentally evoked long-forgotten state-dependent memories during the natural-phase transitions of pregnancy and childbirth (Rossi & Cheek, 1988; Rossi & Ryan, 1986). Erickson, for example, was consulted by a woman who ostensibly wanted hypnosis to help her recover memories of giving birth to her first child. In this case, which was carefully recorded verbatim, Erickson demonstrated his indirect approach to facilitating a *passive state of receptivity* so that the woman would become more sensitive and receptive to the state-dependent memories she was looking for. He began his hypnotherapeutic induction with these words (Erickson & Rossi, 1979, p. 284): *"Will you sit back in your chair with your feet flat on the floor and your hands on your thighs. The hands not touching each other, and just look at one single spot here. You don't need to talk. You don't need to move. You don't even need to listen to me. Your unconscious mind is close enough to me to hear me. And that's the only important thing."*

This hypnotherapeutic approach facilitated a state of passive receptivity that matched to some degree the drug-induced state of "twilight sleep" during which she gave birth. This psychobiological matching presumably optimized the probability that she could actively experience her problem (Principle VI) and access the state-dependent memories she was seeking (Principle V). With this approach, the woman was successful in recovering some significant details of the birth of her first child three months earlier. This case is particularly interesting because in the process of the revivification of these memories of childbirth, she also "accidentally" recovered previous traumatic life experiences she had forgotten for many years. As she recovered the experience of these early traumas, she was able to reorganize a significant portion of her emotional life in a meaningful manner that led to a surprising maturation of her personality.

This was a clear example of what Erickson (1948/1980) described as the deeply emotional experiential "reassociation," "reorganization," and "resynthesis" of inner life that led to problem solving and healing as follows.

> The induction and maintenance of a trance serve to provide a special psychological state in which the patient can reassociate and reorganize his inner psychological complexities and utilize his own capacities in a manner in accord with his or her own experiential life ... Therapy results from an inner resynthesis of the patient's behavior achieved by the patient himself. It's true that direct suggestion can effect an alteration in the patient's behavior and result in a symptomatic cure, at least temporarily. However, such a "cure" is simply a response to suggestion and does not entail that reassociation and reorganization of ideas, understandings, and memories so essential for actual cure. It is the experience of reassociating and reorganizing his own experiential life that eventuates in a cure, not the manifestation of responsive behavior, which can, at best, satisfy only the observer.

As we shall soon see, Erickson's view of the "reassociation" and "resynthesis" as the essence of psychotherapy has new support from recent neuroscience research on novelty and life-enriching experience in facilitating neurogenesis (new brain growth).

### Case Two: Psychological Shock, Surprise, and Conception

Erickson's early work was considered paradoxical and controversial because of the activating high-phase dynamics he sometimes aroused in his patients. Here is a vivid example that few of us would have the courage to emulate today (Rossi, 1973).

A 30-year-old university professor attended a university dance and saw a 30-year-old woman on the other side of the room. She saw him and they rapidly gravitated toward each other. Within a month, they had planned their future and were married. Three years later, they appeared in Erickson's office and told their sad story. In telling it, they were extremely prudish and embarrassed and used almost stilted, formal wording. In essence, their complaint was that even before marriage, they had planned to have a family and because of the fact that both were 30 years old, they felt they should not delay doing so. But after three years, they were still childless despite medical examinations and advice. They were both present in the office and, in describing their problems, the man said, "In my thinking and that of my wife, we have reached the conclusion that it is more proper that I give voice to our trouble in common and state it succinctly. Our problem is most distressing and destructive of our marriage. Because of our desire for children, we have engaged in the marital union with full physiological concomitants each night and morning for procreative purposes. On Sundays and holidays, we have engaged in the marital union with full physiological concomitants for procreative purposes as often as four times a day. We have not permitted physical disability to interfere. As a result of the frustration of our philoprogenitive desires, the marital union has become progressively unpleasant for us, but although it has not interfered with our efforts at procreation, it distresses both of us to discover our increasing impatience with each other. For this reason, we are seeking your aid since medical aid has failed."

At this point, Erickson interrupted and said to the man, "You have stated the problem. I would like to have you remain silent and have your wife state her opinion in her own words." In almost exactly the same way with even greater embarrassment than her husband had shown, the wife voiced their complaint. Erickson said, "I can correct this for you but it will involve shock therapy. It will not be electric shock or physical shock but a matter of psychological shock. I will leave you alone in the office for 15 minutes so that the two of you can exchange views and opinions about your willingness to receive a rather severe psychological shock. At the end of 15 minutes, I will come back into the office and ask your decision to abide by it." Note how Erickson was using the chronobiology of the typical 15–20-minute period creative work presented in Principle IV (Rossi & Nimmons, 1991).

Erickson left the office, returned 15 minutes later, and said, "Give me your answer." The man said, "We have discussed the matter both objectively and subjectively and we have reached the conclusion that we will endure anything that might possibly satisfy our philoprogenitive desires."

Erickson asked the wife, "Do you agree fully?" She answered, "I do." Erickson explained that the shock would be psychological, involve their emotions, and be a definite strain on them. "It will be rather simple to administer, but you will both be exceedingly shocked psychologically. I suggest that you sit there in your chairs and reach down under the sides of your chairs and hang on tightly to the bottom of the chair and listen well to what I say. After I have said it, and as I am administering the shock, I want the two of you to maintain absolute silence. Within a few minutes, you will be able to leave the office and return to your home 40 miles from here. I want the two of you to maintain absolute silence all the way home, and during that silence you will discover a multitude of thoughts rushing through your minds. Upon reaching home, you will maintain silence until after you have entered the house and closed the door. You will then be free! Now hang on tightly to the bottom of your chairs because I am now going to give you the psychological shock. It is this: For three long years you have engaged in the marital union with full physiological concomitants for procreative purposes at least twice a day, and sometimes as often as four times in 24 hours, and you have met with defeat of your philoprogenitive drive. Now why in the hell don't you f--- for fun and pray to the devil that you [the wife] aren't knocked up for at least three months. Now please leave."

As the man described later, they maintained silence all the way home, thinking "many things." Then, when they finally got inside the house with the door shut, "We found we couldn't wait to get to the bedroom. We just dropped to the floor and we didn't 'engage in the marital union.' We had fun, and now the three months are barely up and my wife is pregnant." Nine months later a baby girl was born. When Erickson called on them to see the baby, he found that formal speech and polysyllabic words and highly proper phrases were no longer necessary in their conversations.

Needless to say, this radically unconventional approach to shock, surprise, and creative moments in high-phase hypnotherapy that was published a generation ago is *not* recommended for contemporary practice. It is presented here only to break through the misconception that hypnosis is always mediated by the sleeplike state of relaxation and comfort of low-phase hypnosis. This case illustrates how a therapeutic process can be facilitated by high-phase hypnosis leading to an extreme of emotional arousal. Research is now needed to assess the neuropeptide hypothesis (Principle II) that would predict that high-phase hypnosis is associated with an initial sympathetic system activation and then a shift from a peak in cortisol to a peak in beta-endorphin during the critical phase transition of the creative process as explained in more detail elsewhere (Rossi, 1996).

## FUTURE DIRECTIONS IN THE PSYCHOBIOLOGY
## OF CREATIVE WORK

In what direction will Ericksonian psychotherapy evolve in the new millennium? It has been proposed that the naturalistic psychobiology of creative work in general, and of Ericksonian approaches to high-phase hypnosis in particular, may be mediated by immediate-early genes (Rossi, 1997, 1998). Immediate-early genes (IEGs) are the newly discovered mediators between nature and nurture (Merchant, 1996; Tölle, Schadrack, & Zieglgansberger, 1995). Sometimes called "primary response genes" or "third messengers," they act as transducers, allowing strong signals of stress, emergency, and arousal from the external environment to regulate genes within the internal matrix of the nucleus of life itself. These IEGs can initiate a series of molecular-genetic transformations that can transduce relatively brief signals of arousal from the environment into enduring changes in the physical structure of the developing nervous system, as well as its plasticity in the form of memory and learning throughout life (Tölle, Schadrack, & Zieglgansberger, 1995). C-fos, for example, is an IEG that is turned on by arousing or stressful environmental stimuli to activate neurons of the brain, where it leads to the production of a protein called "fos." Fos can then bind to the DNA molecule, where it can turn on other genes. C-fos, in combination with other IEGs, such as those in the jun family, can regulate, and be regulated by, other families of genes that are involved in the material, energetic, and informational dynamics of the cell in response to psychosocial, as well as physical, stress and trauma. Although more than 100 IEGs have been reported, many of their functions remain unknown. The complex range of interrelated biological and psychological functions that IEGs are already known to serve, however, recommends a central role for these genes in the psychobiological foundations of hypnotherapy.

In the neurons of the CNS, for example, IEGs are now recognized as general or universal transducers responding to many classes of noxious environmental stimuli by inducing adaptive changes in gene transcription to facilitate the healing of stress and trauma due to mechanical or physical injury, severed neurons, epilepticus, spreading cortical depression, viral and bacterial infections, drug intoxication, and so on (Merchant, 1996). Studies of the role of *c-fos* are currently changing the face of pain research in both acute and chronic pain, phantom-limb pain, hyperalgesia, and allodynia. Most drugs that deal with pain—as well as related addictive drugs, such as cocaine, amphetamine, and the opiates—are also mediated by IEGs. The implication is that IEGs are central in moods and behavioral addictions (Tölle, Shadruck, & Zieglgansberger, 1995).

Most arousing environmental stimuli that have been studied can induce IEGs within minutes, their concentrations typically peak within 15 to 20 minutes, and their effects are usually over within an hour or two. These are the same time parameters of the general model of mindbody communication and hypnotherapeutic work proposed in Principle IV. Changes in the orchestration of patterns or complexes of gene transcription and new protein formation initiated in this time frame can lead to lasting changes in the CNS by converting short-term memory to long-lasting learning by long-term potentiation (Bailey, Bartsch, & Kandel, 1996; Tully, 1996). The IEGs are now used as markers or indicators of changes in neuronal activity in such psychopathological conditions as schizophrenia. Antipsychotic drugs are currently being designed to modulate the effects of IEGs on pathways leading to the production and utilization of neurotransmitters, such as dopamine, serotonin, and noradrenaline, in the "dopamine hypothesis" of schizophrenia (Merchant, 1996).

There are as yet no studies of the effects of hypnosis or any other approach to creative work on IEGs. Recent research on the relation of the IEGs *c-fos* and nerve-growth-factor-induced A (NGFI-A) in the wake–sleep cycle, however, suggests how they may be related to the activity–passivity dimension of high- and low-phase hypnotherapy. It has been found "that the expression of *c-fos* during waking is strictly dependent on the level of activity of the noradrenergic system ... high levels of *c-fos* during forced and spontaneous waking and ... low levels during sleep" (Cirelli, Pompeiano, & Tononi, 1998, p. 46). It is tempting to speculate that such stimulation of the noradrenergic system and IEG expression may be the molecular-genetic basis of Braid's (1855/1970) "psychophysiology of fascination" as the major pathway to healing in hypnosis. This leads to an interesting idea that builds a bridge between the traditional spiritual approaches of complementary medicine and modern psychobiological research and Ericksonian psychotherapy on the cellular-genetic level.

*Principle VII: A positive sense of novelty, wonderment, and fascination, variously described as experiences of numinosity, spirituality, highest hope and expectation, focused attention and absorption in creative moments of art, music, drama, and humor, as well as individual and cooperative human endeavor, can evoke the immediate-early gene cascade to facilitate the synthesis of healing proteins to optimize mindbody communication, neurogenesis, and healing.*

The entire history of hypnotherapy, including ancient spiritual rituals, exorcism, shamanism, fire walking, and modern but still "mysterious methods" of acupuncture, body work, therapeutic touch, and biofeedback that evoke a sense of wonder and expectation, is the empirical database for this hypothesis about fascination, healing, and hypnosis. We speculate that psychobiological healing by the religious experience of the "numinosum," consisting of a combined sense of fascination, the mysterious and the tremendous (Otto, 1923/1950), has much in common with traditional and modern rituals of healing associated with the mysterious expectations of hypnotherapy. We hypothesize that just as negative states of emotional arousal can stimulate the neuroendocrine system and messenger molecule receptor psychosomatic network to initiate an IEG cascade leading to the synthesis of stress proteins and illness, so can positive experiences of the numinosum initiate a cascade of healing at the IEG protein level. This implies that the experience of positive fascination, mystery, surprise, and insight experienced in hypnotherapy (Rossi, 1973) could access and facilitate an IEG cascade, leading to the synthesis of healing proteins.

*Principle VIII: Placebos entrain pathways of mindbody communication between positive psychosocial expectation and the state-dependent dynamics of the CNS and the psychosomatic network that trigger immediate-early gene cascades leading to the synthesis of proteins at the structural, energetic, and informational levels of mindbody healing.*

It is now well established that in mature mice and primates the experience of novelty and environmental enrichment can initiate IEG cascades, leading to the formation of new proteins, synapses, and dendrites in the hippocampus of the brain that encode new memory and learning (Kempermann, Kuhn, & Gage, 1997). When combined with voluntary exercise, such as running, the number of new cells is doubled (Van Praag, Kempermann, & Gage, 1999). Neurogenesis (the growth of new neurons) is now documented as taking place in the adult human hippocampus as well (Eriksson, Pefilieva, Björk-Ericksson, et al., 1998; Kempermann & Gage, 1999). The significance of such neuroscience research is that it provides a new rationale for understanding Erickson's use of positive emotional arousal, surprise, and fascinating paradox in his therapeutic work. The prospect of using the entire panorama of Erickson's innovations to optimize neurogenesis in the human brain is a heady prospect for psychotherapy in the new millennium.

Squire and Kandel (1999) provide the most engaging and accessible overview of research on the conditions leading to neurogenesis in the human brain. They describe how neurogenesis takes place in the hippocampus and associated structures during "declarative" knowledge. Declarative, or conscious, explicit memory, learning, and behavior are available to a person's conscious will and voluntary control. "Nondeclarative" or nonconscious, implicit memory, learning, and behavior, in contrast, are acquired by the automatic and more unconscious reflex mechanisms of classical conditioning, particularly emotionally based fear conditioning associated with trauma, stress, and mindbody symptoms. From this perspective, the essential task of Ericksonian psychotherapy is to access and transform symptoms encoded by the nondeclarative mechanisms of implicit memory with the declarative processes of voluntary consciousness (Rossi, 1986/1993, 1996, 2000). In my early work with Erickson, I described this as the use of "psychological implication" (Erickson, Rossi, & Rossi, 1976, pp. 59–62) as follows: "For Erickson, psychological implication is a key that automatically turns the tumblers of a patient's associative processes into predictable patterns without awareness of how it happened. The implied thought or response seems to come up autonomously within patients, as if it were their own inner response rather than a suggestion initiated by the therapist. Psychological implication is thus a way of structuring and directing patients' associative processes when they cannot do it for themselves ... It is important in formulating psychological implications to realize that the therapist only provides a stimulus; the hypnotic aspect of psychological implications is created on an unconscious level by the listener. The most effective aspect of any suggestion is that which stirs the listener's own associations and mental processes into automatic action. It is this autonomous activity of the listener's own associative and mental processes that creates hypnotic experience." This early description of the essence of Ericksonian work, together with current neuroscience research, suggests a more general principle about the relationships between nondeclarative (the patient's implicit, inner creative resources) and declarative conscious processes in evoking gene/protein cascades during many psychosocial rituals and the placebo response.

Placebo research is consistent in finding that about 30% of subjects report themselves as experiencing a therapeutic benefit (Harrington, 1997; Quitkin, McGrath, & Stewart, 1996). With psychiatric drugs, such as the selective serotonin uptake inhibitors, there is a relapse rate of 45% after one year. This means that 55% of the patients reported a significant placebo response after one year (Moller & Volz, 1996). Is such a healing placebo response merely a positive phenomenological experience of hope and wishful thinking on the cognitive-emotional level, or does it reflect some form of healing that is measurable on the cellular-genetic-protein level as well? The "novelty effect" is a common observation about the apparent value of the placebo response. Throughout history, it has been noted that new medicines are surprisingly effective when they are new and first introduced, but their therapeutic value is reduced and then lost completely after their novelty value wears off. Why should this be? Since it is now known that novelty can generate an IEG response, we propose that a "novelty immediate-early gene protein effect" could generate an IEG cascade leading to the formation of proteins that are the bottom line of healing at the cellular level (Rossi, 1997). We hypothesize that a heightened, positive sense of fascination, emotional arousal, and expectation associated with a novel, brightly colored sugar pill can be just as effective as a new and mysterious therapeutic ritual introduced by a healer coming from a far country. Just as increased corticotropin-releasing factor, CRF mRNA, appears in the paraventricular nucleus of the hypothalamus to initiate an adaptive arousal response within minutes of experiencing an acute physical or psychological stressor, we propose that a positive psychological placebo can initiate and entrain the chronobiological parameters of a "healing response" at the cellular-genetic level. This accounts for the fact that the placebo response appears within minutes, but disappears when its novelty effect wears out—just as is the case when the CRF cascade is metabolized out when the stressor is removed.

How should the therapist respond regarding an illness that medicine does not know how to cure entirely (e.g., cancer, rheumatoid conditions) when the patient asks about a treatment that the doctor suspects is a placebo? The following is an adaptation of the type of therapeutic suggestion that is true to the facts while maintaining the possibility of enhancing a strong placebo for the patient who believes in it (Brown, 1998). The italicized words in the following placebo prescription empower the patient's positive expectations while still allowing the therapist to speak wisely to the realities of the human condition.

*A Placebo Prescription*

*"Yes, it is true that some people have responded well to the alternative treatment you are asking about.* I usually do not recommend it to my patients because medical science has not yet documented if or how it works. *Your interest and hopes about the value of this treatment suggest you may benefit from it,* however, *if you are really sincere in wanting to try it.* You have a number of options in this situation. You can begin by *taking the medication I usually recommend because it does help,* even though it is not a complete cure and it does have some side effects we will have to monitor carefully. Or you can begin by trying *your alternative treatment first to find out how well it works for you.* We are all different on many levels and *the very special person you are might work wonders with this very special alternative treatment* you are asking about. *Medical miracles do seem to happen!* Still, it would be important to monitor the effectiveness of your alternative treatment carefully if you really would like to give it a trial. How long a trial do *you believe would be right for you?* Would you like to try your alternative approach by itself at first or in combination with the medication I usually recommend?"

The sense of self-empowerment and self-efficacy that is enhanced by allowing patients reasonable choices in their treatment plan has been shown to be a highly significant factor in health and well-being (Antonovsky, 1992).

## SUMMARY AND CONCLUSIONS

A careful consideration of the history of hypnosis, as well as current research, reveals that there is a universal psychobiological foundation for all forms of creative work, psychotherapy, and hypnotherapy. The psychobiological aspects of Ericksonian approaches to psychotherapy, in particular, may be conceptualized in a series of basic principles that outline the entire process of mindbody communication and healing, from the spiritual and psychosocial levels to the cellular-genetic-protein levels. The implications of current neuroscience research suggest that many of Erickson's innovative approaches to hypnosis and psychotherapy will find practical applications in facilitating neurogenesis in the hippocampus of the human brain in the new millennium.

---

### Practical Approaches to the
### Psychobiology of Ericksonian Healing and Hypnosis

- Utilize the patient's ongoing behavior in the therapy session to *access a state-dependent reexperiencing of the source of his or her problems*, as well as inner resources for solving the problems in his or her own way.
- Facilitate the patient's understanding of the "symptoms" as mind-body signals that the patient needs to reduce the psychopathological dynamics of stress engendered by chronic interference with the patient's own *natural quasi-periodic circadian and ultradian rhythms of creative work and healing.*
- Utilize *high-phase (emotional arousal) and low-phase (traditional relaxation) hypnosis* to access the cellular-genetic-protein levels of healing in hypnosis.
- Utilize a *placebo prescription* to facilitate the patient's own belief system in the spiritual and naturalistic efficacy of healing and creative problem solving in psychotherapy.
- Facilitate healing and brain growth by evoking the *novelty immediate-early gene protein effect* by utilizing the patient's *numinous sense of wonder and fascination.*

---

### References

Aldrich, K., & Bernstein, D. (1987). The effect of time of day on hypnotizability. *International Journal of Clinical & Experimental Hypnosis, 35,* 141–145.

Antonovsky, A. (1992). Can attitudes contribute to health? *Advances, 8,* 33–49.

Bailey, C., Bartsch, D., & Kandel, E. (1996). Toward a molecular definition of long-term memory storage. *Proceedings of the National Academy of Sciences USA, 93,* 13445–13452.

Barber, T. (1984). Changing unchangeable bodily processes by (hypnotic) suggestions: A new look at hypnosis cognitions, imagining, and the mindbody problem. *Advances, 1,* 7–40.

Bernheim, H. (1886/1957). *Suggestive therapeutics: A treatise on the nature and uses of hypnotism.* Westport, CT: Associated Booksellers.

Black, S. (1963). Inhibition of immediate-type hypersensitivity response by direct suggestion under hypnosis. *British Medical Journal,* 925–929.

Braid, J. (1855/1970). The physiology of fascination and the critics criticized. In M. Tinterow (Ed.), *Foundations of hypnosis.* Springfield, IL: C. C. Thomas.

Brewerton, D. (1992). *All about arthritis.* Cambridge, MA: Harvard University Press.

Brown, P. (1991a). Ultradian rhythms of cerebral function and hypnosis. *Contemporary Hypnosis, 8,* 17–24.

Brown, P. (1991b). *The hypnotic brain: Hypnotherapy and social communication.* New Haven, CT: Yale University Press.

Brown, W. (1998). The placebo effect. *Scientific American, 278,* 90–95.

Brush, F. R., & Levine, S. (1989). *Psychoendocrinology.* San Diego, CA: Academic Press.

Cahill, L., Prins, B., Weber, M., & McGaugh, J. (1994). B-Adrenergic activation and memory for emotional events. *Nature, 371,* 702–704.

Cirelli, C., Pompeiano, M., & Tononi, G. (1998). Immediate early genes as a tool to understand the regulation of the sleep-wake cycle: *In situ* hybridization, and antisense approaches. In R. Lydic (Ed.), *Molecular regulation of arousal states.* New York: CRC Press.

DeBenedittis, G., Cigada, E., & Gosi-Greguss, A. (1994). Autonomic changes during hypnosis. *American Journal of Clinical Hypnosis, 42,* 140–152.

De Wied, D. (1990). *Neuropeptides: Basics and perspectives.* New York: Elsevier.

Erickson, M. (1948/1980). Hypnotic psychotherapy. In E. Rossi (Ed.), *The collected papers of Milton H. Erickson, Vol. IV* (pp. 35–48). New York: Irvington.

Erickson, M. (1958/1980). Naturalistic techniques of hypnosis. In E. Rossi (Ed.), *The collected papers of Milton H. Erickson on hypnosis. Vol. I. The nature of hypnosis and suggestion* (pp. 168–176). New York: Irvington.

Erickson, M. (1959/1980). Further clinical techniques of hypnosis: Utilization techniques. In E. Rossi (Ed.), *The collected papers of Milton H. Erickson on hypnosis. Vol. I. The nature of hypnosis and suggestion* (pp. 177–205). New York: Irvington.

Erickson, M., Rossi, E., & Rossi, S. (1976). *Hypnotic realities.* New York: Irvington.

Eriksson, P., Perfilieva, E., Björk-Ericksson, T., Alborn, A.-M., Nordborg, C., Peterson, D., & Gage, F. (1998). Neurogenesis in the adult human hippocampus. *Nature Medicine, 4,* 1313–1317.

Ewin, D. (1986). Emergency room hypnosis for the burned patient. *American Journal of Clinical Hypnosis, 29,* 7–12.

Freeman, W. (1995). *Societies of brains.* New York: Erlbaum.

Glaser, R., Kennedy, S., Lafuse, W., Bonneau, R., Speicher, C., Hillhouse, J., & Kiecolt-Glaser, J. (1990). Psychological stress-induced modulation of interleukin 2 receptor gene expression and interleukin 2 production in peripheral blood leukocytes. *Archives of General Psychiatry, 47*, 707–712.

Glaser, R., Lafuse, W., Bonneau, R., Atkinson, C., & Kiecolt-Glaser, J. (1993). Stress-associated modulation of proto-oncogene expression in human peripheral blood leukocytes. *Behavioral Neuroscience, 107*, 525–529.

Gorton, B. (1957). The physiology of hypnosis, I. *Journal of the American Society of Psychosomatic Dentistry, 4*, 86–103.

Gorton, B. (1958). The physiology of hypnosis: Vasomotor activity in hypnosis. *Journal of the American Society of Psychosomatic Dentistry, 5*, 20–28.

Harrington, A. (Ed.). (1997). *The placebo effect.* Cambridge, MA: Harvard University Press.

Harris, R., Porges, S., Clemenson Carpenter, M., & Vincenz, L. (1993). Hypnotic susceptibility, mood state, and cardiovascular reactivity. *American Journal of Clinical Hypnosis, 31*, 15–25.

Hull, C. (1933/1968). *Hypnosis and suggestibility.* New York: Appleton-Century-Crofts.

Iranmanesh, A., Veldhuis, J., Johnson, M., & Lizarralde, G. (1989). 24-hour pulsatile and circadian patterns of cortisol secretion in alcoholic men. *J. Androl., 10*, 54–63.

Izquierdo, I., Netto, C., Dalmaz, D., Chaves, M., Pereira, M., & Siegfried, B. (1988). Construction and reconstruction of memories. *Brazilian Journal of Medical and Biological Research, 21*, 9–25.

Kempermann, G., & Gage, F. (1999). New nerve cells for the adult brain. *Scientific American*, 48–53.

Kempermann, G., Kuhn, G., & Gage, F. (1997). More hippocampal neurons in adult mice living in an enriched environment. *Nature, 386*, 493–495.

Kirsch, I., & Lynn, S. (1995). The altered state of hypnosis: Changes in the theoretical landscape. *American Psychologist, 50*, 846–858.

Kleitman, N. (1969). Basic rest-activity cycle in relation to sleep and wakefulness. In Kales (Ed.), *Sleep: Physiology and pathology* (pp. 33–38). Philadelphia: Lippincott.

Kleitman, N., & Rossi, E. (1992). The basic rest-activity cycle—32 years later: An interview with Nathaniel Kleitman at 96, by E. Rossi. In D. Lloyd & E. Rossi (Eds.), *Ultradian rhythms in life processes: A fundamental inquiry into chronobiology and psychobiology* (pp. 303–306). New York: Springer Verlag.

Lippincott, B. (1992). Owls and larks in hypnosis: Individual differences in hypnotic susceptibility relating to biological rhythms. *American Journal of Clinical Hypnosis, 34*, 85–192.

Lloyd, D., & Rossi, E. (Eds.). (1992). *Ultradian rhythms in life processes: A fundamental inquiry into chronobiology and psychobiology.* New York: Springer Verlag.

Lloyd, D., & Rossi, E. (1993). Biological rhythms as organization and information. *Biological Reviews, 68,* 563–577.

Mann, B., & Sanders, S. (1995). The effects of light, temperature, trance length and time of day on hypnotic depth. *American Journal of Clinical Hypnosis, 37*(3), 43–53.

McGaugh, J. (1989). Involvement of hormonal and neuromodulatory systems in the regulation of memory storage. *Annual Reviews Neuroscience, 12,* 255–287.

Merchant, K. (1996). *Pharmacological regulation of gene expression in the CNS.* Boca Raton, FL: CRC Press.

Moller, H., & Volz, H. (1996). Drug treatment of depression in the 1990s: An overview of achievements and future possibilities. *Drugs, 52,* 625–638.

Naish, P. (Ed.). (1986). *What is hypnosis? Current theories and research.* Philadelphia: Open University Press.

Olness, K., Culbert, T., & Uden, D. (1989). Self-regulation of salivary immunoglobulin by children. *Pediatrics, 83,* 66–71.

Osowiec, D. (1992). Ultradian rhythms in self-actualization, anxiety, and stress-related somatic symptoms. Ph.D. dissertation, California Institute of Integral Studies.

Otto, R. (1923/1950). *The idea of the holy.* New York: Oxford University Press.

Papez, J. (1937). A proposed mechanism of emotion. *Arch. Neur. Psych., 38,* 725–744.

Pardue, M., Feramisco, J., & Lindquist, S. (1989). *Stress induced proteins.* New York: Alan Liss.

Pert, C., Ruff, M., Spencer, D., & Rossi, E. (1989). Self-reflective molecular psychology. *Psychological Perspectives, 20,* 213–221.

Pert, C., Ruff, M., Weber, R., & Herkenham, M. (1985). Neuropeptides and their receptors: A psychosomatic network. *Journal of Immunology, 135,* 820s–826s.

Quitkin, F., McGrath, P., & Stewart, J. (1996). Chronological milestones to guide drug change: When should clinicians switch antidepressants? *Archives of General Psychiatry, 53,* 785–792.

Rainville, P., Ducan, G., Price, D., Carrier, B., & Bushnell, C. (1997). Pain affect encoded in human anterior cingulate but not somatosensory cortex. *Science, 277,* 968–871.

Rossi, E., (1973). Psychological shocks and creative moments in psychotherapy. *American Journal of Clinical Hypnosis, 16,* 9–22.

Rossi, E. (1982). Hypnosis and ultradian cycles: A new state(s) theory of hypnosis? *American Journal of Clinical Hypnosis, 25,* 21–32.

Rossi, E. (1986). Altered states of consciousness in everyday life: The ultradian rhythms. In B. Wolman & M. Ullman (Eds.), *Handbook of altered states of consciousness* (pp. 97–132). New York: Van Nostrand.

Rossi, E. (1986/1993). *The psychobiology of mind-body healing.* New York: Norton.

Rossi, E. (1990). From mind to molecule: More than a metaphor. In J. Zeig & S. Gilligan (Eds.), *Brief therapy: Myths, methods and metaphors* (pp. 445–472). New York: Brunner/Mazel.

Rossi, E. (1992). Periodicity in self-hypnosis and the ultradian healing response: A pilot study. *Hypnos, 19,* 4–13.

Rossi, E. (1996). *The symptom path to enlightenment: The new dynamics of self-organization in hypnotherapy.* Pacific Palisades, CA: Palisades Gateway.

Rossi, E. (1997). The symptom path to enlightenment: The psychobiology of Jung's constructive method. *Psychological Perspectives, 36,* 68–84.

Rossi, E. (1998). Mindbody healing in hypnosis: Immediate-early genes and the deep psychobiology of psychotherapy. *Japanese Journal of Hypnosis, 43,* 1–10.

Rossi, E. (2000). *Dreams, consciousness and spirit. The quantum dynamics of self-reflection and co-creation.* Malibu, CA: Palisades Gateway.

Rossi, E., & Cheek, D. (1988). *Mind-body therapy: Ideodynamic healing in hypnosis.* New York: Norton.

Rossi, E., & Nimmons, D. (1991). *The twenty minute break: Using the new science of ultradian rhythms.* Pacific Palisades, CA: Palisades Gateway.

Rossi, E., & Ryan, M. (Eds.). (1986). *Mindbody communication in hypnosis.* Vol. 3. *The seminars, workshops, and lectures of Milton H. Erickson.* New York: Irvington.

Routtenberg, A., & Meberg, P. (1998). A novel signaling system from the synapse to the nucleus. *Trends in Neurosciences, 21,* 106.

Ruzyla-Smith, P., Barabasz, A., Barabasz, M., & Warner, D. (1995). Effects of hypnosis on the immune response: B-cells, T-cells, helper & suppressor cells. *American Journal of Clinical Hypnosis, 38,* 71–79.

Saito, T., & Kano, T. (1992). The diurnal fluctuation of hypnotic susceptibility. *Japanese Journal of Hypnosis, 37,* 6–12.

Scharrer, E., & Scharrer, B. (1940). Secretory cells within the hypothalamus. In *Research Publications of the Association of Nervous and Mental Diseases.* New York: Hafner.

Selye, H. (1976). *The stress of life.* New York: McGraw-Hill.

Smith, G., & McDaniel, S. (1983). Psychologically mediated effect on the delayed hypersensitivity reaction to tuberculin in humans. *Psychosomatic Medicine, 46,* 65–73.

Sommer, C. (1993). Ultradian rhythms and the common everyday trance. *Hypnos, 20,* 135–140.

Soreq, H., & Friedman, A. (1997). Images of stress in the brain. *Discovery*, 19–20.

Spiegel, D. (1998). Hypnosis and implicit memory: Automatic processing of explicit content. *American Journal of Clinical Hypnosis, 40*, 231–240.

Squire, L., & Kandel, E. (1999). *Memory: From mind to molecules.* New York: Scientific American Library.

Sturgis, L., & Coe, W. (1990). Physiological responsiveness during hypnosis. *International Journal of Clinical Hypnosis, 38*(30), 196–207.

Tinterow, M. (1970). *Foundations of hypnosis.* Springfield, IL: Charles C. Thomas.

Todorov, I. (1990). How cells maintain stability. *Scientific American, 263*, 66–75.

Tölle, T. R., Schadrack, J., & Zieglgansberger, W. (1995). *Immediate early genes in the CNS.* New York: Springer Verlag.

Tully, T. (1996). Discovery of genes involved with learning and memory: An experimental synthesis of Hirschian and Benzerian perspectives. *Proceedings of the National Academy of Sciences USA, 93*, 13460–13467

Turner, J., Dewerth, M., & Fine, T. (1993). Effects of flotation REST on salivary Iga: Presented at the Fifth International Conference on REST investigation, Seattle, WA, February.

Van Praag, H., Kempermann, G., & Gage, F. (1999). Running increases cell proliferation and neurogenesis in the adult mouse dentate gyrus. *Nature Neuroscience, 2*, 266–270.

Wagstaff, G. (1986). Hypnosis as compliance and belief: A socio-cognitive view. In P. Naish (Ed.), *What is hypnosis? Current theories and research* (pp. 57–84). Philadelphia: Open University Press.

Wallace, B. (1993). Day persons, night persons, and variability in hypnotic susceptibility. *Journal of Personality and Social Psychology, 64*, 827–833.

Wallace, B., & Kokoszka, A. (1995). Fluctuations in hypnotic susceptibility and imaging ability over a 16-hour period. *International Journal of Clinical and Experimental Hypnosis, 16*, 7–19.

Weinstein, E., & Au, P. (1991). Use of hypnosis before and during angioplasty. *American Journal of Clinical Hypnosis, 34*, 29–37.

Woody, E., and Farvolden, P. (1998). Dissociation in hypnosis and frontal executive function. *American Journal of Clinical Hypnosis, 40*, 206–216.

# 10

# Caveat Therapist:
# Ethical and Legal Dangers in
# the Use of Ericksonian Techniques

*Alan W. Scheflin*

To neophyte psychology, psychiatry, or counseling students, the therapeutic theories and techniques they encounter must seem as numerous as the stars in the firmament. Of course, some of those stars shine with a familiar brightness. The psychoanalytic theories of Freud, although recently somewhat tarnished and battered, remain viable. The client-centered warmth of Carl Rogers has spawned a variety of modern humanistic approaches to mental and social maladjustments. Other stars appear suddenly in the heavens and blaze boldly, like EMDR, but no one can yet predict how long their light will continue to shine.

In this constellation of counseling concepts there are ideas and theories that run the gamut of the human imagination. Some of our leading healers have urged therapists to concentrate on the client's *unconscious* mind through techniques of free association. Other theorists argue with equal persuasion that the *conscious* mind is the proper arena for change by talking the client out of self-doubts. Still others maintain that the therapist does not talk the client *out of* self-doubts, but rather *into* new frames of reference. Many counselors dispute the necessity of working with the mind at all, preferring instead to concentrate on behavior. Those who adopt this view might choose to arrange certain stimuli to produce new behavioral responses. Or they might arrange new rewards to create new behaviors. Some may request that their clients learn about new behaviors through role-play. Other healers do not concentrate on the patient, but on the system or network of relationships involving the patient. Different theorists focus on affect, or imagination, or nonverbal communication, or any one of the basic premises of quite literally hundreds of theoretical schools of therapy.

Yet in this vast cosmos of unique and differing curative notions, none is perhaps quite so unusual and intriguing as the method of healing pioneered and practiced by Dr. Milton H. Erickson. One's first encounter with his techniques is reminiscent of Alice's trip through the looking glass into a world where everything is topsy-turvy and the rules of life somehow seem to have become reversed. When Ericksonian therapists communicate with each other, in person or through books and articles, they describe how they urge their clients to worsen their symptoms, or to reverse an apparent therapeutic gain by suffering a relapse! In the world of this truly paradoxical therapy, certain clients are encouraged to falter, or to fail. Cooperative clients are told to resist, and resistant clients are told to resist even more (Haley, 1973). Some clients are given therapeutic prescriptions that actually provide alternatives that are worse than what the client is now facing. Ordeal therapy, which forms an important part of Ericksonian methodology, prescribes physically and mentally discomforting activities as curative (Haley, 1984).

Milton H. Erickson (1902–1980) was a physician, a psychologist, and a psychiatrist. He is generally acknowledged to be the most gifted hypnotist, and one of the most extraordinary healers, of the 20th century. His Sherlock Holmesian powers of observation, and his ingenious and fanciful cures of the most bizarre ailments, are already legends. What is most remarkable, however, is that he achieved success mostly by doing exactly the opposite of prevailing psychiatric orthodoxy.

When Erickson was an infant, his family traveled *east* by covered wagon (Haley, 1993a). From that auspicious beginning, he never stopped traveling against the current.

In a moving tribute to his late friend, therapist Jay Haley has written that "Erickson's cases were as distinctive as a Picasso painting" (Haley, 1993b). His solutions to his patients' disturbances were so unique that therapists immediately recognized Erickson's imprint on them. Ordeal therapy is just one small part of Erickson's achievement.

Whereas most psychiatrists followed strict rules about dual relationships, Erickson would frequently have social contacts with patients outside the therapy room. Indeed, he would often arrange social situations to have a beneficial impact on his patients. For example, he would have friends, family members, or other patients participate in therapeutic cures.

While other psychiatrists studiously avoided making direct suggestions to patients, Erickson could be quite authoritarian. The opposite is even more true. Part of Erickson's acknowledged genius was in his ability "indirectly" to influence people around him. He could hypnotize selected people in a room without their, or anyone else's, realization. He could hypnotize a person while that person was bragging that he or she could not be hypnotized. He developed an unending array of "conversational" inductions that put people in trance during an ordinary chat. At professional conferences, he would demonstrate his ability to induce trance during an ordinary handshake.

Haley has effectively shown that Erickson's contributions to hypnosis and therapy are so unique that they appear to have no predecessors. No one worked the way Erickson worked. He used hypnosis 30 years before medical associations validated the technique; he applied family therapy procedures decades before family therapy was created; he utilized techniques of sex therapy and systems therapy that were not officially recognized until long after he had developed them; he concentrated on quick solutions rather than long-term psychoanalysis; he attached great significance to presenting problems rather than searching for historical causes; he rejected the negative image of the unconscious and instead made it an ally in the healing process; and he developed techniques that even today are beyond the comprehension of psychiatry's most gifted practitioners.

Erickson's powers of observation were so acute that he often left people with a feeling that he had read their minds. What is especially remarkable is the fact that he was so observant despite being tone-deaf, color-blind, and incapacitated by two different strains of polio. Although he possessed an extraordinary talent for getting people to do what he wanted them to do in their therapy, they were never left with an uncomfortable feeling that he had manipulated them, even as they were aware of being manipulated.

In addition to an active psychiatric practice, Erickson found time to coauthor five books and over 130 professional articles. During his lifetime, he was the acknowledged master of hypnosis and communication. Since his death, his legend has grown to mythic proportions. A "cult of Erickson" has arisen—true believers who deify him as a wizard, sorcerer, or guru with miraculous powers and magical cures. Erickson would have found this worship distasteful, as do many of those who have kept his work preserved at professional conferences (Hammond, 1984). Zeig is correct in noting, "Ericksonian methods are probably the fastest-growing field of psychotherapy in the Western world" (Zeig, 1985a, p. 31).

Therapists swap Erickson stories with the gusto of young boys trading baseball cards. "Did you hear about the time he had that man urinate through a tube?" "How about the time he had the mother sit on her son?" "And the phobic man who had to ride in an elevator with a very seductive young woman?" And the stories go on because there are so many of them. There are so many of them because Erickson brought ingenuity and humor to his cases. He disliked using the same approach twice, and he carefully tailored his cure to the individual idiosyncrasies of the particular patient.

One of the more fascinating Erickson cures involved a man who had been institutionalized for many years because he claimed to be Jesus Christ. The staff and psychiatrists had no success with him. Despite their pills and procedures, he continued to insist that he was Jesus. What could Erickson do that had not already been tried?

Erickson's solution displayed his manner of working. One day, Erickson walked up to the young man and said, "I understand that you are a carpenter." The young man had to acknowledge this point. "Well," Erickson continued, "could you build me a bookcase? I will pay you. Come to my office so we can take measurements." Surely, if the young man was a carpenter, he could make a bookcase. After taking the measurements, he did just that. Another psychiatrist saw it and asked Jesus to build him one. Soon, Jesus was so busy building bookcases, and acquiring a genuine mastery of his craft, that he gave up being Christ and opened a carpentry business. Erickson's solution was, in Haley's felicitous phrase, "typically Erickson." He respected the client's presenting problem and worked with it constructively to a positive outcome.

## WHAT A DIFFERENCE A DECADE MAKES

Aside from his obvious genius, his intense research and prolific scholarship, his dedication to his profession and his patients, and his warmth and humanity, Erickson had another advantage—he worked in an era when therapists were not sued for their talking cures. Up until 1980, when Erickson died, there had not been a single appellate legal decision in all of the country involving a lawsuit against a therapist for the manner in which the therapy had been conducted, excluding cases of inappropriate physical contact or sexual intimacy (Alexander & Scheflin, 1998; Scheflin & Spiegel, 1998). Horowitz (1984) has observed that:

> . . . it is still the case that virtually no reported decisions exist in which a psychotherapist has been successfully sued for negligence in what was said to a client during the therapeutic process. As long as therapists restrict their practice to talk, interpretation, and advice, they will remain nearly immune from suit, no matter how damaging their comments, or how incorrect their interpretations. (p. 1638)

In the 1980s, however, the legal climate turned inhospitable to the practice of therapy. By the 1990s, nearly 1,000 lawsuits had been filed against psychiatrists, psychologists, social workers, and other mental health professionals, challenging the therapies practiced, and even the realm of psychotherapy itself (Brown, Scheflin, & Hammond, 1998). Virtually every element of Erickson's inspiration and technique for healing is now under legal assault, especially his beloved hypnosis.

### Hypnosis

In 1923, while Erickson was a sophomore at the University of Wisconsin, his hypnosis experiments came to the attention of a professor of psychology, Clark Hull. Hull, himself now recognized as one of this century's most significant psychology researchers, realized the importance of young Erickson's work and held a postgraduate seminar on hypnosis that addressed Erickson's experiments. The work that began in Hull's classroom in 1923 culminated in the publication exactly 10 years later of Hull's classic book, *Hypnosis and Suggestibility* (1933). It was this book that liberated hypnosis from the confines of stage entertainment and mysticism. Hull's work made the scientific study of hypnosis respectable.

Erickson's genius was in recognizing that hypnosis was a pattern of communication that provided clues to human behavior that could be used therapeutically without a formal hypnotic trance. Would it be possible to place a person in a trance without using a formal direct hypnotic induction? If so, this would be especially useful with resistant clients. Erickson explored techniques of "indirect induction" and achieved a success that bordered on the mythical. In describing his feats, Jay Haley has written that Erickson "can hypnotize one person while talking with another, he can give a lecture and induce a trance in a particular person in the audience by emphasizing certain words, and often he will work with a person who only later, if at all, realizes that he was hypnotized" (Haley, 1973).

As he refined his art with a perfectionist's precision, Erickson noticed that the strongest indirect induction techniques utilized the client's own behaviors and experiences. What was even better, if the client resisted, this very behavior could be used to induce trance!

What factors produce such an intense and highly focused concentration? Erickson found that if the conscious mind could be distracted with a task requiring all its attention, the unconscious mind would have more freedom in which to operate and would be more available for communication. To distract the conscious mind, Erickson developed countless dramatic and entertaining techniques to shock it, confuse it, challenge it, or send it on an extensive memory search. In any of these situations, the conscious mind will react with intense concentration, thus leaving the unconscious more accessible for messages, and ultimately trance.

If the conscious mind could be distracted by confusion, what could be more confusing than having a therapist completely agree with a client's resistance? Let's take a simple illustration. A client agrees to try hypnosis, but when you, as the therapist, say that the client may feel his hand is getting lighter and lighter, the client responds that his or her arm is actually getting heavier and heavier. Erickson would reply to the client by saying that the arm could get heavier and heavier still. Now the client is in a bind. If the arm gets heavier, the client is no longer resisting. Yet if the arm gets lighter, the client is still cooperating, but this time with the earlier suggestion that the arm *may* get lighter. For the client, all paths of resistance have now become paths of cooperation. This is so confusing to the conscious mind that it is distracted enough to permit access to the unconscious. The client's resistance, which has been fully accepted, becomes the vehicle for hypnotic induction.

Erickson's brilliance in developing and utilizing indirect inductions stemmed from his belief that hypnosis was not a separate distinct entity, but a part of the overall network of communication systems operating simultaneously in each piece of every person's behavior. This viewpoint had an important consequence for Erickson—obtaining informed consent was unnecessary. As long as hypnosis could be seen as benign and therapeutic, informed consent would be a needless formality.

In 1980, the Minnesota Supreme Court became the first state tribunal to declare that hypnosis was so dangerous that anyone hypnotized for the purpose of memory recollection was disqualified from testifying in court about anything remembered during or after the hypnosis (*State v. Mack*, 1980). Within the next few years, most courts stampeded in the direction of harsh antihypnosis rules (Scheflin, 1996; Scheflin & Shapiro, 1989). As pointed out in Scheflin (1997a):

> According to the ... position supporting the *per se* exclusion rule for hypnotized witnesses, a person who has been lobotomized can testify in court, a person who has received massive electroshock treatments can testify in court, a person who has taken enormous dosages of mind-altering psychiatric drugs or psychedelics can testify in court, a person who has suffered substantial organic brain damage can testify in court; but a person who had been competently hypnotized by an experienced licensed professional who carefully followed strict guidelines to avoid undue suggestions cannot testify in court. (p. 160)

During the last 20 years, courts have grown highly suspicious of hypnosis and the alleged capacity to use it to distort the mind (Scheflin, 1999a). Hypnosis has become the primary target in the false memory debate with claims that it is an experimental, dangerous, and unduly suggestive procedure. Given today's judicial climate, therapy with hypnosis may expect a cool reception from judges. Failure to use informed-consent forms when working with hypnotically refreshed memory may expose the therapist to malpractice liability (Hammond, Garver, Mutter, et al., 1995; Scheflin, 1993). Indirect induction techniques may raise questions of lack of informed consent that are now becoming the basis of civil litigation.

I have described the assaults on the use of hypnosis elsewhere (Scheflin, 1997b, 1995). Unless judicial opinions concerning hypnosis are reversed, therapists will have difficulty explaining its therapeutic value.

## Informed Consent

In medicine, the doctrine of informed consent preserves an individual's autonomy concerning body and mind. No one may interfere with a person's body without that person's consent. The tort of battery is defined as a touching of the body without consent. Especially since the Nuremberg Code was passed in 1948, informed consent has been the concept structuring the relationship between healer and patient (Annas & Grodin, 1992).

Informed consent to physical procedures that affect the mind, such as electroshock therapy, psychosurgery, or drug therapy, is a precondition for the use of those procedures. Is there also a requirement that the patient must give informed consent to nonphysical techniques used to influence the mind? Smith (1991) has observed that "informed consent to medical treatment has received considerable attention in recent years, but its application to psychotherapy has not been fully defined" (p. 218).

Should the doctrine of informed consent apply to psychotherapy situations as well? In a classic thought-provoking article, Zeig (1985b) makes the argument that the medical model, where informed consent works nicely, differs substantially from the mental model, where it does not appear to fit well at all:

> The patient has a right to successful treatment. Psychotherapy cannot be tailored to the Procrustean bed of antiquated ethical strictures that are impossible to follow.
>
> It is ill-advised to require psychologists to fully inform consumers and/or to require overt consent. Requiring overt consent does not have sufficient scope to cover modern strategic and Ericksonian approaches. Providing full information and demanding direct consent can intrude into the clinical situation.

Although Zeig agrees that the patient has a right to receive some information on which to base responsible choices, he notes the danger attendant on a fully informed consent:

> However, the patient's right to self-determination cannot be com-

promised. Patients must be afforded freedom of choice. While fully informing patients of the nature of treatment is impossible and based on an antiquated linear conception of human functioning, patients should generally be informed of inherent risks of treatment.

In the courts, the primary purpose of the doctrine of informed consent is to maintain the patient's right to self-determination by providing information about inherent risks of procedures. ... To reflect that philosophy, the APA Code of Ethics could be amended to state, "Psychologists *inform consumers as to the inherent risks* of an evaluation, treatment, educational or training procedure. ..." This wording provides a concept that can be operationalized, researched and applied.

The doctrine of informing the patient of risks cannot be applied indiscriminately, because a therapist will not be merely providing information; he or she will also be influencing the patient. ...

For example, if the therapist tells the patient that the potential risk of treatment is divorce, not only is a fact being stated, but a suggestion is also being made. As experts in communication, therapists should be sensitive to the multileveled structure of communication and responsible for its effect in all aspects of the therapy, including those involving ethics.

As psychologist Michael Yapko (1983) has pointed out: "Maneuvering the client into a position of accepting offered suggestions is evidence of the skilled use of hypnosis." Just as a patient needs to be made ready for surgery, a patient also needs preparation for effective psychotherapy. This preparation is often outside the awareness of the patient.

Zeig's position is now at odds with a growing movement to demand a new, specialized form of informed consent before any therapy is undertaken. Legislators in Arizona are debating a bill entitled "Mental Health: Consumer Protection." Activity concerning this proposed legislation may be found at

http://www.azleg.state.az.us/legtext/44leg/1r/bills/hb2416p.htm.

Should this bill pass, consumers will be so protected that mental health treatment will become a virtual impossibility. Earlier versions of this bill were condemned by the American Psychological Association (1995) and by commentators (Brown, Scheflin, & Hammond, 1998; Saunders, Bursztajn, & Brodsky, 1995; Simon, 1995). Under this new informed-consent concept, patients must be informed about outcome studies scientifically demonstrating the effectiveness of the treatment they will receive. According to the Arizona bill, "Large series of single-case designs and anecdotal reports are not sufficient to meet this standard." Because the clinical literature is weighted heavily with these single-case and anecdotal studies, clinicians will be forced to run long-term scientific experiments in order to validate their treatment modalities and to satisfy informed-consent requirements. Thus, clinicians must become laboratory experimentalists. Most of the great body of work penned by Erickson would be inadmissible in court. Failure to meet these requirements would constitute actionable fraud under the Arizona bill's terms.

But Arizona is not alone in contemplating these antitherapy restrictive pieces of legislation masquerading as consumer protection laws. The Congress and several states are considering similar proposals. Unless defeated, such bills could threaten Ericksonian therapy's continuing vitality.

## Suggestion and Influence

Influence is all around us. We are bombarded by countless suggestions every day of our lives. Some suggestions motivate us; others repel us. We follow some suggestions, but ignore most of them. Why some suggestions attract our attention and influence our lives, whereas others are unpersuasive and leave us unaffected, is one of the mysteries of life. This idea is beautifully captured by Peter Shaffer in his Tony Award–winning play "Equus," about a psychiatrist's attempt to understand why a 17-year-old stableboy who loved horses should suddenly blind six of them. The psychiatrist says:

A child is born into a world of phenomena all equal in their power to enslave. It sniffs—it sucks—it strokes its eyes over the whole uncomfortable range. Suddenly one strikes. Why? Moments snap together like magnets, forging a chain of shackles. Why? I can trace them. I can even, with time, pull them apart again. But why at the start they were ever magnetized at all—just those particular moments of experience and no others—I don't know. *And nor does anyone else.* Yet, *if* I don't know—if I can never know that—then what am I doing here? (p. 88)

Critics of therapy have argued that it is a process of undue influence whereby overly persuasive, charismatic, or authoritarian leaders are able to manipulate and control their vulnerable, suggestible patients (Singer & Lalich, 1996; Ofshe & Watters, 1994). These critics liken therapy to brainwashing and mind control. As noted by Singer and Lalich (1995):

> Thus, thought reform is a concerted effort to change a person's way of looking at the world, which will change his or her behavior. It is distinguished from other forms of social learning by the conditions under which it is conducted and by the techniques of environmental and interpersonal manipulation that are meant to suppress certain behavior and to elicit and train other behavior. (p. 62)

Such criticism puts therapists in an unusual bind. To defend against these claims, it is natural to oppose them by saying that therapists do not work with influence or suggestion. Rather, they create independence and freedom of choice in their patients. A more compelling response, however, acknowledges that therapy, as well as every interpersonal encounter, is naturally a product of suggestive influences. As noted by Corrigan, Dell, Lewis, and Schmidt (1980):

> Virtually all human relationships involve persons attempting to influence each other. Although much of the influence may be exerted inadvertently, deliberate, purposeful influence is common when people attempt to do things with, for, or to each other. In the counseling relationship, counselors attempt to help clients attain some change in their behavior, attitudes, values, or views of the world. These attempts might be construed as purposeful influence whether or not the counselor or client conceptualize the events as such. (p. 395)

As Howard and Conway (1986) similarly have noted:

> Why do humans behave in the ways they do? This question represents one of the most enduring puzzles of intellectual history. The possibility that science might partially illuminate answers to this mystery is the promissory note on which all of the human sciences are based.

The error of critics is readily identifiable. They make the assumption that everything a therapist says or does is an irresistible suggestion that is not in the best interests of the patient. Furthermore, they ignore the fundamental point of Erickson's work—that every person is a unique individual. Instead, critics assume that all patients are highly suggestible and manipulated against their will. When rigid scientific demands are placed on critics to justify their opinions, the critics' cases evaporate (Brown, Scheflin, & Whitfield, 1999).

In essence, no one comes to therapy and says, "I am perfect the way I am. Do not change me." Instead, people come to healers because they have been unable to cure themselves. It is precisely suggestion and influence that they want and need, provided the therapist acts in the best interests of the patient and not according to some hidden agenda.

## CONCLUSION

Ericksonian therapy is a rich body of technique based on respect for the individuality of the patient and the complexity of human communication. After enjoying unfettered freedom to develop and grow, its central tenets are now threatened by an antitherapy movement sweeping across the country with the vengeance of a Texas twister. Fundamental ethical and forensic issues have arisen in the last decade that demand new responses. Unless these challenges are met, the grandeur of what Erickson taught us about healing will be needlessly tarnished.

---

### Five Practical Ideas

- Be aware of your state's legal restrictions on hypnotically refreshed recollection.
- Make use of informed-consent forms to protect yourself and your patients.
- Be familiar with the literature of suggestion and suggestibility in order to avoid undue influence.
- Use objective testing instruments wherever possible to provide scientific data about the patient.
- Maintain detailed notes that validate the choice of treatment, the alternatives rejected, and the results.

# References

Alexander, G. J., & Scheflin, A. W. (1998). *Law and mental disorder.* Durham, NC: Carolina Academic Press.

American Psychological Association (1995). APA resolution on "mental health consumer protection" acts (February 18).

Annas, G. J., & Grodin, M. A. (1992). *The Nazi doctors and the Nuremberg code.* Oxford: Oxford University Press.

Brown, D., Scheflin, A. W., & Hammond, D. C. (1998). *Memory, trauma treatment, and the law.* New York: Norton.

Brown, D., Scheflin, A. W., & Whitfield, C. L. (1999, Spring). Recovered memories: The current standard of evidence in science and in the courts. *Journal of Psychiatry & Law, 27,* 5–156.

Corrigan, J. D., Dell, D. M., Lewis, K. N., & Schmidt, L. D. (1980). Counseling as a social influence process: A review. *Journal of Counseling Psychology Monograph, 27*(4), 395–441.

Haley, J. (1973). *Uncommon therapy: The psychiatric techniques of Milton H. Erickson, M.D.* New York: Norton.

Haley, J. (1984). *Ordeal therapy.* San Francisco: Jossey-Bass.

Haley, J. (1993a). Milton H. Erickson: A brief biography. In *Jay Haley on Milton H. Erickson* (pp. 1–8). New York: Brunner/Mazel.

Haley, J. (1993b). Typically Erickson. In *Jay Haley on Milton H. Erickson* (pp. 176–199). New York: Brunner/Mazel.

Hammond, D. C. (1984). Myths about Erickson and Ericksonian hypnosis. *American Journal of Clinical Hypnosis, 26,* 236–245.

Hammond, D. C., Garver, R. B., Mutter, C. B., Crasilneck, H. B., Frischholz, E., Gravitz, M. A., Hibler, N. S., Olson, J., Scheflin, A. W., Spiegel, H., & Wester, W. (1995). *Clinical hypnosis and memory: Guidelines for clinicians and for forensic hypnosis.* Des Plaines, IL: American Society of Clinical Hypnosis Press.

Horowitz, S. (1984). The doctrine of informed consent applied to psychotherapy. *Georgetown Law Journal,* 1637–1663.

Howard, G. S. & Conway, C. G. (1986). Can there be an empirical science of volitional action? *American Psychologist, 41*(11), 1241–1251.

Hull, C. L. (1933). *Hypnosis and suggestibility: An experimental approach.* New York: Appleton-Century-Crofts.

Ofshe, R., & Watters, E. (1994). *Making monsters: False memories, psychotherapy, and sexual hysteria.* New York: Scribner's.

Saunders, L. S., Bursztajn, H. J., & Brodsky, A. (1995). Recovery of memory and managed care: HB 236's post-*Daubert* "science" junket. *TBN, 17* (Spring).

Scheflin, A. W. (1993, August). Avoiding malpractice liability. *American Society of Clinical Hypnosis Newsletter, 34*(1), 6.

Scheflin, A. W. (1995). The current assaults on hypnosis and therapy. Canadian Society of Clinical Hypnosis, Alberta Division, *News & Views* (Fall/Winter).

Scheflin, A. W. (1996). Commentary on *Borawick v. Shay*: The fate of hypnotically retrieved memories. *Cultic Studies Journal, 13*, 26–41.

Scheflin, A. W. (1997a). False memory and Buridan's ass: A response to Karlin and Orne. *Cultic Studies Journal, 14*(2), 207–289.

Scheflin, A. W. (1997b). Ethics and hypnosis: Unorthodox or innovative therapies and the legal standard of care. In W. Matthews & J. H. Edgette (Eds.), *Current thinking and research in brief therapy: Solutions, strategies, narratives* (pp. 41–62). New York: Brunner/Mazel.

Scheflin, A. W. (1999a). Hypnosis and the courts: A study in judicial error. *Journal of Forensic Psychology Practice* (in press).

Scheflin, A. W. (1999b). The evolving standard of care in the practice of trauma and dissociative disorder therapy. *Bulletin of the Menninger Clinic* (in press).

Scheflin, A. W., & Shapiro, J. L. (1989). *Trance on trial*. New York: Guilford.

Scheflin, A. W., & Spiegel, D. (1998, December). From courtroom to couch: Working with false/repressed memory and avoiding lawsuits. *Psychiatric Clinics of North America—Diagnostic Dilemmas Part II, 21*(4), 847–867.

Shaffer, P. (1974). *Equus*. New York: Avon Books.

Simon, J. (1995, Fall). The highly misleading "Truth and Responsibility in Mental Health Practices Act": The "false memory" movement's remedy for a nonexistent problem. *Moving Forward, 3*, 11–21.

Singer, M. T., & Lalich, J. (1995). *Cults in our midst: The hidden menace in our everyday lives*. San Francisco, CA: Jossey-Bass.

Singer, M. T., & Lalich, J. (1996). *"Crazy" therapies: What are they? Do they work?* San Francisco: Jossey-Bass.

Smith, S. R. (1991). Mental health malpractice in the 1990s. *Houston Law Review, 28*, 209–283.

*State v. Mack* (1980). 292 N.W. 2d 764 (Minn.).

Yapko, M. (1983). A comparative analysis of direct and indirect hypnotic communication styles. *American Journal of Clinical Hypnosis, 25*, 270–276.

Zeig, J. K. (1985a). *Experiencing Erickson: An introduction to the man and his work*. New York: Brunner/Mazel.

Zeig, J. K. (1985b). Ethical issues in hypnosis: Informed consent and training standards. In J. K. Zeig (Ed.), *Ericksonian psychotherapy, Vol. I: Structures* (pp. 459–473). New York: Brunner/Mazel.

# 11

# Revisiting the Question:
# What is Ericksonian Hypnosis?

*Michael D. Yapko*

I n 1986, I wrote a chapter entitled "What is Ericksonian Hypnosis?" to
appear in *Hypnosis: Questions and Answers*, edited by Zilbergeld, Edelstein, and Araoz. As a well-structured collection of chapters on a wide
variety of topics in the realm of hypnosis written by respected clinicians
and researchers, the book provided numerous insights into many important aspects of the skilled utilization of hypnosis.

Now, more than a dozen years later, I have been asked to update and
expand that original chapter in which I attempted to give some structure
to the modality known as "Ericksonian hypnosis." The task has grown
even more complicated because, in 1986, although the innovative work of
Milton H. Erickson was already quite popular, it was still in its infancy in
terms of the depth of understanding of his contributions to clinical practice. Much of the Ericksonian philosophy and methodology had not been
articulated, and very little had been done by way of researching Erickson's underlying assumptions and the efficacy of his methods. Even now,
although the relevant clinical and research literatures continue to grow,
much remains to be better understood about the diverse methods that
have come to be termed Ericksonian. However, I will attempt—once
again—to provide a succinct overview of Ericksonian hypnosis. In so

doing, I will also attempt to refute some of the common misconceptions about Ericksonian approaches.


## OVERVIEW

Milton H. Erickson (1901–1980) was a gifted clinician who evolved unique perspectives about, and highly creative applications of, clinical hypnosis and strategic psychotherapies. At a time in the early history of psychotherapy when most psychotherapists were practicing relatively crude hypnotic rituals and long-term psychodynamic therapies, Erickson was developing a style of treatment that differed radically, both in its aims and in its methods. He thought therapy should be brief, result oriented, multidimensional, and tailored to the needs of the individual rather than bound to some elaborate theory that the clinician happens to favor. Erickson's work has inspired a new generation of clinicians to become interested in hypnosis and the valuable applications it can have in various clinical contexts (Haley, 1985, 1996).

The Milton H. Erickson Foundation, established in Phoenix, Arizona, in 1979, was organized to advance the awareness of Erickson's pioneering methods through clinical training and research. The Foundation holds triennial meetings at which the latest developments in Ericksonian approaches are presented. These meetings are enormously popular; each is typically attended by 1,000 to 2,000 professionals, making them the largest meetings ever held on the subject of clinical hypnosis. (The latest on December 8–12, 1999, celebrated the Foundation's 20th anniversary.) The interest in and appreciation of Erickson's influence on the fields of hypnosis and psychotherapy are truly remarkable. Consider comments about Erickson from colleagues he inspired, each considered a major contributor to the field in his own right.

*Jay Haley, M.A.:* "The contemporaries of Erickson thought of him as the best among equals. [I] thought of him as a man who knew his business as a therapist. He worked at it, he practiced it, he experimented with it, and he innovated remarkable procedures" (Personal communication, 1988; see Haley, 1996; Yapko, 1990).

*William Kroger, M.D.:* "Erickson was a very modest man; he was never looking for self-aggrandizement. I attribute the success of his tech-

niques to a profound knowledge of human nature, a solid eclectic psychology on the nature of everyday living. He could take a patient into
his heart; that was his secret, the patient could feel the empathy" (Personal communication, 1987; see Yapko, 1990).

*André Weitzenhoffer, Ph.D.*: "The really skilled people—good hypnotists—
are quite skilled. They have skills that are other than just giving a suggestion. They have skills in interpersonal relations, ability to empa-
thize, to establish rapport ... Milton Erickson was marvelous at those
things and that is why he was so good. He had some real skills" (Personal communication, 1988; see Yapko, 1990).

*Jeffrey K. Zeig, Ph.D.*: "There was something extraordinary about Erickson: Perhaps his profound effect was due to his acute sensitivity, respect for the individual, intensity, verve, uniqueness, and joie de vivre
in the face of adversity. I saw him struggle to bring out the best in
himself and it inspired me to want to do the same" (Zeig, 1985, p.
167).

What is it about Erickson's work that has generated so much contro-
versy and inspired so much interest in (and devotion to) a less traditional
style of clinical practice? The answer to this seemingly simple question is
actually very complex. Scores of books have been written about Erickson
the man, Erickson the innovative theorist (who, paradoxically, advocated
a theory about the reasons not to have theories), and Erickson the genius
and creator of remarkable clinical interventions. Thus, it is well beyond
the scope of this chapter to provide an in-depth analysis of Erickson or
his legacy. Instead, I will focus on several basic Ericksonian principles and
elaborate on the relevant issues and techniques.

## THE NATURALISTIC PERSPECTIVE

Arguably, the most influential contribution Erickson made to the field of
clinical hypnosis was his emphasis on what he termed the "everyday
trance." What made this contribution radical at the time was the prevailing wisdom in the field that held hypnosis to be a "special state" of consciousness, separate and unique in its attributes from "ordinary" states of
consciousness. Traditionalists eschewed the idea of an everyday trance, an

idea that some continue to dislike for its lack of a precise definition. (See Weitzenhoffer's comments on this issue in Yapko, 1990.)

Erickson's ability to observe and demonstrate hypnotic phenomena in people who had not undergone a formal ritual of hypnotic induction became a powerful catalyst for many key developments in the field, including the following.

1.  Research into the state/non-state nature of hypnosis (Chaves, 1997; Coe, 1992; Kihlstrom, 1992; McConkey, 1986; Spanos & Chaves, 1989).
2.  Research into the relative value of direct suggestions as compared with indirect suggestions (Kihlstrom, 1987; Lynn, Weekes, Matyi, & Neufeld, 1988; Matthews & Mosher, 1988; Yapko, 1983, 1990).
3.  Research into the broad range of individual differences between people in response to hypnotic suggestion (Bates, 1993; Council, Kirsch, & Grant, 1996; Evans, 1991; Oakman, Woody, & Bowers, 1996; Orne & Dinges, 1989).
4.  Research into the role of contextual influences on hypnotic responsiveness (Council & Kirsch, 1996; Kirsch & Council, 1992; Nadon, Hoyt, Register, & Kihlstrom, 1991; Spanos, Arango, & de Groot, 1993).

These fruitful areas of research have led to resolution (in a relative, not absolute, sense, of course) of some issues, but not others. In general, Erickson's ideas have fared quite well in the research literature. For example, it is now widely agreed that hypnosis is both an interpersonal and an intrapersonal phenomenon, and that relationship and contextual variables are significant determinants of hypnotic responsiveness, just as Erickson claimed (Lynn & Rhue, 1991). Furthermore, it is now widely accepted that a formal ritual of induction need not take place in order for hypnotic responsivity to occur. Hypnotic phenomena can and do arise spontaneously in a variety of contexts, even complex hypnotic phenomena, such as analgesia (Chaves, 1993; Coe, 1992; Matthews & Edgette, 1997). Although the global term "everyday trance" can be criticized for its lack of defining boundaries, it is clear that Erickson's broader views of hypnotic phenomena were appropriate.

Subject to greater uncertainty is the notion of hypnotizability as a malleable trait, as Erickson seemed to believe. Research has been mixed on the issue, generating some support for hypnotizability both as a fixed trait (Banyai, 1991; Hilgard, 1991) and as a modifiable trait (Bertrand, 1989; Gfeller, 1993). Despite some researchers' doubts that hypnotizability can be modified, many other prominent researchers and clinicians have reported greater responsiveness with individualized and flexible approaches that emphasize positive and realistic expectations of hypnosis (Alman & Lambrou, 1992; Chaves, 1993; Barber, 1991; Spanos, 1986; Spanos, Arango, & de Groot, 1993).

Finally, a major contribution of Erickson's was the possibility of using indirect suggestion as a complement to, or even instead of, direct suggestions. Many people have created an erroneous impression concerning Erickson's work on this topic by suggesting that he was always indirect and metaphorical in his therapies and teachings. This is flatly untrue, and there is no better illustration of how direct and even authoritarian Erickson could be than his own case descriptions and therapy transcripts (Grodner, 1986; Rossi, 1980; Zeig, 1980b).

The issue has never been, as some have incorrectly stated, whether direct suggestions are more or less powerful in their effect than are indirect suggestions. On the basis of this unfortunate dichotomous thinking, an arbitrary and unnecessary polarization evolved in the field of hypnosis; practitioners actually "chose sides" by emphasizing either exclusively direct or exclusively indirect approaches in their teachings and writings. Thus, there evolved an artificial and inhibiting schism separating Ericksonians from traditionalists. There *are* differences in assumptions and methods between models of hypnosis, as I suggest in Table 11.1, but what has now emerged with clarity is that *all types of suggestions are valuable somewhere with someone.* Competent practice involves adapting one's methods to the unique characteristics of one's patient, and is not about what style or approach one prefers (Bloom, 1997; Grodner, 1986). Thus, a skilled clinician would be capable of communicating relevant information and perspectives in a range of structures and styles (Yapko, 1984). This concept represents a cornerstone of the Ericksonian approach called utilization. Jeffrey K. Zeig, founder and Director of the Milton H. Erickson Foundation, succinctly defined utilization in this way: "Utilization is the therapist's posture of readiness to respond strategically to any and all aspects of the patient or the patient's environment" (Zeig, 1997, p. 164).

## ERICKSON'S UTILIZATION APPROACH

Ericksonian hypnosis is based on a number of principles, all of which are implicit in this formula guiding Ericksonian interventions: "Accept and utilize." This is the essence of Ericksonian approaches, collectively known as the utilization approach (Erickson & Rossi, 1979). Table 11.1 presents a comparison of Erickson's approaches with those of traditional and standardized models of hypnosis. The "accept and utilize" formula and its associated principles are described in the remainder of this section.

1. *Each person is unique.* Although all clinicians acknowledge this in principle (Grodner, 1986), the scripting of hypnotic approaches (i.e., the use of the same approach with different patients) precludes this recognition at the level of practice. Ericksonian approaches demand spontaneity and utilization of the patient's unique resources, personal history, and specific responses to the clinician (Yapko, 1985, 1990, 1995). Thus, prepared scripts that are Ericksonian are impossible to create.

2. *The patient's experience is valid for him or her.* Through the acceptance of the patient's experience as a valid product of personal choices, both conscious and unconscious, resistance can be utilized. What is traditionally termed "resistance" in other models is accepted in the Ericksonian approach as useful information describing the limits of the patient's experience. It is respected rather than confronted or interpreted as undesirable.

3. *Each person relates to ongoing experience from his or her own frame of reference.* All people routinely project meaning onto current experiences based on their own range of knowledge and past experiences. Thus, idiosyncratic responses to hypnosis and psychotherapy not only are allowed, but are expected and are considered integral to the treatment process. The patient's unique subjective associations are the focal point of treatment; disrupting undesirable associations and building new, positive associations are the goals of the clinician. Erickson was quite right; subsequent research has shown that it is not hypnosis that is therapeutic, but the new associations in the patient that are generated during hypnosis (Lankton & Lankton, 1983; Fromm & Nash, 1992).

4. *Join the patient at the patient's frame of reference.* One way in which the "accept and utilize" formula is manifested is in the

clinician's accepting the patient's views and experiences and utilizing them in the therapy. Using the language of the patient is another such manifestation.

5. *The unconscious mind has utilizable resources, is capable of generating positive responses, and is patterned from experience.* Unlike
   those views that characterize the unconscious as negative, random,
   and in need of healing, Erickson characterized the unconscious as
   a storehouse of valuable life learnings that could be beneficial to
   a person when properly mobilized (Zeig, 1980b). Thus, he optimistically (and I personally believe *too* optimistically) assumed that
   each person already had within him or her the necessary resources
   for meaningful change (Grodner, 1986). Erickson placed great
   faith in the unconscious mind's capability to guide one's life path
   meaningfully, regulate the flow of information according to what
   one can effectively handle, and otherwise help one to manage
   one's life. Erickson was confident that useful information made
   available to the unconscious through hypnosis could be integrated
   in goal-oriented ways, particularly when that information stimulated the appropriate internal associations, that is, the most meaningful thoughts and feelings, including memories and values
   (Bloom, 1997; Edgette & Edgette, 1995).

### Table 11.1
### Contrasting the Views of the Major Models of Hypnosis:
### General Principles

| Variable | Traditional | Standardized | Ericksonian (Utilization) |
|---|---|---|---|
| Individualized approach? | No | No | Yes |
| Naturalistic concept of hypnosis? | No | No | Yes |
| Naturalistic techniques? | No | No | Yes |
| Hypnotist's demeanor? | Authoritarian | Authoritarian or permissive | Authoritarian or permissive |
| Suggestion style used? | Direct | Direct | Direct or indirect |

## Table 11.1, continued

| Variable | Traditional | Standardized | Ericksonian (Utilization) |
|---|---|---|---|
| Degree of compliance demanded? | High | High | Low |
| How is power in the relationship distributed? | Unequally in favor of the hypnotist | Unequally in favor of the client | Equally |
| Content or process oriented? | Content | Content | Either or both |
| Who can experience hypnosis meaningfully? | Some | Some | All |
| Source of resistance? | Intrapersonal | Intrapersonal | Intra- or interpersonal |
| Reaction to resistance? | Confrontation or interpretation | Confrontation or interpretation | Utilization |
| Emphasizes hypnotic depth? | Yes | Yes | No |
| Makes use of formal suggestibility tests? | Yes | Yes | No |
| Structure of process? | Linear | Linear | Mosaic |
| Relative value of insights? | Low | Low | Low |
| View of the symptoms' intentions? | Negative | Negative | Positive |
| Etiology of symptoms? | Intrapersonal | Intrapersonal | Inter- or intrapersonal |
| Symptomatic vs. dynamic approach? | Either or both | Symptomatic | Either or both |
| Recognition of secondary gains? | No | No | Yes |
| Characterization of the unconscious? | Negative | Negative | Neutral (capable of + or −) |
| Role of the unconscious? | Reactive | Reactive | Active |

## ERICKSONIAN HYPNOSIS

It is difficult to understand Ericksonian hypnosis without considering the larger patterns of Ericksonian psychotherapy that provide the context for their utility. This discussion, however, will focus only on Erickson's use of hypnosis.

Erickson's hypnotic methods have often been described as indirect. In fact, as discussed earlier, many of Erickson's methods were indirect, but not exclusively so. Erickson could be, and often was, very direct and authoritarian in his manner, particularly when his patients were open and responsive to him (Yapko, 1983, 1990, 1995). In general, however, Erickson's methods tended to be less direct because his typical goal was simply to allow for the possibility of a response rather than directly demanding one (Zeig, 1980b). Thus, he would suggest ways in which the patient might meaningfully respond, and then accept and utilize whatever the patient offered as responses (Erickson & Rossi, 1979, 1981).

Ericksonian approaches to hypnosis have been characterized as naturalistic (i.e., conversational). In employing this approach, there is no need to identify the onset of the hypnotic procedure overtly; rather, the clinician simply may involve the patient in an interaction that is absorbing, helping him or her to build an internal focus on his or her potentials, resources, and whatever subjective associations happen to arise during the process. This is the phase of hypnotic induction, with underlying goals of facilitating less reliance on conscious processes (thereby altering one's usual frame of reference) and building further hypnotic responsiveness. Strategically guiding the patient's experience in therapeutic ways through the deliberate and careful introduction of new information, new viewpoints, and other pattern-interrupting methods becomes the therapy phase, or hypnotic utilization phase (Erickson & Rossi, 1979, 1981). In actual clinical practice, the phases of hypnotic interaction are much less clearly defined than in more traditional, structured approaches (Haley, 1973; Yapko, 1990, 1995, 1996).

Evident in most of Erickson's hypnotic patterns is the facilitation of both the hypnotic state and the various hypnotic phenomena through his naturalistic method. In terms of actual technique, this involves describing interesting yet routine contexts in which hypnotic responses may typically arise without the patient's having previously thought about them in that way. The clinician using a conversational approach to induction might simply, but meaningfully, describe a situation in which one spontaneously enters hypnosis. Concurrent with the verbalizations, the clinician can nonverbally emphasize certain ideas (a process known as the "marking" or "embedding" of suggestions) through the use of gestures or changes in rhythm or tonality. As an example, the entrancing qualities of watching a fire are described in the following conversational induction process.

> ... This past winter was such a cold one ... and I often found myself so grateful for the simple pleasure of having a fireplace ... fireplaces are so soothing in the wintertime ... you may know that from your own experience ... for *you can feel so warm and so comfortable* ... when you *take time to just sit quietly and know that you can relax deeply* ... and *be so comfortable* ... and you know how to feel good ... and a fire can be so beautiful to watch ... and watching for hours can seem like minutes ... because the colors are so absorbing ... and the patterns of the wood burning at different rates in different spots is so soothing to watch ...

Building an internal focus and inspiring increased responsiveness to the clinician's guidance are primary goals of the hypnotic induction. These may be accomplished through a variety of methods, such as (1) the revivification of previous informal hypnotic experiences, as in the fireplace example; (2) the revivification of previous formal hypnotic experiences ("You can recall in vivid detail what your most satisfying experience with hypnosis was like ... how you were sitting, which relaxing images you saw," etc.); and, (3) the use of negative suggestions when wanting to utilize the resistance of a patient responding in a contrary manner ("You don't have to sit comfortably ... and you don't even need to think about allowing yourself the soothing experience of closing your eyes and letting your mind drift," etc.) (Yapko, 1990).

To facilitate a particular hypnotic phenomenon, one might simply describe a natural context in which the desired type of response occurs, creating the possibility of that response in the patient as he or she is encouraged to relate experientially to the description (Edgette & Edgette, 1995; Zeig, 1980a, 1980b, 1982). To facilitate age regression, for example, one might offer the patient the following.

> ... Recently, I had the experience of visiting the town in which I grew up ... and it was so very interesting to *go back in time and*

*reexperience important memories from childhood* ... memories that had been long forgotten drifted into awareness ... and it was such a good feeling to *remember happy experiences* ... an early birthday party ... a friend in school ... an important event that had a big impact on the kind of person I am today ... and *you can experience what that must be like* ...

In this example suggesting the possibility of an age regression, the patient is gently oriented to past experience in a way that is not personally threatening, thus reducing or eliminating the need for defensive reactions. The possibility is created that the patient may think of early childhood memories. Which specific memory then becomes a focal point for interaction is a product of personal choice that is derived from a combination of personal, interpersonal, and situational factors (Yapko, 1990, 1995). The patient's choice is accepted, and the information is utilized in whatever ways the clinician sees fit.

As a general strategy for acquiring skills in doing Ericksonian hypnosis, recognizing hypnotic phenomena as they arise in the course of daily living will provide numerous possibilities for naturalistically facilitating such phenomena with patients (Edgette & Edgette, 1995). Absorbing descriptions of the sensory details of the context in which the hypnotic response is evident can stimulate unconscious associations in the patient, allowing him or her to relate to the experience in a personal and experiential way (Watzlawick, 1978; Zeig, 1980b). Erickson was an advocate of the notion that people have many valuable resources within themselves into which they might tap, if they could just be "connected" to them. Hypnosis is a strategic means for facilitating this process (Bloom, 1997; Grodner, 1986; Lankton, 1986; Lankton & Lankton, 1989).

The primary vehicle for Erickson's indirect methods was the anecdote, commonly addressed in the literature on Erickson as the "therapeutic metaphor." Evident in the previous sample induction and utilization, the anecdotal method involves the telling of a story that can contain meaningful messages on multiple levels of awareness (Barker, 1985). Erickson observed that when patients present their problems to clinicians, they inevitably communicate on various levels; there is the surface meaning of their chosen words, but there is also an underlying reality concerning what the patient "really" means or what the symptom "really" symbolizes (Zeig, 1980a, 1980b).

Erickson believed that instead of solely attempting to promote awareness of the deeper-level meanings of patient communications, thereby restricting oneself to only one level (and, in his view, the most limited level) of the individual, the clinician can also communicate on multiple levels, including some outside of conscious awareness (Zeig, 1980b). This is the conceptual basis for Erickson's anecdotal methods. Furthermore, the use of anecdotes to make a point allows the patient to absorb the point experientially, by placing the relevant learning in an interesting, and usually realistic, context of human experience, thus making it far more real and emotionally significant for the patient. Emotionally significant learnings afford a greater opportunity for the integration of information than do less significant ones (Lankton, 1986).

Anecdotes (1) encourage the patient to identify actively with the story, since it is introduced in a way that suggests it is relevant to the patient's needs; (2) encourage the patient to learn actively from others' experiences; (3) may diminish resistance, because the patient is encouraged to respond to the anecdote in whatever way is desired without the demand for a specific response; and (4) provide a memorable and meaningful way to integrate new learnings (Barker, 1985; Lankton & Lankton, 1989; Zeig, 1980b).

Anecdotes can be used to induce hypnosis, to facilitate specific hypnotic phenomena, to suggest resolutions to problems, and to address a problem's unconscious underlying dynamics without necessarily encouraging or promoting insight, as well as a variety of other meaningful applications. Lankton (1986) encouraged the use of metaphors to restructure attitudes, to encourage affective release and greater emotional flexibility, and to facilitate behavior change. He likewise described using of open-ended suggestions to create possibilities, rather than closed-ended suggestions, which may be unnecessarily restrictive.

Whereas the indirect, anecdotal method is certainly one of Erickson's key contributions to hypnotic procedure, there are other uniquely Ericksonian hypnotic patterns that are also worthy of consideration. These include the interspersal approach and confusion methods.

The interspersal approach involves the use of specific words or phrases in the larger context of a routine conversation or therapeutic metaphor that, through repetition, are designed to facilitate the building of new associations within the patient (Erickson, 1966; Erickson & Rossi, 1979, 1981; Otani, 1990). If, for example, a clinician wants to facilitate an expectation of positive changes ("building expectancy"), the clinician can intersperse suggestions leading the patient in that direction, as in the following.

> ... You came here hoping that I might say or do something that would ... make it possible to feel better ... and you'd like to and *you can look forward to feeling better* ... and *having things improve surprisingly soon* ... and you didn't know just what I would say ... or what I would do ... and you forgot that you have already gone through *so many positive changes you're capable of remembering* ... and *change is inevitable* ... and you can't stop progress ... you know you have changed ... and *you can expect more changes* ... without even working at it ... you have *a change of mind* ... a *change of heart* ... a *change* of luck ... and *changes on even deeper levels* ...

Interspersed in this example are multiple references to the possibility and probability of change, attempting to build a therapeutic momentum based on positive expectations. Also evident in this example are other verbal strategies, such as presupposition, dissociation, indirect posthypnotic suggestions, truisms, and open-ended suggestions (Erickson & Rossi, 1979, 1981; Yapko, 1990). Such strategies are typical of the Ericksonian approach, which emphasizes the creative use of verbal as well as nonverbal patterns. Nonverbal patterns include the "marking" of suggestions, modeling (behaving in the manner desired by the hypnotized patient, for example, unmoving, fixed attention, or the deliberate matching or mismatching of patient nonverbals), and the use of varied voice dynamics to facilitate the integration of verbal messages (Yapko, 1990, 1995).

The confusion methods are designed to disrupt the patient's usual patterns for processing experience (Erickson & Rossi, 1979; Gilligan, 1987). It is well known that when one is certain about something, it is very difficult to induce a change of attitude. Confusion methods are designed to create a state of uncertainty in the patient as a means of introducing the possibility of change (Erickson, 1964). Such methods may involve sensory overload (i.e., the use of multiple, complex ideas or sources of input that overwhelm the patient's ability to sort consciously through it all), or pattern interruption (introducing a new behavior or idea that disrupts the patient's usual sequence of responding, making it difficult or impossible for the person to attain his or her usual, undesirable outcome). Confusion methods typically disorient the person, facilitating an inward search (and thus their utility in either hypnotic induction or hypnotic utilization) in an attempt to make meaning of presumably meaningful yet confusing ideas or demands (Gilligan, 1987). As the patient focuses on the language of the clinician, the deeper meanings of embedded suggestions can take effect. The clinician can intersperse meaningful suggestions throughout the confusing ramblings, giving those more important suggestions greater clarity and significance by creating a contrast with their confusing background. In the following example, a confusion method is employed for the purpose of facilitating a structured hypnotic amnesia.

> ... and after learning what you've learned about yourself today ... you have an opportunity to decide at a deeper level ... how much you'd like to remember ... and your conscious mind can know at one level ... and your unconscious can know at a deeper level ... and you can remember what you'd like to remember ... and *remember to forget* what you'd like to ... and when you *remember to forget* what you'd like to *forget to remember* ... you can remember to forget what you've forgotten to forget when you realize deeply that remembering to *remember to forget* that no one has to remember to learn what they came here to learn by *forgetting to remember* the memory of insignificant and forgotten learnings that can mean a lot ...

As the patient attempts to sort through the confusing suggestions surrounding remembering and forgetting, those very processes are accessed. The patient can choose what degree of remembering and forgetting will be the most beneficial for him or her. And, as the research shows quite clearly, spontaneous amnesia is an uncommon response, suggesting that people can and do remember their hypnotic experiences if they choose to do so (Simon & Salzberg, 1985).

## CONCLUSION

Erickson did not promote a specific and detailed theoretical model of personality or clinical intervention. His view was a theoretical one that emphasized the need to respond to the uniqueness of each individual. Thus, "Ericksonian hypnosis" as a style may be more easily characterized by the flexibility of the general "accept and utilize" formula than by any specific hypnotic or psychotherapeutic approach.

In this description of Erickson's work, emphasis has been placed on the clinician's assuming a flexible, yet active, role in guiding the course of treatment in a solution-oriented direction, even when indirect methods are judged to be the most likely to succeed. The broad range of Ericksonian patterns of hypnosis involves a sophisticated use of linguistic and cognitive structures that are increasingly well described in the clinical and research literature. This literature requires an open-minded, careful analysis by the serious practitioner of clinical hypnosis.

The creative verbal and nonverbal strategies used by modern clinicians that are derived from Erickson's work, and his many insights concerning hypnotic phenomena that paved the way for our greater understanding of hypnosis, provide lasting evidence of Erickson's importance to the entire field.

## References

Alman, B., & Lambrou, P. (1992). *Self-hypnosis: The complete manual for health and self-change* (2nd ed.). New York: Brunner/Mazel.

Banyai, E. (1991). Toward a social-psychobiological model of hypnosis. In S. Lynn & J. Rhue (Eds.), *Theories of hypnosis: Current models and perspectives* (pp. 564–598). New York: Guilford.

Barber, J. (1991). The locksmith model: Accessing hypnotic responsiveness. In S. Lynn & J. Rhue (Eds.), *Theories of hypnosis: Current models and perspectives* (pp. 241–274). New York: Guilford.

Barker, P. (1985). *Using metaphors in psychotherapy*. New York: Brunner/Mazel.

Bates, B. (1993). Individual differences in response to hypnosis. In J. Rhue, S. Lynn, & I. Kirsch (Eds.), *Handbook of clinical hypnosis* (pp. 23–54). Washington, DC: American Psychological Association.

Bertrand, L. (1989). The assessment and modification of hypnotic susceptibility. In N. Spanos & J. Chaves (Eds.), *Hypnosis: The cognitive-behavioral perspective* (pp. 18–31). Buffalo, NY: Prometheus.

Bloom, P. (1997). How does a non-Ericksonian integrate Ericksonian techniques without becoming an Ericksonian? In W. Matthews & J. Edgette (Eds.), *Current thinking and research in brief therapy: Solutions, strategies, narratives* (pp. 65–77). New York: Brunner/Mazel.

Chaves, J. (1993). Hypnosis in pain management. In J. Rhue, S. Lynn, & I. Kirsch

(Eds.), *Handbook of clinical hypnosis* (pp. 511–532). Washington, DC: American Psychological Association.

Chaves, J. (1997). The state of the "state" debate in hypnosis: A view from the cognitive-behavioral perspective. *International Journal of Clinical and Experimental Hypnosis, 45*(3), 251–265.

Coe, W. (1992). Hypnosis: Wherefore art thou? *International Journal of Clinical and Experimental Hypnosis, 40*, 219–237.

Council, J., & Kirsch, I. (1996). Explaining context effects: Expectancy and consistency. *Contemporary Hypnosis, 13*, 29–32.

Council, J., Kirsch, I., & Grant, D. (1996). Expectancy, imagination, and hypnotic susceptibility. In R. Kunzendorf, B. Wallace, & N. Spanos (Eds.), *Imagination and hypnosis* (pp. 41–65). Amityville, NY: Baywood.

Edgette, J., & Edgette, J. (1995). *The handbook of hypnotic phenomena in psychotherapy*. New York: Brunner/Mazel.

Erickson, M. (1964). The confusion technique in hypnosis. *American Journal of Clinical Hypnosis, 6*, 183–207.

Erickson, M. (1966). The interspersal hypnotic technique for symptom correction and pain control. *American Journal of Clinical Hypnosis, 8*, 198–209.

Erickson, M., & Rossi, E. (1979). *Hypnotherapy: An exploratory casebook*. New York: Irvington.

Erickson, M., & Rossi, E. (1981). *Experiencing hypnosis: Therapeutic approaches to altered states*. New York: Irvington.

Evans, F. (1991). Hypnotizability: Individual differences in dissociation and the flexible control of psychological processes. In S. Lynn & J. Rhue (Eds.), *Theories of hypnosis: Current models and perspectives* (pp. 144–168). New York: Guilford.

Fromm, E., & Nash, M. (Eds.). (1992). *Contemporary hypnosis research*. New York: Guilford.

Gfeller, J. (1993). Enhancing hypnotizability and treatment responsiveness. In J. Rhue, S. Lynn, & I. Kirsch (Eds.), *Handbook of clinical hypnosis* (pp. 235–249). Washington, DC: American Psychological Association.

Gilligan, S. (1987). *Therapeutic trances: The cooperation principle in Ericksonian hypnotherapy*. New York: Brunner/Mazel.

Grodner, B. (1986). Learning Erickson's methods. In B. Zilbergeld, M. Edelstein, & D. Araoz (Eds.), *Hypnosis: Questions and answers* (pp. 248–251). New York: Norton.

Haley, J. (1973). *Uncommon therapy*. New York: Norton.

Haley, J. (1985). *Conversations with Milton H. Erickson, M.D.* (Vols. I–III). New York: Triangle Press.

Haley, J. (1996). *Jay Haley on Milton H. Erickson.* New York: Brunner/Mazel.

Hilgard, E. (1991). A neodissociation interpretation of hypnosis. In S. Lynn & J. Rhue (Eds.), *Theories of hypnosis: Current models and perspectives* (pp. 235–249). Washington, DC: American Psychological Association.

Kihlstrom, J. (1987). The cognitive unconscious. *Science, 237,* 1445–1452.

Kihlstrom, J. (1992). Hypnosis: A sesquicentennial essay. *International Journal of Clinical Hypnosis, 40,* 301–314.

Kirsch, I., & Council, J. (1992). Situational and personality correlates of hypnotic susceptibility. In E. Fromm & M. Nash (Eds.), *Contemporary hypnosis research* (pp. 267–291). New York: Guilford.

Lankton, C., & Lankton, S. (1983). *The answer within: A clinical frame of Ericksonian hypnotherapy.* New York: Brunner/Mazel.

Lankton, C., & Lankton, S. (1989). *Tales of enchantment: Goal-oriented metaphors for adults and children in therapy.* New York: Brunner/Mazel.

Lankton, S. (1986). Choosing the right metaphors for particular clients. In B. Zilbergeld, M. Edelstein, & D. Araoz (Eds.), *Hypnosis: Questions and answers* (pp. 261–267). New York: Norton.

Lynn, S., & Rhue, J. (Eds.). (1991). *Theories of hypnosis: Current models and perspectives.* New York: Guilford.

Lynn, S., Weekes, J., Matyi, C., & Neufeld, V. (1988). Direct versus indirect suggestions, archaic involvement, and hypnotic experience. *Journal of Abnormal Psychology, 97*(3), 296–301.

Matthews, W., & Edgette, J. (Eds.). (1997). *Current thinking and research in brief therapy: Solutions, strategies, narratives.* New York: Brunner/Mazel.

Matthews, W., & Mosher, D. (1988). Direct and indirect hypnotic suggestion in a laboratory setting. *British Journal of Experimental and Clinical Hypnosis, 5*(2), 63–71.

McConkey, K. (1986). Opinions about hypnosis and self-hypnosis before and after hypnotic testing. *International Journal of Clinical and Experimental Hypnosis, 34,* 311–319.

Nadon, R., Hoyt, I., Register, P., & Kihlstrom, J. (1991). Absorption and hypnotizability: Context effects re-examined. *Journal of Personality and Social Psychology, 60,* 144–153.

Oakman, J., Woody, E., & Bowers, K. (1996). Contextual influences on the relationship between absorption and hypnotic ability. *Contemporary Hypnosis, 13,* 19–28.

Orne, M., & Dinges, D. (1989). Hypnosis. In H. Kaplan & B. Sadock (Eds.), *Comprehensive textbook of psychiatry* (5th ed., pp. 1501–1516). Baltimore: Williams & Wilkens.

Otani, A. (1990). Structural characteristics and thematic patterns of interspersal techniques of Milton H. Erickson: A quantitative analysis of the case of Joe. In S. Lankton (Ed.), *Ericksonian monographs, no. 7: The broader implications of Ericksonian therapy* (pp. 40–50). New York: Brunner/Mazel.

Rossi, E. (Ed.). (1980). *The collected papers of Milton H. Erickson on hypnosis* (Vols. I–V). New York: Irvington.

Simon, M., & Salzberg, H. (1985). The effect of manipulated expectancies on posthypnotic amnesia. *International Journal of Clinical and Experimental Hypnosis, 33*, 40–51.

Spanos, N. (1986). Hypnosis and the modifications of hypnotic susceptibility: A social-psychological perspective. In P. Naish (Ed.), *What is hypnosis? Current theories and research* (pp. 85–120). Milton Keynes, England: Open University Press.

Spanos, N., Arango, M., & de Groot, H. (1993). Context as a moderator in relationships between attributed variables and hypnotizability. *Personality and Social Psychology Bulletin, 19*, 71–77.

Spanos, N., & Chaves, J. (1989). Hypnotic analgesia, surgery and reports of nonvolitional pain reduction. *British Journal of Experimental and Clinical Hypnosis, 6*, 131–139.

Watzlawick, P. (1978). *The language of change.* New York: Basic Books.

Yapko, M. (1983). A comparative analysis of direct and indirect hypnotic communication styles. *American Journal of Clinical Hypnosis, 25*, 270–276.

Yapko, M. (1984). Implications of the Ericksonian and neurolinguistic programming approaches to responsibility of therapeutic outcomes. *American Journal of Clinical Hypnosis, 27*, 137–143.

Yapko, M. (1985). The Erickson hook: Values in Ericksonian approaches. In J. Zeig (Ed.), *Ericksonian psychotherapy, Vol. 1: Structures* (pp. 266–281). New York: Brunner/Mazel.

Yapko, M. (1986). What is Ericksonian hypnosis? In B. Zilbergeld, M. Edelstein, & D. Araoz (Eds.), *Hypnosis: Questions and answers* (pp. 223–231). New York: Norton.

Yapko, M. (1990). *Trancework: An introduction to the practice of clinical hypnosis* (2nd ed.). New York: Brunner/Mazel.

Yapko, M. (1995). *The essentials of hypnosis.* New York: Brunner/Mazel.

Yapko, M. (1996). Hypnosis: Treatment in a trance. *Encyclopedia Britannica Medical and Health Annual*, 366–370.

Zeig, J. (1980a). Symptom prescription and Ericksonian principles of hypnosis and psychotherapy. *American Journal of Clinical Hypnosis, 23*, 16–22.

Zeig, J. (Ed.). (1980b). *A teaching seminar with Milton H. Erickson.* New York: Brunner/Mazel.

Zeig, J. (Ed.). (1982). *Ericksonian approaches to hypnosis and psychotherapy*. New York: Brunner/Mazel.

Zeig, J. (1985). *Experiencing Erickson: An introduction to the man and his work*. New York: Brunner/Mazel.

Zeig, J. (1997). Experiential approaches to clinician development. In J. Zeig (Ed.), *The evolution of psychotherapy: The third conference* (pp. 161–177). New York: Brunner/Mazel.

# 12

# The Philosophical Position of the Ericksonian Psychotherapist

*Michele K. Ritterman*

In the seven years I traveled frequently to Phoenix to study with Milton Erickson, I was most interested in the principles that guided his work, particularly his philosophy of life. In this chapter, I highlight what I extracted of those values, sharing with the reader vignettes of my interactions with Dr. Erickson that revealed his assumptions about human nature.

It was in my initial meeting with Erickson that I received my first philosophy lesson. Prior to that visit, I had done my homework. I had read everything my teacher, Jay Haley, had published on Erickson's work; I studied Herb Lustig's video of an Erickson session; and I adapted his approaches to the clients I treated as an intern at the Philadelphia Child Guidance Clinic. Finally there, in his little office in Phoenix, facing him, I was confronted with his first direct question. "Why have you come to see me?" I found myself responding, "What impresses me most about you is your philosophy of life. No matter what case is before you, you are so positive! I'd like to be like that." "Young lady," he answered, inhaling deeply and looking at me with his steady, penetrating gaze, "I'm neither an optimist nor a pessimist, but a realist, which means that into every life a little rain must fall. Therefore, it behooves us to enjoy the sunshine."

Years later, after Milton Erickson died, his youngest daughter, Kristina, shared with me a variation on that theme. I was then working with torture survivors, people whose bodies and personalities had been shattered by abuse. She said, "I think my father would like you to know something he understood from his having suffered nearly total paralysis caused by polio. He used to say to me, 'Kristina, I find that to *do anything* is pleasing.' "

Combining these ideas, I began to recognize a principle underlying Erickson's work: Start with whatever ray of light, shred of hope, or crumb of real positivity is at hand and help the client to make a realistic step that will enable that person to create further openings from the confines of his or her own mental limitations.

Since initially I had come to Milton Erickson as a psychotherapist and a student of Haley's, rather than as a young woman seeking personal counsel, he asked me to begin our discussion by defining my theory of psychotherapy. This conversation revealed Erickson's ideas about transformation in therapy. I proudly rattled off a few sentences about how I worked to change people, rather than analyze them. Unimpressed, he reminded me: "In psychotherapy, the therapist changes absolutely nothing. We create the circumstances under which an individual can respond spontaneously and produce his or her own change. Heartened by the possibility of change—no matter how small, positive, or negative—that person will naturally go on to make other changes."

As our interaction progressed, and I went deeper into trance, Erickson asked me what I would really like to talk about. To my surprise, a flood of emotions poured forth, and I began talking about wanting to have a child. Immediately afterward, I was embarrassed, and he said, "Now, we can talk about whatever you like. Tell me about one of your cases." He then demonstrated with me, to me, and for me, that whatever the therapist and client are talking about, they are always addressing what is most important to the unconscious mind, even though it might be in a coded language. He was demonstrating his belief that the human being tips his or her hand or reveals himself or herself in everything he or she does. He loved holograms, because a hologram conveys the essential idea that the whole can be seen from any part. Although known for indirection, Erickson, in fact, worked very directly, but through whatever personal code the client wished to provide.

If a person spoke to Erickson in body language, for example, he communicated directly in body language in return, matching whatever content or format in which the person wished to speak. He accepted clients' frames of reference. He did not project onto them. He did not analyze them from the perspective of a particular theory of personality. Erickson emphasized that you can know where people are by understanding their unique perspectives. I remember using this wisdom during a horseback riding lesson. I knew absolutely nothing about horses. My teacher was irresponsible. It was nighttime and my second lesson. "This horse is in heat," I complained to my teacher. "How do you know that?" the teacher asked. My reply: "She's ignoring your instructions and paying all her attention to what is going on out the pasture." The horse, like a man or woman having an affair, was distracted. Erickson believed that therapists ought not try to get clients to speak the therapist's language, but rather, should speak directly to clients in their language and about whatever content they choose to use to express their problems.

Erickson had no mentor or teacher, it is said. I disagree. Pain was his teacher. If anything can get a person to focus on practical matters, it's the question of what to do about pain. On one visit, we spent seven hours eyeball to eyeball. He said that as long as he was in trance, he could feel no discomfort, but once the trance was broken, he felt as if someone had been rolling a baseball bat up and down his spine.

Much of Erickson's work can be understood by looking at how he learned to deal with excruciating pain. The kind of pain he suffered taught him, for example: "If you want to destroy something, analyze it." Of course, he was enjoying a dig at psychoanalysis, but he was also teaching that the way to confront symptoms is to see them in their parts, to decompose them. In this broken-down state, big troubles become manageable ones. He taught that many pains have a "before," a "during," and an "after." He wrote a beautiful paper[1] about how to work with pain in those three stages.

His use of paradox related to his observation that people don't like to be told what to do. They don't like you to tell them to stop a problem behavior! It tends to make them dig in their heels and persist. Tell them to keep on doing what they are doing, and even improve on doing it, and they will rebel. If he hoped for a client to carry out an assignment on a

---

[1] "An introduction to the study and application of hypnosis for pain control." In J. Lassiter (Ed.), *Proceedings of the International Congress on Hypnosis and Psychosomatic Medicine*. Berlin, Heidelberg, New York: Springer Verlag. Reprinted from *College of General Practice of Canada Journal*.

Wednesday, he'd said: "Your mother might prefer you do this on Monday or Tuesday. I, myself, am hoping for Thursday or Friday, and I'm certain your husband would be pleased for it to occur on the weekend." He observed human behavior and from those general observations developed techniques tailored to the unique individuals at hand.

Erickson also taught that it is okay if your client thinks you are God, but you'd better not get confused by that. People make mistakes. He said that the Navajo weave an error into every rug to show that only God is perfect. He disliked it when therapists or doctors told people what they were capable of in terms of recovery. His resentment of this attitude dated back to the day when a doctor told his mother that her son would be dead by the next morning. Paralyzed, he was able to get his mother to position a dresser mirror so that he could watch the sunrise from his bed. He managed to be fully conscious at sunrise, long enough for his mother to see that the doctor was wrong, before he lapsed into a coma for several days. He had made his point to his mother.

When Kay Thompson and I talked at a workshop in Italy about her amazing recovery from a major accident, she explained that were it not for Milton Erickson's philosophy, she wouldn't have dared envision a physical healing that the doctors said was impossible.

Just before that workshop, I had been thrown from the thoroughbred racing horse in heat that my teacher had put me on, and had crushed a bone in my elbow. I was told I'd never straighten that arm again. "How dare you tell me what my arm is capable of doing?" I protested. When the physician wanted to leave the arm in a bent position in a cast after surgery, I knew the arm needed to come out of the cast to prevent it from healing in that position. I had to consult three different doctors before I could find one who would listen to my body. If I had not known Erickson, I would not have believed in my own body and its special healing powers. My arms now are symmetrical.

Erickson took his practical understandings of visceral pain and applied them to many other human dilemmas. Troublesome patterns people suffer, such as the abuse cycle, are subject to being broken down into before, during, and after phases. We know from Erickson that each of those three phases of any symptom pattern—whether an individual's mental set or a family's sequences of interaction—gives therapists that many clinical opportunities to enter in, and help to create, a circumstance in which the person can respond spontaneously and change. Working with abuse in this manner—treating the fighting, the forgiveness, the building of tensions—helps to destroy the entire symptom pattern. Few psychological symptoms are continuous and nonstop. Erickson learned many of the aforementioned lessons from physical pain.

Erickson also learned that some pains, insufferable in one body part, can be tolerated when transferred to another body part: Someone getting a shot, for example, can soften the pain of the needle by digging a fingernail into the fleshy part of the palm. That digging affords control over the pain. Erickson learned that part of what hurts about pain is that it is out of the person's control and, therefore, surprising, and even humiliating. We know that people can change by moving a problem from one facet of life to another where it is less bothersome, but can still keep the problem. Other therapies are less innovative because they are based on theory rather than on the tangibles and practicalities of urgent human suffering.

Along with one of Erickson's daughters, I once sat on a panel whose members were asked to discuss their relationship with him. His daughter and I said the same thing: We felt accepted by him. Erickson did not try to change people because they were having trouble, whereas the goal of many therapies is to make better people of clients or to get clients to conform to a prescribed model of mental health. Erickson liked to watch minds open like flowers blooming in the sun. He didn't compare a rose with a sunflower. Despite his reputation as a supreme manipulator, he actually meddled less than any other clinician with whom I've studied. He did as little as necessary because he really did accept people for who they were.

Erickson said to me, "You are as unique as your fingerprints. There never has been, and never will be, anyone exactly like you. So you have the right to be that, fully. There are things you can change, but other things are like your fingerprints. You can't change them. So just accept them." He helped people to acquire "the wisdom to know the difference." He also conveyed a complete acceptance of a person's uniqueness.

Accepting individuality in part established the basis for his paradoxical work. He said that when, as a teenage athlete, he had been totally paralyzed, except for the use of one eye, he became a keen observer of human behavior. Paradox and other methods came to him simply by observing how people actually work—not by hypothesizing about their childhoods, but by watching them in motion. He noticed that if you ask someone who is running to an appointment to tell you the time, when the person starts off again, it may be in the wrong direction. This observation formed the basis for his distraction techniques in psychotherapy.

Erickson added to this his observation that if you want a baby to put down a knife, you give it something else to pick up and the baby will let go of the knife. Otherwise, that baby will hold on, as if for dear life, to the dangerous object. Likewise, in child rearing in general, and in treating human problems, distraction can allow the mind to open to something new.

One of Erickson's favorite tricks was to show highly educated people that their broad and deep studies had not prevented them from suffering a philosophically rigid mental set. He had a lot of ways to shake up minds. One was his brain-teaser puzzle: "A farmer plants five rows of trees, four trees in each row, for a total of ten trees. How is this possible?" I watched him present this riddle to a variety of visitors from around the world. Everyone I saw was stumped by it. I'll leave the reader with this one. Milton didn't give the answer. He once said to me, "You're in your 30s and want to think you know it all right now. If your theory of life were right and mine wrong, life would be deadly dull. I'm in my 70s and I learn something new every day."

In summary, Milton Erickson helped me to form a pragmatic and yet intriguing philosophy of psychotherapy. To condense some of the basic ideas, we can consider the eight principles.

---

### The Eight Principles

- Principle One. Be neither a pessimist nor an optimist, but a realist: Help your client to go through the best door that is open.
- Principle Two. Therapists create the circumstances in which change can occur. It is the client who makes the changes.
- Principle Three. Therapists need to speak in the client's language, not the other way around.
- Principle Four. Let (your own) pain be your teacher.
- Principle Five. Accept the things you cannot change.
- Principle Six. Observe human behavior. Let those observations, and not some theory, guide your interventions for each unique situation.
- Principle Seven. Therapists are not gods, but guides.
- Principle Eight. Therapists don't need to provide answers, they need to provide mind-openers.

# PRACTICE

# 13

# A Goal-Directed Intervention for Decisive Resolution of Coping Limitations Resulting from Moderate and Severe Trauma

*Stephen R. Lankton*

T he world of therapy offers abundant approaches to every imaginable human problem. Most of these solutions are explained in terms rooted in jargon that is part of a particular theory. In the case of trauma resolution, writers speak about such vague concepts as "working through" and "redistributing cathexis." But many of these approaches simply reexplain various common problems as seen through the lens of that theory. If my favorite theory explains the mysteries of every ailment from ADD to MPD, and from OCD to obesity, then there are workshops to be given, books to be written, and money to be made in the field of therapy. Unfortunately, certain therapists can be very clever at solving certain problems owing to their unique intuitions, not to their unique education. And most theoretical approaches are the same wine in new bottles.

This chapter focuses on a method to help clients decisively resolve traumatic reactions in very brief, often one-session, therapy. Victims of trauma can suffer in significantly different ways before ever seeking therapy. They can be recent victims who are primarily experiencing a great

deal of anxiety and disorientation, as is often the case with victims of auto-
mobile and public transportation accidents. Or they may have suffered for
years from the effects of earlier life trauma and present themselves in
therapy with defense mechanisms that limit their experience in terms of
joy, sense of self, intimacy, security, livelihood, and more. These two
extremes describe vastly different clients and problems and illustrate that
total recovery from the effects of trauma, for many people, will not happen in one session. This chapter is not about solving all of a client's problems that may have resulted from trauma. It is not about resolving the
grief from loss. It is not about relearning new habits and perceptions to
fill learning deficits, and it is not about the social changes that rehabilitation may require. What it is about is overcoming the major limitation to
growth that trauma creates. It is about the most decisive technique for
getting on with growth and learning in the case of both mild and severe
traumas. In some cases, especially patients with recent traumas that have not
become part of a lifestyle, this intervention may make up most of the therapy. In other cases, those of long-standing trauma, it will serve as the ground-
work to make the journey to more pervasive growth and change possible.

The techniques listed here derive from a complex association and dissociation paradigm. Because the literature on trauma often suggests that
therapists must assist victims in some type of reliving and abreaction, an
explication of the similarities and differences between association/dissoci-
ation techniques and techniques of reliving/abreaction is offered. But I
will begin with a global comparison to clarify the major differences in the
approaches.

## SUMMARY OF RESEARCH

A traditional view of trauma states that the boundary between ego and
the outside world is obstructed. Victims lose some of their ego strength
and/or potential development as a result. The therapeutic goal of such
treatment is the constructing of ego boundaries (Berghold, 1991). The
common approach to accomplish ego strengthening for PTSD often uses
regression, recall, abreaction, and a subsequent "reintegrate." It was
shown that this method is correlated with hypnotizability (Evans, 1991).
Thus, the use of abreaction following age regression has become a popular
approach to treatment (Pickering, 1986). In fact, it is often expected that
the same "reliving" of the experience should take place, after hypnosis, in

the waking state. In the treatment of war neurosis, it is suggested that there is an absolute need to "revivify and develop a psychodynamic understanding of the precipitation stress in the hypnotic state and repeat this in conscious state" (Balson, 1980).

The therapy of trauma contains elements related to the treatment of phobia, and we can look to research also related to that condition. Several approaches to the treated phobia have been measured and found to be essentially equal in effectiveness: relaxation, approach fantasy, abreaction, and posthypnotic suggestion (Horowitz, 1970).

The idea that abreaction may not be necessary for successful treatment is an orientation that fits the Ericksonian approach. Other clinical research shows that hypnosis is a valuable tool to replace shame with autonomy relating to factors regarding the cure (Eisen, 1992). These include making meaning of the experience, framing the identity of the abuser, and defining levels of regained autonomy. This may be attributable to the manner in which the hypnotic state can operate to block the feedback system maintaining conscious control (Spivak, 1990) and in some manner protect the conscious mind from pain both during and after hypnosis.

## The Use of Hypnosis

It may be that those individuals who suffer most from traumatic situations are those who are most responsive to hypnosis. A high correlation among stress-dissordered victims was found with 313 subjects according to the Stanford Hypnotic Suggestibility Scale (Stutman et al., 1985). This type of correlation makes hypnosis a quite logical tool. Hypnosis is shown to be a good technique for accessing and working through the dissociated trauma memory (Spiegel, 1986, 1990). PTSD may be seen as a defense against memory and experience recalled by the event itself. In order to treat this defensive dissociative reaction, Spiegel (1988) recommends what he calls the "8-Cs": confrontation, condensation, confession, consolation, consciousness, concentration, control, and congruence. Some researchers have found that memory content can be changed to aid in the reduction of traumatic experience (Lamb, 1985).

But the treatment of trauma needs to go hand in hand with therapy focusing on the *process*, not on the content (Kingsbury, 1992). This brings us to elements of association and dissociation created by both traumatic events and therapy. Even the simple pairing or associating of relaxed breathing, relaxing, and distraction by counting can reduce the fears and be used as an effective bridge to uncover trauma (Malon, 1987).

The context of storytelling, sometimes called therapeutic metaphor, has even been shown to aid in the therapeutic process of shifting the variables of association to fear or pain. For example, the use of metaphor with children and associating safety; sharing imagination; introducing reality events; addressing issues of loss, love, and trust; and reducing guilt has been effective for victims of sexual abuse (Rhue, 1991).

The overall scope of treatment in the case of traumas should not be confined to helping a client alter memory or emotional experience. Rather, treatment needs to help victims form relationships, transform the memory into meaningful experience, take action to overcome helplessness (VanderHart et al., 1990b), and deal with the various sequelae of guilt and grief or mourning (VanderHart et al., 1990a).

## ERICKSON'S APPROACH

Erickson's clinical cases were often used to illustrate several interventions, but not the entire treatment of a client with regard to grief, stress on the family, and other life readjustments. As a result, there are few examples of trauma cases in his collected papers, and of those included, each deals with the recovery of repressed memories using hypnosis. There are brief references to cases of obsessive personality (Erickson, 1980, III, p. 251), hysterical amnesia (Erickson, 1980, II, p. 277), criminal activity (Erickson, 1980, III, p. 221), blood phobia (Erickson, 1980, II, p. 188), and the two cases discussed below. There are only a few detailed cases where Erickson used hypnosis to help unravel the mysteries of people plagued by previous traumas, and all of these involve institutionalized individuals. One case described a man who had repeated outbursts and Erickson used a complicated series of hypnotically induced dreams. The dreams became increasingly less symbolic so that, over a short time, the man was able consciously to interpret them. In this manner, he progressively informed himself of his trauma of incestuous victimization at the hands of his parents (Erickson, 1980, IV, pp. 58–70).

In another case, a woman was induced to use symbolic writing in trance so that communication to Erickson could take place that she seemed unable to face either consciously or unconsciously (Erickson, 1980, IV, pp. 163–167).

Both of these cases used a complicated method of communication within trance: from an unknowing part of the unconscious, through the conscious mind, and, finally, to the therapist. This type of communication was difficult for Erickson, and possibly even more tedious for other therapists and their clients. To employ the same ideas shown in Erickson's cases, but to make the process amenable to those of us (and our clients) who are less talented, I devised an approach that relies on communication between visual mediators of unconscious resources.

## COMPARISON BETWEEN
## DISSOCIATION AND ABREACTION

Consider that you have come to therapy because of the continued tension and anxiety you have experienced since you were on an Amtrak train that derailed and killed many persons and from which you narrowly escaped with some minor medical problems, all of which have been corrected and are healed. The therapist you visit has two major ideas for your therapy.

Reliving and abreaction require that you mentally, emotionally, and experientially return to the disaster. You will be encouraged to verbalize and release your emotions freely for all aspects of the incident. You will be expected, encouraged, and supported in the expression of fear, anger, shock, confusion, panic, helplessness, sadness, dependency, and so on, as the explication of the scene is relived and verbalized. Perhaps you might also be a candidate to express anger and other types of aggression. The major goal of this emoting is to help you rediscover your true feelings and adaptive response mechanisms, to own the emotions you concealed, and to grow in ego strength gained by acquiring previously denied parts of yourself. Your success in reaching some of these goals depends largely on the skill the therapist provides. There will usually be some major resistance to this approach on your part, the client, primarily a general reluctance to show emotions before the therapist and a reluctance actually to experience the unpleasant incident again.

Abreaction can produce a corrective emotional experience, attitude change, and redistribution of psychic energy, and most likely will result in an increased focus on the past as it encourages regression and reduces the use of denial. There is an unfortunate risk of retraumatizing the client during the reliving. More worrisome, perhaps, is the possibility of increasing reliance on the therapist, and becoming alienated from the family of origin (in the case of family-created trauma) or actually reconstructing a past of false traumas in the process of "therapy."

With association/dissociation techniques, by contrast, you can still experience a corrective emotional experience and attitude change, but the focus is on the present and future of your life. There is no risk of reexperiencing the trauma or of increasing dependency on therapists. You can build additional adaptive defenses, learn to use the parts of yourself lost in the trauma, and increase your self-support and personal resources.

In either case, these interventions are not being suggested as the only interventions necessary for a full and complete recovery. They are being used as the major interventions for regaining the ability to cope, function, be creative in living, and recognize that the trauma is behind you and you are improving radically. This association/dissociation model is being offered as an effective, viable, and preferable alternative to abreaction methods. (See table 13.1.)

### THREE CATEGORIES OF TRAUMA IMPACT

Results of trauma are divided here into three discrete categories. These are intuitively logical groups that are all-inclusive and, for the most part, mutually exclusive. These three categories dictate three types of increasingly complex interventions. The categories are "type 1—simple," "type 2—complex," and "type 3—state-bound" traumatic reactions. Discussing clients who have psychological and sometimes physical results of trauma requires that we differentiate levels of severity or hurt that might have come from events of the past. A continuum from "type 1—simple reaction" to "type 2—complex reaction" to "type 3—state-specific reaction" facilitates this process. Two of the approaches are discussed in the following and the complex association/dissociation "type 2" is illustrated with a case. Although the personal impact of traumatic events obviously is unique in every situation, the general limiting effects of trauma have some recognizable similarities. Some attempts have been made to assess PTSD in several areas: alterations in sense memory, repetitive behavior, trauma-specific fears, and changed attitudes. Indeed, the range of events from memory, to experience, to relationship change needs to be addressed for effective treatment. It needs to help victims form relationships, transform the memory into meaningful experience, and take action to overcome helplessness (VanderHart et al., 1990b).

**Table 13.1**

**Continua of the Trance Phenomena**

|                                         | Association/Dissociation | Abreaction |
|-----------------------------------------|:------------------------:|:----------:|
| Be a corrective emotional experience    | Can                      | Can        |
| Foster attitude change(s)               | Yes                      | Can        |
| Focus on past                           |                          | Yes        |
| Focus on present/future                 | Yes                      |            |
| Redistribute energy                     | Can                      | Can        |
| Encourage regression                    |                          | Yes        |
| Reduce denial                           | Can                      | Yes        |
| Risk pain of re-trauma                  |                          | Yes        |
| Build additional defense                | Yes                      |            |
| Learn to accept part of self            | Can                      | Can        |
| Learn to use part of self               | Yes                      |            |
| Intrapsychic                            |                          | Yes        |
| Intersocial                             | Yes                      |            |
| Risk distancing family of origin        | Can                      | Yes        |
| Risk distancing self                    | Can                      |            |
| Increase stress on current system       |                          | Can        |
| More likely to be resisted              |                          | Yes        |
| Build self-support                      | Yes                      |            |
| Risk increased reliance on therapist    |                          | Yes        |
| Construct the reality of the past       | Can                      | Can        |
| Connect with personal resources         | Yes                      | Yes        |

## Type 1 Trauma

"Simple trauma" refers to the unavailability of resources in certain needed situations. In simple trauma, an individual has been inhibited from learning certain experiences. Consider that the aim of a healthy person is to be able to associate to needed experiences and resources in each unique life situation. However, in the course of suffering a trauma in growth, the victim cannot organize or associate to or retrieve experiences needed in particular situations. For instance, experiences commonly called confidence are needed (or at least are very useful) in public speaking. A simple trauma has occurred when a specific event prevents experiences of confidence from being vividly remembered (or experienced) in the context of public speaking *and* the person is still able to operate in some other area of his or her life with confidence, and even sometimes amble through events that call for public speaking. Public speaking is not impossible for victims of this simplest kind of trauma, but the act of public speaking would result in considerable distress if it could not be avoided. There is not a significant loss of muscle flexibility, there are no significant attitudinal alterations about the world, and the person is likely to be resourceful enough to be quite successful in almost all areas of his or her life.

### Type 2 Trauma

"Complex trauma" refers to outcomes that constitute developmental learning problems. In these situations, the effect of the traumatic situation was sufficiently severe to render the person impaired over a *specific developmental area of coping* that would seem otherwise to be within the person's behavioral repertoire. The client with this type of trauma will usually show fairly severe use of denial, have many attitudinal and perceptual changes related to avoiding, and have much tension, which is used to prevent the breakdown of such defenses as reaction formation and denial. There may be frequent outbursts, child abuse, or anxiety attacks as efforts fail to maintain defense mechanisms. For example, a person may be unable to be in a position of speaking to the public and would arrange things so that this situation would never happen. Not merely uncomfortable, public speaking would be such a threat that even the thought of it would cause severe panic attacks. More usually, the events to be avoided are such things as sexual experiences, use of machinery, travel, love, and other major commitments and responsibilities.

Coping skills may be diminished, defensive attitudinal disposition may become a major problem that results in the person's moving away from choices in life, intrusive memories break into consciousness, and the person may experience a major loss of certain muscle groups (such as sexual organs). The panic that can be felt is often handled by alcoholism, avoidance of family members, occasional collapse, institutionalization, and so on.

## Type 3 Trauma

"State learning" refers to situations in which the troubling mind-set is very persistent. Being immersed in a state from which one can't recover is often referred to as state-specific, and this is consistent for severely traumatized individuals. A person who experiences this type of reaction to trauma is severely limited by compartmentalized ego states. There are problems for these individuals in *nearly all areas of development* that follow the traumatic event(s). They may show excessive fear, may have amnesia for large areas of their past, and usually feel helpless, not just in the area related to the trauma, but in life in general. They often use the defense of identification with the aggressor that may result in self-harming long after the traumatic events are over. Musculature, perception, attitude, emotional growth, and social skills are all impaired. Severe war traumas and severe child-abuse trauma, including seeing siblings murdered, for instance, may give rise to this reaction.

### SOLVING THE EFFECTS OF TRAUMA

The goal of brief therapy is to promote increased and sufficient functioning as soon as possible. To accomplish this, clients need to look at present and future goals, become involved with loved ones and other support, and replace doubt and worry with permission to feel positive. Therapy needs to associate current resources to future tasks, reframe perceived failures, provide posthypnotic suggestions for future success, and train clients in self-image thinking to reassess their skills and strengths.

Successful therapy identifies strengths and stimulates attitude change. In addition, it will increase self-nurturing by retrieving safety, comfort, rehearsal, self-talk, and self-acceptance by helping the often disowned self cast off shame.

Finally, there will be an ego-strengthening that comes from grieving, building new boundaries, and developing feedback loops to become self-sustaining in many ways. Other dynamic problems and social problems might also be solved, especially when it can be seen that personal or social situations have been limited by the historical impact of the trauma, or that clients, originally troubled in these areas, were in some ways predisposed to the traumatic effects that they suffered. In most cases, it is effective to involve other family members to help clients cope with helplessness (Moore, 1981).

## "COMPLEX ASSOCIATION/DISSOCIATION" PARADIGM FOR TYPE 1 AND TYPE 2 TRAUMA

The rationale for this paradigm is that the conscious mind is capable of noticing representations of internal communications and changes that can remain mostly out of awareness. Therapists merely need a way in which this communication and those representations can be set up. Most people will immediately accept a metaphorical framework of "talking" to other, usually younger, parts of the self, owing to the commonality we all have of family, community, and the ability to use that metaphor to sort experiences in terms of age and size. Once established, this metaphor of dissociative review makes it possible to associate to other needed resources of cognitive, perceptual, attitudinal, and emotional experience. Therefore, by accepting the metaphor of the older self talking to the younger self, clients' needed resources will become available in their experience as they think about and remember bits of traumatic memories. That is, they will have experiences that had been eliminated in the context of recalling bits of their traumas. The detailed outline for establishing and conducting this intervention follows.

## STEPS IN THE "COMPLEX ASSOCIATION/DISSOCIATION" PARADIGM

1. Complex association/dissociation: if clients cannot recall the known trauma or resource or if it is an extremely "volatile" memory:

   A. Establish a safe environment.
   B. Retrieve necessary resources.
   C. Ask the client to imagine a "grown self" in the room.

      i. This self is usually a representation of the current aware and resourceful self.
      ii. This self is usually the same age and has the same characteristics.

      In some cases, this representation will be of a self from the future, when the problem has been solved. The future self may be presupposed to be years or only hours into the future.

      iii. This self is conscious and knows what the conscious mind knows.

          a. Presuppose a position of observation toward the conscious mind.
          b. This conscious mind of the client will communicate with this part of the client.
          c. Client imagines communication taking place between these parts in an unspecified manner (by feeling, words, etc.).
          d. Ideomotor signaling is established for the therapist to continue with more intricacy. This is usually a head nod from the client indicating that agreement has occurred between the self and this resourceful part.

D. Ask client to ask the projected part to further dissociate.

      i. The projected part (part 1) is asked to see another part (part 2), which is younger.
      ii. This second part (part 2) is often not seen by the client.
      iii. Part 2 represents the more unconscious self and can communicate via the ties with part 1. This part is also usually chosen from all possible younger selves because of some special strengths or resourcefulness.
      iv. Part 1 and part 2, therefore, become buffers between any memories created by part 2 and the real client.

E. Have the client ask part 1 to ask part 2 to review the traumatic events from a comfortable distance. Part 2 would see the trauma happen to a third part, part 3.

      i. Suggest that only by means of dialogue or signaling (such as seeing the "head nods") from the imaginary part 2 to part 1, and then from part 1 to the client, can the client know what is occurring to part 3 in the mind or memory of part 2.
      ii. Conduct a careful elaboration of part 2, reviewing the scenes about part 3 and sharing with part 1 only that

which it is safe to share. Have part 2 communicate the review to part 1 by ideomotor signals so that part 1 can report the communication to the client and, likewise, the client can report to the therapy (all by ideomotor signals, such as head nods).

iii. This presupposes that the memory of the trauma to part 3 exists and is known to some part of the self (at least to part 2).

iv. The client's conscious report of "not knowing" is expected. In this way, even poorly recalled traumas (to part 3) can be reviewed by the dissociated part 2. In fact, forgotten traumas presumably can be reviewed and overcome in this manner.

F. Repeatedly review and communicate with self from past.

i. Continually request and guide the client to instruct part 1 to ask part 2 (only) to review the trauma that occurred to the younger part 3 with words and pictures only. Thus, part 2 continues to be at a distance from the trauma that is being seen as it happens to the younger part 3.

ii. Help the client instruct part 1 to instruct part 2 to accomplish (essentially) a simple association/dissociation with part 3. Part 2 should watch the events, see them take place in speeded-up time, watch them unfold in chronological sequence, even watch them unfold in reverse order—all the while verifying that part 1 and part 2 and the client are safe and secure during the process.

G. Remove the intermediate parts gradually and integrate the learning and resources.

i. It is possible for parts 2 and 1 to be gradually removed after the client accepts the presupposition of the safety and security and other desired resources occurring as the traumatic memory is reviewed.

ii. The client must repeat the above steps until it is presupposed that he or she can handle the awareness and have the resources—and possibly even use the bits of memories as signals that desired resources are available and can be experienced and used.

iii. As each part collapses into the neighboring part, one at a time, the client eventually creates the situation of the client in a simple association/dissociation.

iv. Finally, there can be a merging of the secure part with the youngest traumatized part. In doing this, the secure client can be directed to reassure and nurture that younger part. This constitutes a reframing of the role the client has played to the role of self care-giver, nonvictim, resourceful, and empowered. The client, in this way, learns a role that generates strength and maturity any time the traumatized self is remembered in this way. It should also be said that the chances of the client's taking this empowered role in the future are quite high because there has been no other adaptive role mapped out for the client since the trauma. Therefore, this intervention will represent a decisive turning point for the client's growth.

H. Provide posthypnotic associations for the client to find and use these learnings and resources in the future.

It will be especially important to help the client think through possible future times that might have resembled the traumatic event or might have been avoided due to the old traumatized self-image.

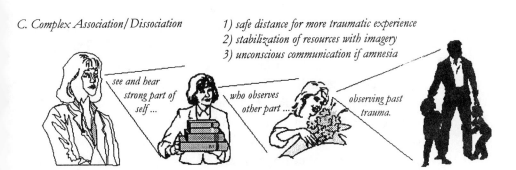

*C. Complex Association/Dissociation*

1) *safe distance for more traumatic experience*
2) *stabilization of resources with imagery*
3) *unconscious communication if amnesia*

*see and hear strong part of self ...*

*who observes other part ...*

*observing past trauma.*

Figure 13.1

After this intervention is used (usually a full one- or two-session event), therapy can proceed to deal with any other issues that have arisen for the client. These might include changes in family life, recreation, self-care, grieving, intimacy, sexual functioning, educational or occupational goals, or learned awareness of physical pain. Each client will have unique needs in these areas. It is most likely that clients for whom the trauma was recent will have few maladjustments to correct and clients for whom the trauma has been long-standing will have far more difficulties that have arisen during the years of avoidance, excuses, lower self-esteem, and so on.

The following case illustrates the actual wording for setting up this intervention. This case was a single-session intervention and is useful as an example in that it demonstrates this intervention in isolation and since it shows how to follow the outline while still modifying it slightly in some creative ways to accommodate the client's unique situation. Specifically, this client reported that no part of herself was without fear and anxiety. Therefore, the representation of the self (part 1) was constructed as a presupposed self from the future who was expected to be free of the anxiety. Part 2 was a teenage self who existed before the trauma. Of course, the most distant self (part 3) was the client's self from the disaster. Her head nods indicated the recognition of the relation of part 3 to part 2, if not of her (real self), and an agreement with various swapping of resources and attitudinal self-nurturing comments recommended by the therapist from the real and future self to part 3.

CASE EXAMPLE OF
COMPLEX ASSOCIATION/DISSOCIATION

The "Mobile Amtrak Disaster" refers to an accident in the latter half of the 1990s in which an Amtrak train bridge collapsed and resulted in the death of several passengers trapped in a submerged Amtrak car. This client, "Mary," came to my office within a week after the disaster and was unable to speak about the incident in any way without collapsing into heavy tears and fear. Since the accident had happened only a week earlier, it did not make sense to ask Mary to place an image of two remembered selves in between her traumatic memory *that she had gained since the trauma.* Instead, I asked her to recall an earlier self that was surprisingly strong and a future self that had totally recovered from the effects of the incident. These then were used as imagined mediators in the intervention.

She was asked to have the future self (51 years old) communicate with another, mediating image (that of a 17-year-old), who, in turn, communicated with the Mary who was in the disaster. In this manner of imagining, Mary (48 years old) was asked to review the events of the disaster from the distance of these two imagined intermediaries. The following excerpt comes from 20 minutes into the session and illustrates some of the more difficult communication that typified the heart of the session.

Ask Mary, who is 51 years old, to pass along to that adolescent Mary that she is from the future, that she lived through and overcame the fears and helplessness of the train disaster. Then, have the 51-year-old tell the teen that she is going to help her review the incident of last week—in words and pictures only—when the 48-year-old experienced the train crash. And add that each of you—the 48-, 51-, and 17-year-old—will hold on to the secure and resourceful experiences you each have now.

I want you, the 48-year-old, to tell the 51-year-old to tell the teen that the four of us will figure out how we are going to use the next few minutes cooperatively to overcome fears that have occurred. Ask the 51-year-old to help you by telling the teen that you want very little of her. Ask the 51-year-old to tell the teen that you just want her to stay in communication, if she would, and nod her head when she complies. Ask the 51-year-old Mary to ask the teen to nod her head as a signal that she understands and is willing to participate in that way. And when the 51-year-old sees the head nod, have her nod her head to you. In turn, when you see the 51-year-old nod her head to you, nod yours to me as a signal that we can proceed. And remember, you, the 48-year-old, don't need to watch for or see the teen or the incident she will soon review. Yes, let the 51-year-old see the teen, and when she does, have her nod her head to you.

Usually, it is possible to see smaller nods that seem to represent the client's experience of the series of communications between all the "selves" represented in imagination. I wait for the more exaggerated head nod from the client, which is intended for me. After receiving the affirmative signal of the nod, I continue this rather laborious and careful manner of speaking as I proceed with the steps outlined above. It is important to remember and to remind clients that they do not need to see and hear the trauma, but rather just see and hear that the other "part of themselves" is seeing and hearing it in review. They only need to see the mediating part or parts signal the beginning and ending of the review done by the most remote part of the self. In this regard then, some clients will report that they did not see and hear the review and some will report that they did. In a few cases, clients have even completed this process without ever consciously knowing what was reviewed and what the content of the trauma actually was. Nevertheless, such measures as the reduction of avoidance behavior suggest that the procedure has been successful in dissociating negative emotional limitations and associating to necessary and desired experiences. Thus, the similarities to Erickson's progressive symbolic dreaming and cryptic automatic writing (cited above) are obvious. This procedure appears to offer a method for parts of the unconscious to communicate to other parts of the unconscious, and ultimately to the conscious mind in progressive steps. However, the procedure is far easier for both clients and therapists than in the examples offered by Erickson.

A client has to be quite focused on internal representations to complete the review. Because the representations are symbols of resources the client has not been able to associate to as a result of the trauma, an ego-strengthening occurs. In terms of classical conditioning, we might say that the client has associated desirable experiences to the cognitive images of the trauma. Thus, the memories of the trauma no longer leave clients feeling helpless and without coping skills.

In cases where one of the representations is of a person from the future, as we saw here, the client creates a presupposition of successfully being cured of the traumatic reaction. The power of this presupposition is not trivial and deserves serious research. It appears that the creation of a positive presupposition of success directs people to seek and find desired resources over time. The more that people find their desired resources in contexts in which they need them, the less they report being troubled, having problems, and needing help or therapy.


## CONCLUSION

This intervention was absolutely pivotal in the change process as it supplied the means for the client, Mary, to keep her desired experiences in the foreground so she could begin to function immediately in the real world. It also allows clients the increased capability to become more creative and responsible for themselves in the remainder of therapy work. Most notable in this case is that Mary, when she came into the office, had been completely unable to talk about the traumatic incident *at all* without crying, sometimes uncontrollably. However, only one week following the single session of intervention described here, she was interviewed on a national television "talk" show. The hostess made sure to ask all the touchy questions possible during the televised interview. She even played the panicked voices on the audio recording of the 911 emergency call from that fateful night. However, Mary was able to describe and explain the entire incident and answer all questions in detail. Not once did she collapse into tears during the program.

After this single-treatment intervention has been used, most clients describe more energy, greater availability of resources, good reality orientation, more self-support, an integration with earlier emotional strengths, and adaptive, creative behavior. The process is not resisted and defensive mechanisms are replaced by adaptive mechanisms. This procedure works well for traumas that are type 2 or type 1 reactions. In fact, type 1 traumas can succeed with fewer intermediaries in the imagination chain. Type 3 traumas, however, are not likely to be suitable for this procedure and therapists are recommended to refrain from the use of this tool for such persons. A process that involves a greater stabilization of normal waking state, conscious focus, and secure experiences is recommended for type 3 trauma victims.

Total therapy for Mary, or for any client reacting to a trauma, should be expected to require several sessions. Future sessions concentrate on social, occupational, self-image, and other issues, in older traumas, where learned limitation had taken a toll over time. Finally, dealing with grief and self-forgiveness is sometimes essential for a full recovery.

---

**Practical Ideas**

- Divide trauma clients on the basis of severity and sequelae.
- Identify representations of past experiences that contain strong resources.
- Help clients make visual representations of the past "selves."
- Arrange the imaginations of past "selves" so that clients rely on signals from each.
- Verbalize to clients in such a way as to stimulate a review by a distant "self" in words and pictures only.
- Continue to suggest that a series of selves communicate about and conduct the review of the trauma so that the client does not need to review it directly.

---

# References

Balson, P. (1980). Treatment of war neurosis from Vietnam. *Comprehensive Psychiatry, 21*(2), 167–175.

Berghold, J. (1991). The social trance. *Journal of Psychohistory, 19*(2), 221–243.

Eisen, M. (1992). The victim's burden. *Imagination, Cognition & Personality, 12*(1), 65–88.

Erickson, M. H. (1980). The clinical and therapeutic applications of time distortion. In E. Rossi (Ed.), *The collected papers of Milton H. Erickson, M.D. on hypnosis. Vol. II: Hypnotic alteration of sensory, perceptual and psychophysical processes* (pp. 266–290). New York: Irvington.

Erickson, M. H. (1980). Negation or reversal of legal testimony. In E. Rossi (Ed.), *The collected papers of Milton H. Erickson, M.D. on hypnosis. Vol. III: Hypnotic investigation of psychodynamic processes* (pp. 221–230). New York: Irvington.

Erickson, M. H. (1980). The permanent relief of an obsessional phobia by means of communications with an unsuspected dual personality. In E. Rossi (Ed.), *The collected papers of Milton H. Erickson, M.D. on hypnosis, Vol. III: Hypnotic investigation of psychodynamic processes* (pp. 230–260). New York: Irvington.

Erickson, M. H. (1980a). Hypnosis: Its renascence as a treatment modality. In E. Rossi (Ed.), *The collected papers of Milton H. Erickson, M.D. on hypnosis, Vol. IV: Innovative hypnotherapy* (pp. 52–75). New York: Irvington.

Erickson, M. H. (1980b). Special techniques of brief hypnotherapy. In E. Rossi (Ed.),

*The collected papers of Milton H. Erickson, M.D. on hypnosis, Vol. IV: Innovative hypnotherapy* (pp. 149–173). New York: Irvington.

Evans, B. (1991). Hypnotizability in posttraumatic stress disorder: Implications for hypnotic interventions in treatment. *Australian Journal of Clinical & Experimental Hypnosis, 19*(1), 49–58.

Horowitz, S. (1970). Strategies within hypnosis for reducing phobic behavior. *Journal of Abnormal Psychology, 75*(1), 104–112.

Kingsbury, S. (1992). Strategic psychotherapy for trauma. *Journal of Traumatic Stress, 5*(1), 85–95.

Lamb, S. (1985). Hypnotically induced deconditions: Reconstruction of memories in treatment of phobia. *American Journal of Clinical Hypnosis, 28*(2), 56–62.

Malon, D. (1987). Hypnosis with self-cutters. *American Journal of Psychotherapy, 41*(4), 531–541.

Moore, C. (1981). Hypnosis: An adjunct to pediatric consultation. *American Journal of Clinical Hypnosis, 23*(3), 211–216.

Pickering, J. (1986). Use of age regression in a case of traumatization during late childhood and adolescence. *Australian Journal of Clinical & Experimental Hypnosis, 14*(2), 169–172.

Rhue, J. (1991). Story telling, hypnosis and treatment of sexually abused children. *International Journal of Clinical & Experimental Hypnosis 39*(4), 198–214.

Shapiro, M. (1988). Hypno-play therapy with adults: Theory, method, and practice. *American Journal of Clinical Hypnosis, 31*(1), 1–10.

Spiegel, D. (1986). Dissociation damage: Special issue: Dissociation. *American Journal of Clinical Hypnosis, 29*(2), 123–131.

Spiegel, D. (1988). Dissociation and hypnosis of posttraumatic stress disorder. *Journal of Traumatic Stress, 1*(1), 17–33.

Spiegel, D. (1990). New uses of hypnosis in the treatment of posttraumatic stress disorder. *Journal of Clinical Psychiatry, 51*(1), 39–43.

Spiegel, D. (1991). Disintegrated experience. *Journal of Abnormal Psychology, 100*(3), 366–378.

Spivak, L. (1990). Neurophysiological correlates of altered states of consciousness. *Human Physiology, 16*(6), 405–410.

Stutman, R., et al. (1985). Posttraumatic stress disorder, hypnotizability and imagery. *American Journal of Psychiatry, 142*(6), 741–743.

VanderHart, O., et al. (1990a). Hypnotherapy for traumatic grief: Janetian and modern approaches integrated. *American Journal of Clinical Hypnosis, 32*(4), 263–271.

VanderHart, O., et al. (1990b). Pierre Janet's treatment of posttraumatic stress disorder. *Journal of Traumatic Stress, 2*(4), 379–395.

## Suggested Readings

Dolan, Y. (1985). *A path with a heart: Ericksonian utilization with resistant and chronic patients*. New York: Brunner/Mazel.

Dolan, Y. (1991). *Resolving sexual abuse: Solution-focused therapy and Ericksonian hypnosis for adult survivors*. New York: Norton.

Lankton, C., & Lankton, S. (1989). *Tales of enchantment: Goal-oriented metaphors for adults and children in therapy*. New York: Brunner/Mazel.

Lankton, S. (1988). *A children's book to overcome fears: The blammo–surprise book!* New York: Brunner/Mazel.

Lankton, S., & Lankton, C. (1983). *The answer within: A clinical framework of Ericksonian hypnotherapy*. New York: Brunner/Mazel.

Lankton, S., Lankton, C., & Matthews, W. (1991). Ericksonian family therapy. In A. Gurman & D. Kniskern (Eds.), *The handbook of family therapy (Vol. 2)*. New York: Brunner/Mazel.

Mills, J., Crowley, R., & Ryan, M. (1986). *Therapeutic metaphors for children and the child within*. New York: Brunner/Mazel.

# 14

# Anxiety Disorders

*R. Reid Wilson*

T he anxiety disorders constitute a set of problem areas that are prevalent, debilitating, and costly. Over 14% of the adult population of the United States (27 million) will have a clinically diagnosed anxiety disorder at some point in their lives (Regier & Robins, 1991). The social and economic costs of anxiety disorders totaled more than $65 billion in 1994, representing 32% of the total costs for all mental disorders. And without proper treatment, the anxiety disorders tend to be chronic. Concurrently, behavioral-health-care costs have declined by 54% over the past 10 years (Hay Group, 1998). These simple but staggering facts demand that mental health providers redouble their efforts to study and apply the most efficient noninvasive methods of relieving the suffering of those with phobias, panic disorder, obsessive-compulsive disorder (OCD), posttraumatic stress, and generalized anxiety.

The gold standard of psychotherapeutic treatment in this field today is cognitive-behavioral therapy (CBT). Research has shown that treatment paradigms incorporating graduated exposure to feared situations, tolerance of discomfort, and applied mastery of relaxation skills, combined or independent, can relieve long-standing anxiety symptoms (Abramowitz, 1997).

In what way do these CBT methods coincide with Ericksonian principles? How can heightened awareness of Ericksonian practices strengthen the clinician's application of these proved techniques? Those questions will be explored in this chapter. Although Ericksonian methods are relevant to all the anxiety disorders, the treatment of panic disorder and OCD will serve as illustrative models.

## TREATMENT OF PANIC DISORDER

The individual suffering from panic disorder experiences sudden episodes of intense and overwhelming fear that seem to come on for no apparent reason. Physical symptoms may include racing heart, chest pain, difficulty in breathing, a sensation of choking, lightheadedness, tingling, or numbness, while the accompanying thoughts relate to fear of impending doom, such as humiliation, physical illness, or death.

Exposure treatment, in which the patient is instructed to remain in feared situations for prolonged periods, is well documented as a treatment approach for panic disorder (Marks, 1987). Cognitive therapy, with its focus on confronting negative schemata, is gaining support in the literature (Hoffart, 1993). The combination of these approaches, with their overlapping protocols and outcomes, will likely prove to be the most efficacious treatment.

A brief review of the theory of panic maintenance and the standard treatment of panic can support this proposal. Panic sufferers are sensitized to their anxiety response. Once they become aware of low-grade physical sensations, or consider entering a situation known for its association with panic, they tend to brace psychologically and physically for panic. They also fear that any anxiety, once initiated, will increase in intensity, resulting in panic, and will last an interminable time. Their coping strategies include the belief that the only way to manage the symptoms is to avoid them or escape. Thus, they develop elaborate defensive solutions to stop the noxious feelings.

To gain mastery over the anxiety symptoms of panic, three events must occur. First, patients' fear structures must be activated: They need to face their frightened feelings directly for prolonged periods without turning away or blocking. Second, they must discover that their predicted catastrophic outcome (such as that the symptoms will last forever) fails to occur. And third, they need to acquire self-efficacy, Bandura's (1977) term, whereby they conclude that their specific actions led to the less than horrible outcome. It is this specific type of exposure that results in habituation.

A simple application of treatment theory does not always mean a successful outcome in clinical practice. Physical and cognitive avoidance during exposure (such as sitting near an exit, sitting down when dizzy, carrying benzodiazepine, or thinking of escape plans) can blunt the effects of exposure by inhibiting the fear activation and habituation processes. The patient thinks, "If I hadn't done *that*, the symptoms would have been too much to handle." Thus, such avoidance during exposure interferes with the habituation process (Grayson, Foa, & Steketee, 1982). Misattributing the results of the experiments, especially by assuming the external locus of control, will similarly mute habituation. When patients conclude, "I didn't panic because the mall wasn't crowded enough" (or ". . . because it just happened to be a good day"), then exposure practice will not serve as a reinforcer for a new therapeutic cognitive set.

## Reframing and the Paradoxical Approach

Strategic and Ericksonian principles are the driving forces behind clinician interventions for panic disorder. When effective, they move the therapeutic goals forward (to face fearful situations and gain self-efficacy) and circumvent patients' defensive strategies (physical or cognitive avoidance and misattribution of success).

Incorporating aspects of a patient's behavior, perceptions, skills, and abilities into the therapeutic intervention was a signature approach for Erickson (1958). In this model, the clinician views the strategies of panic patients—to avoid threatening situations, fear the worst outcomes, and attempt to block the eruption of physical symptoms—as legitimate reflections of their inner states and models of the world. By intervening while respecting this deeper level of meaning, therapeutic changes can begin to break down the fortress built by the fear of panic, and these changes can stabilize over the long term. As Erickson stated, "Sometimes—in fact, many more times than is realized—therapy can be firmly established on a sound basis only by the utilization of silly, absurd, irrational, and contradictory manifestations" (Erickson, 1965, p. 59).

Watzlawick and his colleagues were the first to define reframing as altering patients' perceptions of the problem, its solutions, or their resources in such a way as to reinforce therapeutic interventions. "What turns out to be changed as a result of reframing is the meaning attributed to the situation, and therefore its consequences, but not its concrete facts" (Watzlawick, Weakland, & Fisch, 1974, p. 95).

Reframing is essential here and is a central principle of cognitive therapy (Clark, 1986). Panic sufferers must create a new interpretation of their discomforting symptoms, both as to what is causing them and where they are leading. A panic attack takes place when the person interprets harmless physical sensations (tachycardia, dizziness) or psychological experiences (racing thoughts, fear of death) as dangerous. It is this catastrophic judgment that leads to a rapid escalation of anxiety, which, in turn, intensifies symptoms and produces the panic episode. In cognitive therapy, the clinician confronts the catastrophic misinterpretation of these physical and psychological sensations experienced either before or during panic attacks (either induced or spontaneous). Behavioral experiments challenge patients' hypotheses of feared outcomes. These provide exposure to anxiety-provoking external situations and introceptive exposure to feared bodily sensations (such as dizziness from purposeful hyperventilation). In this manner, the therapist proposes an alternative hypothesis that the patient's somatic and psychic reactions are not the first signs of a heart attack or fainting, but are manifestations of anxiety, which will gradually dissipate. This is a prime example of reframing: to change the interpretation of a particular situation for therapeutic gain.

At the same time, the task of interrupting the ongoing cognitive set can be daunting, because the fear structure is so hardy. Gentle, step-by-step protocols that encourage weeks of relaxation training followed by incremental exposures to specific stressors can lead to minimal results since the criteria for habituation go unmet. The clinician must maintain the perspective that direct and prolonged exposure, with minimal defenses in place, gives patients their most powerful tool for healing. Rossi (1986, p. 82) reminds us of this: "Avoiding, resisting, or blocking a problem, however, only prevents one from accessing and therapeutically reframing it. When a problem or symptom 'haunts' a patient, it is only because mind and nature are attempting to bring it up to consciousness so it can be resolved." It is this viewpoint that helps the clinician to elevate behavioral experiments to a place of highest priority within and between sessions.

It is essential that the patient and clinician join forces in the therapeutic endeavor. This requires that patients adopt a paradoxical view of the recovery process for panic disorder. Once they embrace this framework, it is common for patients to generate homework assignments and other behavioral experiments independently of clinician directives.

The most straightforward method of reaching this stage of patient ownership of the recovery process is to propose a brief set of therapeutic directives as treatment is initiated. Adopting these directives and acting on them will bring an immediate transformation of the power dynamic, because panic-related symptoms shift from involuntary, dissociated actions to voluntary action. Typical patients enter treatment using the following imperatives: fear the symptoms, resist and defend against them, prevent them from getting worse or being noticed, worry to stay in control, brace yourself, and avoid threatening situations.

Commitment to a paradoxical orientation is often a "missing link" when the treatment of panic tends to fail. That is, one can attempt to face symptoms using a "proper" technique, but remain wedded to the need to resist and be frightened. A patient's disposition is usually, "This technique had better work, because I can't tolerate any more symptoms!" The following four paradoxical stances reflect the basic foundation upon which all behavioral experiments rest. They are introduced during the initial treatment sessions and remain in the forefront throughout all CBT sessions.

1. Seek out and accept discomfort.
2. Don't just do something, stand there.
3. It's O.K. if this doesn't work.
4. I want more symptoms now.

Note that each stance confronts a natural, instinctual reaction to panic symptoms. We all seek comfort. When scared, our urge is to take action; our minds race and we want to move. All strategies we invoke are for the express purpose of ending our suffering; we want them to work! And the least likely item on our wish list is to begin feeling even worse than we do.

### Hypnosis and Visual Rehearsal

At any stage of the treatment process, hypnosis can enhance therapeutic goals by exploring outside a patient's usual frame of reference. Hypnotic phenomena, whether in or out of formal trance, increase the patient's sense of control and, therefore, responsibility for the circumstances. They enhance the patient's receptivity to new ideas, build confidence, and limit certain patterns of response while expanding others (Wilson, 1985). The types of hypnotic phenomena and their benefits are broad, including:

1. *Dissociation*—to view an anxiety-provoking scene without discomfort; to rehearse new learnings; to prepare for other trance phenomena.

2. *Age regression*—to access previous significant events and learn to retrieve resources; to go back in time before fearfulness.

3. *Hypermnesia*—to gather diagnostic information; to clarify details of a past event; to prepare for a speech/test/event.

4. *Time distortion*—to decrease the length of panic or anxiety; to increase comfortable time; to prepare for age regression or pseudo-orientation in time.

5. *Pseudo-orientation in time*—to think, feel, and believe differently in the face of an old memory; to change portions of a problematic imagery; to go to the future and experience success; to plan "backward" from a successful future; to access resources from the future; to rehearse learnings.

6. *Positive hallucination*—to intensify a resource; to rehearse new learnings.

7. *Negative hallucination*—to not notice uncomfortable stimuli (crowds, feared objects).

8. *Amnesia*—to protect from past trauma, for posthypnotic suggestions; to forget past anxiety attacks.

One of the most productive hypnotic phenomena is age progression. This workhorse not only is an essential tool for rehearsing skills for a future behavioral task, but it helps embed a sense of long-lasting success in a healthy future. Most panic patients are competent students in the art of future progression. Their difficulty lies in the fact that 100% of their images are commonly of failure.

Hypnotic age progression focuses patients' attention in the direction of a therapeutic response, not a catastrophic one. Suggestions contain a strong psychological implication that the desired response will take place. Its biggest contribution is the disruption of patients' negative cognitive sets. Some patients so strongly believe that their coping abilities will remain inadequate and that task outcomes will continue to be negative that they yield little faith to the therapeutic process. Using binds within age progression addresses this defensive struggle. Erickson, Rossi, and Rossi (1976, p. 63) spoke of double binds as "mild quandaries that provide the patient with an opportunity for growth. These quandaries are indirect hypnotic forms insofar as they tend to block or disrupt the patient's habitual attitudes and frames of reference so that choice is not easily made on a conscious, voluntary level."

A simple bind, added to a common hypnotic task rehearsal, illustrates the benefits. Here is the outline of such a "successful task imagery": "Visualize yourself moving through your task. Let yourself experience two or three episodes in which you have some typical discomfort. Then rehearse what coping skills you want to use to take care of yourself during that discomfort. Imagine those skills *working successfully*." Note that although most elements of the encounter are realistic, the results are not left to chance.

Other binds regarding age progression include experiencing one's self far in the future, having long overcome the problem; floating through the future fearful situation; managing easily; being dissociated from negative feelings; or viewing an elaborate future event, without experiencing any troubles, within a 30-second imagery. Grinder and Bandler (1981) suggested that patients, after reaching the therapeutic goal in trance, experience the future in as much sensory detail as possible. In this process, called future pacing, patients would look back at the intermediate steps that helped them to reach the desired outcome.

## THE TREATMENT OF
## OBSESSIVE-COMPULSIVE DISORDER

Obsessive-compulsive disorder was seen as a chronic illness, unresponsive to treatment (Kringlen, 1965), until the rise of CBT in the early 1980s. Then, a variety of studies showed that both cognitive and behavioral interventions were successful in reducing obsessive preoccupation and in eliminating compulsive rituals (Emmelkamp & Beens, 1991; Emmelkamp, Visser, & Hoekstra, 1988; Van Oppen, de Haan, van Balkom, et al., 1995; Foa, Kozak, Steketee, & McCarthy, 1992; Hoogduin & Duivenvoorden, 1988).

Today, exposure and response prevention (ERP) have gained the most favor as a CBT treatment paradigm. Exposure is the deliberate confrontation with anxiety-provoking situations. Response prevention is the withholding of compulsive rituals. This combination is conducted in a flooding design, where patients provoke their obsessions and maintain their distress over an extended time, leading to habituation. ERP consistently shows long-term efficacy. For instance, O'Sullivan and Marks (1991) conducted a meta-analysis of nine treatment outcome studies. They found that 79% of patients were improved or much improved one to six years after treatment, with an average OC symptom reduction of 60%.

However, ERP, by its very nature, is frightening to patients and leads to avoidance. One study reported that 25% of OCD patients who requested help refused to participate in an ERP program because of this risk (Steketee, Foa, & Grayson, 1982).

Ericksonian principles are not challenges to the basic tenets of ERP, but are enhancements that reduce dropout, boost patient compliance, and so increase the success rate. Strategies within these principles include reframing, the fractional approach, and a variety of pattern disruptions.

## Reframing

Reframing of the OCD symptoms is the initial intervention that sets the tone for all further interventions. Patients learn that their perception of the problem and its solution is maintaining the problem. Four principles offer them a structure within which to view all treatment interventions. Therapists and patients focus attention on comprehending these principles in the initial stages of treatment. Each point, while quite simple, is a direct confrontation of a patient's conscious frame. Therapists maintain attention to these four principles in every session. Behavioral experiments are conducted, stories are told of other patient successes, analogies and metaphors illustrate the concepts—all to reinforce this reframing of the conscious set.

The principles are as follows:

1. Act as though the content of the obsession is irrelevant. In this bind, clinicians need not convince patients that the feared thought is irrational (which, as family, friends, and their previous healing professionals can attest to, is a losing proposition). The treatment goal is simply to act *as though* it is irrelevant.
2. Accept the obsessions instead of resisting them. Here is the first component of the paradoxical approach. All interventions to manipulate the obsessions start with accepting them exactly as they are.
3. Seek out uncertainty. This is a disorder of uncertainty. However, surrendering to that fact is insufficient. Patients must "run toward the roar." Any behavioral experiments they conduct are in the service of their intention to become active in their daily routines while remaining doubtful regarding the obsessive theme.
4. Seek out distress. On the heels of uncertainty comes distress. As patients continue to grasp the fact that they suffer from an anxi-

ety disorder, they comprehend that direct exposure to anxiety is their pathway to relief from OCD.

## The Fractional Approach and Pattern Disruption

Strategic interventions then address the specific obsessions and compulsions. While direct reframing sets up a model for self-help with OCD, the moment-by-moment encounter with distress merits a more careful line of attack. Because the anxiety of impending exposure can erode commitment to behavioral practice, a fractional approach to symptom reduction can lead to greater compliance. Rossi, Ryan, and Sharp (1983, p. 199) summarized Erickson's method: "You approach the correction of psychopathology by a gradual eradication of it, not by attempting to contest it, dispute it, or annihilate it."

The utilization approach of pattern disruption involves encouraging simple alterations in the pattern of a patient's behavior and its surrounding circumstances (Haley, 1973). Erickson wrote of this process as early as the 1930s (Rossi, 1980, vol. 4, p. 254), declaring that the size of the disruption could seem minimal and still effect change. His emphasis on the value of this mechanism continued throughout his career. In 1978, he encouraged the clinician to "try to do something that induces a change in the patient ... any little change, because the patient wants a change, however small, and he will accept that as a change ... And the change will develop in accord with his own needs ... It's much like rolling a snowball down a mountainside ..." (Gordon & Meyers-Anderson, 1981, pp. 16–17).

In this way, obsessions can be disrupted through such techniques as: postponing, singing or writing the obsessions, changing the obsessional image, and structuring daily "worry time" (Foa & Wilson, 1991). Each of these strategies maintains some central components of the obsession while interrupting others. For example, in postponing, patients are allowed to obsess; however, they are to choose the time in which they begin to obsess. Postponing can be for two hours or more, or for as little as 10 seconds; the length is less important than the shift that occurs within the patient. To postpone an obsession instantly turns a long-standing and seemingly intractable, involuntary process into a voluntary one.

Similarly, when patients agree to sing their obsessions, they continue to subvocalize their repetitious, unproductive thoughts, only now they put the words to some simple tune. Not only is it quite difficult to generate anxiety when they are singing, but the willingness to perform this task is a manifestation of at least an initial shift in their belief systems. When a father sings, "I'm going to kill my son, I'll stab him in the heart, I'll never be able to live with that," it is highly likely that he is developing his commitment to the notion that the content of his obsessions is irrelevant.

Strategic techniques for rituals are designed to meet with less patient resistance, and, therefore, promote experimentation and reduce avoidance. As with obsessions, they interrupt the standard process of the compulsion while maintaining significant parts of the compulsive framework. Four procedures prepare patients to give up their rituals: postponing, thinking and acting in slow motion, changing some aspect of the ritual, and adding a consequence (Wilson, 1999). All these interventions, while starting with minimal strategic change, are intended to lead patients to response prevention, where they refuse to engage in the compulsions. Postponing is performed similarly to the way it is used with obsessions, where patients stall the ritual for a designated length of time after their initial urge. The slow-motion procedure is most often applied to checking rituals, where patients replace several repetitions of the same action with one single, long sequence using slow, deliberate physical movements and thinking.

Compulsions are typically rigid structures that patients highly value. When their patterns are disrupted by small, low-threat maneuvers, the rituals become vulnerable to extinction. For example, one young man compulsively squeezed the sponge 10 times after cleaning the kitchen (one of about 16 different rituals in his repertoire). In the first week, he was asked to change hands with each squeeze. In the second week, he was asked to toss the sponge from hand to hand each time. And by the third week, he had enough self-control to squeeze only once, a change that remained stable over time. The patient perceived that passing the sponge from hand to hand was a minor shift in his long-standing ritual. However, the new ritual was only seven days old. The threat of changing a newly created ritual was significantly less than that of changing a four-year ritual.

O'Hanlon (1987, pp. 36–37) listed a series of Erickson's common pattern interventions, each of which can be adapted for use with compulsions. They include changing the order of the pattern, changing the frequency of the repetitions, changing the objects used, and changing the location or conduct of the ritual. For example, if patients have an exact sequence of bedtime rituals, then they can practice performing them by writing the tasks on slips of paper, to be drawn randomly from a jar each night to determine their order. If patients must engage the emergency brake four times, they can start an intervention by applying three sets of two times each. If patients shower for an hour and a half each day, they can commit to stepping out of the shower every 15 minutes, drying off, and leaving the bathroom before returning to the shower for the next 15-minute segment.

Often, patients will react to a compulsion so suddenly that they only become consciously aware of the process in the middle of or just after the behavior. Adding a consequence to the ritual, similar to Haley's ordeal therapy (1984), helps heighten awareness as patients approach future provocative situations. For example, those who perform checking rituals could commit to walking for 35 minutes after work on any day that they catch themselves "accidentally" checking the stove on their way out of the door in the morning. Other common assignments are picking up trash in the park for 30 minutes, placing a dollar in a "donation jar" for each repetition, or copying poetry by hand for 15 minutes. Most patients view such tasks as a game to win and not as "punishment." It is common for a patient to begin a session by smiling broadly and stating proudly, "I only had to walk once this week!"

## Summary and Conclusions

Cognitive-behavioral therapy has been shown to be the most effective current psychotherapy for the anxiety disorders. In this treatment mode, patients need to accept and tolerate distress in various doses, learning that their feared consequences either don't come true or can be tolerated. In this way, they develop self-efficacy, as well as habituation. However, the realities of clinical practice show that to increase their success rate, treatment protocols cannot be rigidly followed. Upon learning of the requirements of CBT, some patients refuse treatment and others drop out prematurely.

Ericksonian methods embellish common techniques of CBT, including reframing and paradoxical interventions, visual rehearsal, and the fractional approach. Just as important, Ericksonian strategies enhance CBT through a commitment to the utilization of patients' ongoing physical, emotional, and perceptual states. Gaining rapport, pacing interventions, generating therapeutic binds, and disrupting patterns not only enhance patient compliance with homework and reduce dropout, but increase the likelihood of interrupting patients' rigid patterns.

For many individuals, the anxiety disorders may surface periodically throughout the life cycle. Brief, specific directives emphasized throughout treatment, can become strategies for relapse prevention, helping to empower patients to maintain their gains over time.

---

**Primary Directives in Panic Disorder**

- Seek out and accept discomfort.
- Don't just do something, stand there.
- It's O.K. if this doesn't work.
- I want more symptoms now.

**Primary Directives in Obsessive-Compulsive Disorder**

- Act as though the content of the obsession is irrelevant.
- Accept the obsessions instead of resisting them.
- Seek out uncertainty.
- Seek out distress.

---

### References

Abramowitz, J. S. (1997). Effectiveness of psychological and pharmacological treatments for obsessive-compulsive disorder: A quantitative review. *Journal of Consulting and Clinical Psychology, 65*, 44–52.

Alon, N. (1985). An Ericksonian approach to the treatment of chronic posttraumatic stress disorder patients. In J. Zeig (Ed.), *Ericksonian psychotherapy, Vol. II: Clinical applications* (pp. 307–326). New York: Brunner/Mazel.

Aronson, E. R. (1987). Ericksonian utilization in shyness intervention with adolescents. In S. Lankton (Ed.), *Ericksonian monographs, no. 2: Central themes and principles of Ericksonian therapy* (pp. 96–118). New York: Brunner/Mazel.

Bandura, A. (1977). Self-efficacy: Toward a unifying theory of behavioral change. *Psychological Review, 84*, 191–215.

Beck, J. G., & Bourg, W. (1993). Obsessive-compulsive disorder in adults. In R. T. Ammerman & M. Hersen (Eds.), *Handbook of behavior therapy with children and adults: A developmental perspective* (pp. 167–185). Boston: Allyn & Bacon.

Clark, D. M. (1986). A cognitive approach to panic. *Behaviour Research and Treatment, 24*, 461–471.

Edgette, J. K. (1985). The utilization of Ericksonian principles of hypnotherapy with agoraphobics. In J. Zeig (Ed.), *Ericksonian psychotherapy, Vol. II: Clinical applications* (pp. 286–291). New York: Brunner/Mazel.

Emmelkamp, P. M. G., & Beens, H. (1991). Cognitive therapy with obsessive-compulsive disorder: A comparative evaluation. *Behavior Research and Therapy, 29,* 293–300.

Emmelkamp, P. M. G., Visser, S., & Hoekstra, R. J. (1988). Cognitive therapy vs. exposure in vivo in the treatment of obsessive-compulsives. *Cognitive Therapy and Research, 12,* 103–114.

Erickson, M. H. (1958). Naturalistic techniques of hypnosis: Utilization techniques. *American Journal of Clinical Hypnosis, 1,* 3–8.

Erickson, M. H. (1965). The use of symptoms as an integral part of therapy. *American Journal of Clinical Hypnosis, 8,* 57–65.

Erickson, M. H. (1980). Pseudo-orientation in time as a hypnotherapeutic procedure. In E. L. Rossi (Ed.), *The collected papers of Milton H. Erickson, M.D.: Vol. 4* (pp. 397–423). New York: Irvington.

Erickson, M. H. (1980). Utilization approaches to hypnotherapy. In E. L. Rossi (Ed.), *The collected papers of Milton H. Erickson, M.D.: Vol. 4* (pp. 147–234). New York: Irvington.

Erickson, M. H., Rossi, E. L., & Rossi, S. I. (1976). *Hypnotic realities: The induction of clinical hypnosis and forms of indirect suggestions.* New York: Wiley.

Feldman, J. (1988). A comparison of Ericksonian and cognitive therapies. In S. Lankton & J. Zeig (Eds.), *Ericksonian monographs, no. 4: Research, comparisons and medical applications of Ericksonian techniques* (pp. 57–73). New York: Brunner/Mazel.

Fisch, R., Weakland, J., & Segal, L. (1982). *Tactics of change.* San Francisco: Jossey-Bass.

Foa, E. B., Kozak, M. J., Steketee, G. S., & McCarthy, P. R. (1992). Treatment of depressive and obsessive-compulsive symptoms in OCD by imipramine and behaviour therapy. *British Journal of Clinical Psychology, 31,* 279–292.

Foa, E. B., & Wilson, R. R. (1991). *Stop obsessing!: How to overcome your obsessions and compulsions.* New York: Bantam Books.

Gordon, D., & Meyers-Anderson, M. (1981). *Phoenix: Therapeutic patterns of Milton H. Erickson.* Cupertino, CA: Meta Publications.

Grayson, J. B., Foa, E. B., & Steketee, G. (1982). Habituation during exposure treatment: Distraction versus attention-focusing. *Behavior Research and Therapy, 20,* 323–328.

Grinder, J., & Bandler, R. (1981). *TRANCE-formations: Neurolinguistic programming and the structure of hypnosis.* Moab, UT: Real People Press.

Haley, J. (1973). *Uncommon therapy: The psychiatric techniques of Milton H. Erickson, M.D.* New York: Norton.

Haley, J. (1984). *Ordeal therapy.* San Francisco: Jossey-Bass.

Hay Group (1998). Health care plan design and cost trends: 1988 through 1997. Prepared for the National Association of Psychiatric Health Systems, Association of Behavioral Group Practices, National Alliance for the Mentally Ill. New York.

Hoffart, A. (1993). Cognitive treatments of agoraphobia: A critical evaluation of theoretical basis and outcome evidence. *Journal of Anxiety Disorders, 7,* 75–91.

Hoogduin, C. A. L., & Duivenvoorden, H. J. (1988). A decision model in the treatment of obsessive-compulsive neuroses. *British Journal of Psychiatry, 152,* 516–521.

Kringlen, E. (1965). Obsessional neurotics: A long-term follow-up. *British Journal of Psychiatry, 111,* 709–722.

Marks, I. M. (1987). Fears, phobias, and rituals. In *Panic, anxiety, and their disorders.* New York: Oxford University Press.

Marks, I. M., Gelder, M. G., & Edwards, G. (1968). Hypnosis and desensitization for phobias: A controlled prospective trial. *British Journal of Psychiatry, 114,* 1263–1274.

O'Hanlon, W. H. (1987). *Taproots: Underlying principles of Milton Erickson's therapy and hypnosis.* New York: Norton.

O'Sullivan, G., & Marks, I. (1991). Follow-up studies of behavioral treatment of phobic and obsessive-compulsive neuroses. *Psychiatric Annals, 21,* 368–373.

Prior, M. (1991). Ericksonian hypnosis in the treatment of clients with examination panic. In S. Lankton, S. G. Gilligan, & J. Zeig (Eds.), *Ericksonian monographs, no. 8: Views on Ericksonian brief therapy, process and action* (pp. 95–105). New York: Brunner/Mazel.

Regier, D. A., & Robins, L. N. (1991). *The NIMH epidemiologic catchment area study.* New York: Free Press.

Rossi, E. L. (1980). *The collected papers of Milton H. Erickson, M.D., Vol. IV.* New York: Irvington.

Rossi, E. L. (1986). *The psychobiology of mind-body healing: New concepts of therapeutic hypnosis.* New York: Norton.

Rossi, E. L., Ryan, M. O., & Sharp, F. A. (1983). *Healing in hypnosis: The seminars, workshops, and lectures of Milton H. Erickson, Vol. I.* New York: Irvington.

Steketee, G. S., Foa, E. B., & Grayson, J. B. (1982). Recent advances in the treatment of obsessive-compulsives. *Archives of General Psychiatry, 39,* 1365–1371.

Van Oppen, P., de Haan, E., van Balkom, A. J. L. M., Spinhoven, P., Hoogduin, K., & van Dyck, R. (1995). Cognitive therapy and exposure in vivo in the treatment of obsessive-compulsive disorder. *Behaviour Research and Therapy, 33,* 379–390.

Watzlawick, P., Weakland, J., & Fisch, R. (1974). *Change: Principles of problem formation and problem resolution.* New York: Norton.

Wilson, R. R. (1985). Interspersal of hypnotic phenomena within ongoing treatment. In J. Zeig (Ed.), *Ericksonian psychotherapy, Vol. II: Clinical applications.* New York: Brunner/Mazel.

Wilson, R. R. (1996). *Don't panic: Taking control of anxiety attacks* (rev. ed.). New York: Harper/Perennial.

Wilson, R. R. (1999). Strategic treatment of obsessive-compulsive disorder. In *Current research and thinking in brief therapy: Solutions, strategies, narratives, vol. III.* New York: Taylor & Francis (in press).

Zeig, J. K. (1980). Symptom prescription and Ericksonian principles of hypnosis and psychotherapy. *American Journal of Clinical Hypnosis, 23*(1), 16–22.

## Suggested Readings

Barlow, D. H., & Cerny, J. A. (1988). *Psychological treatment of panic.* New York: Guilford.

Foa, E. B., & Wilson, R. R. (1991). *Stop obsessing!: How to overcome your obsessions and compulsions.* New York: Bantam Books.

Markway, B. G., Carmin, C. N., Pollard, C. A., & Flynn, T. (1992). *Dying of embarrassment: Help for social anxiety and phobias.* Oakland, CA: New Harbinger.

McNally, R. J. (1994). *Panic disorder: A critical analysis.* New York: Guilford.

Steketee, G. S. (1993). *Treatment of obsessive-compulsive disorder.* New York: Guilford.

Wilson, R. R. (1996). *Don't panic: Taking control of anxiety attacks* (rev. ed.). New York: Harper/Perennial.

Wilson, R. R. (1999). Strategic treatment of obsessive-compulsive disorder. In *Current research and thinking in brief therapy: Solutions, strategies, narratives, Vol. III.* New York: Taylor & Francis (in press).

# 15

# Strategic and Solution-Focused
# Treatment of Depression

*Lynn D. Johnson*

### ABSTRACT

*Depression is a response to a variety of social, psychological, and bio-logical stressors. Treatment is confounded by the fact that a significant number of patients drop out of therapy before resolution of the symptoms. Johnson and Miller (1994) have proposed solution-focused treatment as potentially speeding up response to treatment, which may reduce the failure rate. They proposed an integrative model, utilization formulations of Seligman (1990) and solution-focused interventions of De Shazer (1988) and Berg and Miller (1992). This chapter expands their model and gives an example of a successful brief treatment of depression in a suicidal patient. Relapse issues in the treatment of depression are also addressed.*

There is a story of a carnival operator who found that his customers were staying too long at a particular exhibit and so were clogging up the tent. He wasn't able to sell as many tickets as he wished because of the crowd. He created a sign and placed it over a one-way gate. The sign said, "This Way to the Egress." Of course, many people flocked to see the egress, another word for exit.

When therapists say a patient is "depressed," that label may obscure more than enlighten, and they may find themselves on the outside of the tent of therapeutic effectiveness. In other words, we are captives of our own words. Too often, therapists have been captivated by models of depression that suggest (1) depression is a unitary phenomenon, and the neat categories assigned by the various editions of the *Diagnostic and Statistical Manual of Mental Disorders* (*DSM*) are actual, true representations of literal states; therefore (2) all depressed patients must go through the same process, whether it is restoring putative chemical imbalances, learning to express anger, working through the oedipal neurosis, or correcting faulty thinking processes.

Paul Wachtel (1993) has perceptively pointed out how the concept of "countertransference" may obscure the impact of theory on the therapist. He says:

> The feelings evoked in us by the patient are a function not only of our personal history but of our set as we approach the patient and the therapeutic task. This set, in turn, depends on how we conceptualize the nature of psychological difficulties and the therapeutic process. Whether we experience the patient as manipulative, for example, depends as much on our theory as it does on more personal and idiosyncratic influences. For some therapists, the behavior that might be described as manipulative is understood instead as the patient's trying, imperfectly and largely self-defeatingly, to gain some measure of self-esteem in a life clogged with faulty assumptions about human interaction and consequent unpleasant experiences. Moreover, how manipulative, or resistant, or hostile, or inaccessible the patient feels to the therapist will depend as well on how competent and prepared the *therapist* feels. When one feels competent in the presence of a patient, when one feels one knows what to say and how to be therapeutically effective, the patient is likely to seem more likeable and is easier to empathize with whatever emotions he is manifesting.

As Miller (1993) has noted, the real value of solution-focused theory is not that it clearly improves patient response, but rather that it frees the therapist from theories that can do iatrogenic harm. The assumptions of solution-focused brief therapy (SFBT) of the possibility that a change in the viewing or doing of the problem could immediately resolve any problem leads the therapist to do less harm than does a theory that demands a long working through of repressed material.

Generally, it has been found that brief psychodynamic psychotherapy appears to be less effective than cognitive therapy in very brief therapy (1–12 visits) and equivalent to cognitive therapy in longer therapy of more than 12 sessions (Steenburger, 1994). It has been assumed that the psychodynamic therapists might be seeing more difficult patients and, therefore, need longer to accomplish something of value. In contrast to the position taken by Johnson (1995), there is now evidence (Shapiro, Rees, Barkham, et al., 1995) that with equivalent patients, psychodynamic therapy does not provide as much help in six sessions as does cognitive therapy. However, if patients remained in therapy for 12 sessions, the cognitive and psychodynamic therapies were equivalent. While these data support the notion of common factors being responsible for much of the effect of psychotherapy, they also provide a good argument for time X theory/technique. It would appear that in brief therapy, technique does make a difference. This same argument, that there are fine-grained differences attributable to technique/theory, has been made by others, from psychodynamic to solution-focused work.

The question of whether solution-focused technique actually makes a difference is a vital one, but beyond our scope here. We suspect the focus on immediate changes in perception and behavior makes a good deal of difference, especially in rate of change. In other words, we believe that solution-focused brief treatment may speed up the response to treatment, obviating the supposed advantage of medication, namely, that it works more quickly than does psychotherapy.

This finding has been most forcefully emphasized by the NIMH Collaborative Depression Treatment Research Program. As we have commented elsewhere (Johnson & Miller, 1994), there is a factor that has not been remarked upon by others, namely, that around one-third of the patients failed to complete a course of treatment for depression, and remained depressed and unresponsive to treatment. While more patients dropped out of medication management and placebo/clinical management conditions, even the interpersonal and cognitive therapy conditions had dropout problems.

It is likely that many therapists schooled in long-term treatment models view a patient as dropping out of therapy when, in fact, the patient has achieved what he or she wanted and is terminating, usually with positive feelings about the therapy experience (Pekarik & Wierzbicki, 1986; Talmon, 1990). We are not talking about that here; we are pointing out patients whose depression levels (as assessed by self-ratings via the Beck Depression Inventory or by therapists' ratings, using the Hamilton Depression Rating Scales) had not reduced.

We suspect there are two factors involved in this type of dropout from psychotherapy. First, the therapist may respond inappropriately to the patient, according to the Customer Status relationship. In other words, the depressed patient may be a complainant (or even, conceivably, a visitor, pushed into therapy by concerned family members), and the therapist assigns homework, violating the patient's implicit rules.

Second, the therapeutic process may contain some iatrogenic factors that actually make the patient feel, albeit temporarily, worse. For example, the patient is expected to be evaluated each session, along the lines of the questions necessary to complete the Hamilton. Such assessment procedures may reify the depression in the mind of the patient.

There are certainly other ways of explaining treatment dropouts. One such explanation might be the socialization process that most therapies require. The patient is expected to learn some new ways of thinking, which requires effort and practice. This effort and practice may seem either too difficult or perhaps unrelated to the patient's individual understanding of his or her situation. For example, if the patient feels he or she is depressed because of a biological factor out of his or her control, and if the therapist recommends a particular homework assignment, this implies that the depression is a result of a lack of that particular behavior, and thus not a biological process after all.

The advantage of SFBT is the tailoring of treatment to the mood, attributions, meanings, and behaviors of the patient. Instead of fitting the patient to a Procrustean bed of rigid theory, the therapist tries to match a wide variety of interventions with a specific patient.

However, the therapist must have a theory to guide and inform his or her behavior. It is impossible to intervene in a theory-free way, just as it is impossible to assess a person without simultaneously influencing that person. In this chapter, we assume that the reader is familiar with solution-focused theory and technique (Berg & Miller, 1992; De Shazer, 1988, 1991). At the same time, we believe that an understanding of Milton Erickson and his contributions will empower the brief-solution-focused therapist. And in the contrary case, where a therapist has learned solution-focused therapy without the foundational writings of Erickson, I argue that there is a significant gap in that therapist's understanding—a gap that may, in some very challenging cases, create a situation in which SFBT doesn't have the power to create change.

It may be useful, therefore, for therapists to have a map of possible cognitive schemata that contribute to depression. We do not mean to imply that we should use the schemata to educate the patient, but only to make the therapist's interventions rational and systematic.

The present chapter expands our thinking on the application of solution-focused work to depression. It discusses general protocols of treatment and possible limits to solution-focused treatment and the need for approaches beyond what is in the SFBT literature.

We were favorably impressed with a particular model of depression that seemed to fit well with our views. Such a model of depression emphasizing psychological or cognitive factors as proposed by Seligman (1990) reflects evidence that depression is primarily a reaction to stress, mediated by cognitive predisposing variables (cf. Metalsky & Joiner, 1992; Sweeney, Anderson, & Bailey, 1986). This *stress-diathesis* model posits that an individual's reaction to a stressful event results from whatever frame of reference the person adopts with regard to that event. According to Seligman (1990), there are three polar frames of reference an individual can assume with regard to a negative event: (1) the event is either permanent or temporary; (2) the event is either pervasive or proximal; and (3) the event is caused either personally or externally. Seligman argues that adopting the first choice in each of the three "frames of reference" is predictive of the development of depression, whereas adopting the latter predicts recovery from stressful events.

SFBT techniques appear to address serendipitously the three frames of reference identified by Seligman. In addition, SFBT appears to have the advantage of taking less time to achieve therapeutic impact. Research conducted at the Brief Family Therapy Center across a variety of diagnostic categories has found that with an average of 4.6 sessions, over 80% of clients rated themselves as recovered or as satisfied with therapy outcomes (De Shazer, 1991). Outcome data from the Brief Therapy Center in Salt Lake City are remarkably similar: 26% of patients attend one time; the average number of sessions is 4.1, and, again, patients feel satisfied with their resolution of their problems. The rest of this chapter describes the solution-focused interventions as they correspond with Seligman's three frames of reference.

## SFBT QUESTIONS AND THE SELIGMAN MODEL

Three types of questions in solution-focused therapy appear to address the three negative frames of reference identified by Seligman (1990) as underlying depression: (1) the exception questions, (2) the outcome questions, and (3) the coping and/or externalization questions (Berg & Miller, 1992; De Shazer, 1988; Walter & Peller, 1992). While other types of questions are used by SFBT therapists (such as the scaling questions), these will not be discussed here, so that the focus is kept on the correspondence between Seligman's model and SFBT practices.

### The Exception Questions

Exception questions inquire about times when the problem either was absent, was less intense, or was dealt with in a manner that was acceptable to the client. Calling attention to such times tends indirectly to reframe the meaning frames of depressed clients who have, according to Seligman's model, assumed that a negative or stressful event is *pervasive* rather than proximal. Examples of such questions include:

> "I have a good picture of what happens when there are problems (mention the specific symptoms here). Now, in order to get a more complete picture of your situation, I need to know about when the (specific symptom) does not happen."
>
> "When do you *not* have (symptom)?"
>
> "Tell me about the last time you did *not* have (symptom)?"
>
> "What is different about those times when (the problem does not happen, the problem is less of a problem, you deal with the problem in a way that is acceptable to you)?"
>
> "Tell me about the last time you thought you might have (symptom) and then didn't."

One special type of exception question that is especially relevant to reframing the pervasiveness meaning frame consists of an inquiry about pretreatment change. The pretreatment change exception question asks clients to describe what has changed or improved between the time the patient made the appointment for therapy and attended the first treatment session. For example:

> "Many clients notice that between the time they call for an appointment and their first session things already seem different. What have you noticed about your situation?"

The question can be modified for use during the intake process so that therapeutic intervention can begin even before face-to-face treatment contact. For example, during the intake and scheduling process, clients can be asked actively to look for evidence of pretreatment change while waiting for their scheduled appointment.

Howard, Kopta, Krause, and Orlinsky (1986) estimated that 15% of clients experience positive pretreatment change, but research conducted at the center where SFBT was developed found that as many as two-thirds (66%) of clients will report positive pretreatment change that is related to their goals for treatment, *if asked* about the change by the therapist (Weiner-Davis, De Shazer, & Gingerich, 1987).

Once any exception is identified, detailed information is sought regarding what was different about the time when the exception occurred, as well as how the client may have contributed to the problems being absent, less intense, or dealt with in an acceptable manner. This is accomplished by asking the clients who, what, where, when, and how with regard to the exception period. For example, clients are asked:

> "Who else noticed the time when the problem did not happen?"
> "What would (you/they) say was different about that time?"
> "When and how often did/does this happen?"
> "Where did this happen?"
> "How did this happen?"
> "What would (you/they) say you need to do to make this happen again (or more often)?"

Asking for detailed information serves to amplify and extend the discussion of exception episodes, thereby reframing the depressed client's belief that negative or stressful events are pervasive rather than proximal.

## The Outcome Questions

Outcome questions ask clients to describe what will be different when the problem that brought them to therapy has been successfully treated (Berg & Miller, 1992). By engaging the depressed client in a discussion of how life will be different after the problem is solved, the meaning frame that, according to Seligman's (1990) model, a negative or stressful event is *permanent* rather than temporary is reframed. The most typical form of the outcome question is called the "Miracle Question." Examples include:

> "Suppose tonight, after our session, you go home, go to bed, and fall asleep. While you are sleeping, a miracle happens and the miracle is that the problem that brought you here is *solved*. But because you are asleep you don't know that the miracle has happened. When you wake up tomorrow morning, what will be the first thing that you will notice that will be different that will tell you that the miracle has happened?"

> "Pretend for a moment that our work here together is successful. What will be different in your life that will tell you that treatment has been successful?"

> "What has to be minimally different in your life that will tell you that coming to treatment was a good idea?"

> "Imagine yourself, for a moment, six months or so in the future after you and I have worked together and successfully solved the problem that brings you here today. What will be different in your life six months from now that will tell you the problem has been solved?"

While clients are answering the outcome question, the therapist follows up with questions that shape the evolving description into small, specific, behavioral, positive, situational, interactional, interpersonal, and realistic terms. For example, clients are asked:

> "What will be the *smallest* sign that this is happening?"

> "What will be the *first* sign that this is happening?"

> "I am not quite sure what you mean when you say (happy, light-hearted, or any vague term the client may use to describe the desired outcome). How will others know you have those feelings?"

"If I had a video camera and followed you around when you (were feeling better, had solved this problem, etc.), what would we see you doing on the tape that would tell us that this problem had been solved?"

"When you are no longer (depressed, anxious, drinking, etc.), what will you be doing instead?"

"Where will you be when you first notice this happening?"

"Who will be the first to notice that this is happening?"

"What will be the first thing that others will notice different about you that will tell them this is happening?"

"What do you know about (your past, your self, your situation, others, etc.) that tells you that this could happen for you?"

The follow-up questions serve not only to amplify and extend the discussion of client goals, but also to make the goals more tangible for the client. This is evidenced by the frequent occurrence of clients' spontaneously mentioning exception periods while answering the outcome and related follow-up questions. Throughout the process, the depressed client's belief that negative or stressful events are permanent rather than temporary is further challenged and reframed.

### The Coping and/or Externalization Questions

The coping and/or externalization questions elicit discussion about how the client manages to cope with and endure his or her problem on a day-to-day basis. In the process of answering such questions, the problem becomes a separate and distinct entity *external* to the client (White & Epston, 1990). This, in turn, serves to reframe the meaning frame of depressed clients who, according to Seligman's (1990) model, assume that negative or stressful events are *personally* rather than externally caused. Examples of such questions include:

"This sounds like a very serious problem. How have you managed to cope?"

"Given how (depressed, anxious, etc.) you have been, how do you manage to keep going every day?"

"What have you been doing to fight off the urge to (let yourself be depressed, feel worse, commit suicide, etc.)?"

"How have (you, others) kept things from becoming even worse?"

"What are you doing to keep (anxiety, depression, etc.) from getting the best of you?"

"How did you (know, figure out) that would help?"

"How did you (know, figure out) that was the right thing for you
   to do?"

"If you hadn't been through this experience personally, would you
   have ever thought you had the strength to survive like you
   have?"

"Given how bad things have been, how come things aren't worse?"

Occasionally, in response to externalization/coping questions, clients
report that they engage in coping behaviors that are self-destructive in
nature (e.g., withdrawal, alcohol and drug abuse, self-mutilation). Consistent with Seligman's (1990) formulation, these clients frequently report
that *all* of their strategies are destructive. In other words, they view their
self-destructive coping strategies as pervasive rather than proximal. In
keeping with the SFBT model, questions are posed that focus on the *effect*
that the client achieves from the self-destructive strategy rather than on
the particulars of the strategy. For example, clients would be asked,
"How does it help you when you (withdraw, drink, self-mutilate, etc.)?"
Once the desired effect is described in detail, the treatment professional
return to exception questions to explore for other periods when the client
experienced the same effect *without* having engaged in the self-destructive
coping strategy. For example, the client would be asked, "Tell me about
other times in your life when you (client description of effect) but don't
(self-destructive strategy). What is different about those times?" As previously described, a discussion of exception periods serves to reframe the
depressed client's belief that his or her self-destructive coping strategies are
pervasive rather than proximal.

## CASE EXAMPLE

The following transcript illustrates these principles. This patient was reported to have had a gun in his mouth, threatening suicide the day before
this interview. He called his EAP, who stabilized him over the telephone.
The gun was removed from the house, and he refused offers of inpatient
treatment. He made a no-suicide agreement and the EAP counselor referred him to the author. The patient wears a black leather jacket and

heavy boots, is tattooed with "biker" motifs, has a full beard, and wears sunglasses indoors and outside. His presession Beck Depression Scale raw score was 42.

T:  I talked with you yesterday on the phone. You've been feeling pretty suicidal, but you are still alive.

C:  Yeah.

T:  You said yesterday that things that keep you going are your family, especially your grandchildren ...

C:  That's pretty much it, I don't know what else there would be.

T:  You love your grandchildren a lot.

C:  Very much.

T:  You also said on the phone you have had a lot of anger, depression, and hopelessness for quite a long time. I guess that proves you are a survivor, because somehow you have come through it.

C:  I got to thinking about my obligations, and that keeps me from doing things that I think about a lot.

T:  So you are a person who takes his duty seriously. You don't blow it off.

C:  To my family. Most of the obligations I take seriously. I try not to blow off anything. I get so frustrated because life never works out the way it should. I just plan on the worst possible thing that could happen, and that's what happens.

T:  Nothing works out the way it should, that really gets to you. And I also appreciate the fact that you take things seriously and don't blow stuff off. That shows character, I think. What we do with what happens to us is more important than what happens to us.

C:  Most people would say I don't have any character at all. I am a real quiet person. Once somebody does say something, I clam right up. And sometimes I say the wrong thing. All my life sucks.

T:  Your life does suck now. If it were a little less bad, what would you see that makes you think that life is getting a little better?

C:  Oh! Ah, I don't know. I would have less stomach trouble, that's for sure. Less violence, less anger.

T:  (*Writing*) Less stomach trouble, less violence, less anger. I am impressed that you put those together; when I am angry about things, my stomach hurts, too.

C:     I've had ulcers for years, missed a lot of work because of it. When my stomach acts up, I can't do nothing . . . I hate to have that happen.

T:     That would be a good area to start on, less anger. How is the anger a problem for you?

C:     I get angry a lot, at most every . . . people. Like me and my wife. Oh, she can really get me hotheaded. She expects me to roll over and play dead or sit up and beg like a dog! Don't ever show any emotion at all, like, be a robot! That really gets me mad.

T:     If you do show emotion?

C:     I get ridiculed, all the time. If I stay mad or even talk loud, she snaps back at me and says, "What's your problem?" And she'll shake her head and walk away.

T:     You must love her a lot to stay with her. A lot of men would walk away.

C:     I do love her, but she does get to me.

T:     A lot of people these days, the minute the relationship gets rough, they are out of there, they have no staying power. You have real character to stick out the hard times.

C:     She gets me so wound up that I want to knock her out.

T:     Do you ever hit her?

C:     I almost killed her once when we were first married. Since then I never touch her.

T:     Since then you never touch her, no matter what?

C:     Uh-huh. Even though I want to real bad. I will not do it because I am afraid of what I would do.

T:     Earlier you said something I don't understand. You said some people say you don't have character. But here you recognized it was a bad thing to hit your wife, and you don't do it, even though you want to. There's character there.

C:     That's the way I was raised.

T:     Loyalty. You learned a good rule when you were young, and you are loyal to it. Well, she is not here and you are. Are you willing to work hard to get over your anger? Even if she doesn't change?

C:     Oh, absolutely. I just didn't want her here today because I didn't want her here in the room while you were asking me questions. She could come some other time. I gotta work hard, so I can get my grandkids back.

T:      Who has them now?

C:      The state.

T:      How did that come about?

C:      (Client gives a lengthy explanation of how he was threatening sui-
        cide and his grandchildren were in the room, and the episode was
        reported. His grandchildren have lived with him and their moth-
        er, who is his daughter, all their lives.)

T:      So you are really willing to work damn hard here. Sounds good.
        So what is the first sign the state social workers will see that you
        are getting the help you need?

C:      I made an appointment with you.

T:      Great, you are already on a good path. What's next? What else
        will they be looking for from you?

C:      A home visit, I guess.

T:      What will they see that will tell them you are getting free of this
        anger problem?

C:      I wouldn't be so willing to snap back. I just go in my room a lot,
        and spend a lot of time in my room.

T:      How does that help, to spend time in your room?

C:      I just have to get away, so I don't do something stupid.

T:      So how does that help you, to get away?

C:      I don't know, I just can't stand to be around people when I get
        like that, like it is too much ...

T:      Does it help the family, when you get away into your room?

C:      Not really, because sometimes they bug me about coming out.

T:      If they see you brooding in your room, that worries them?

C:      I'm not doing anything to hurt anybody.

T:      If I think like a social worker on a home visit, and I hear a guy
        goes into his room and broods, I might think he is in there load-
        ing his gun.

C:      I don't have any weapons any more.

T:      How would the social worker think? I am not sure getting away
        from it is the best way to handle that.

C:      I'll have to answer their questions the best I can.

T:      If I am too pushy, you push back. I like it when you push back.
        I have a weakness, I get an idea and push for it, and it might not
        be right for you, so you push back.

C:      You are going good so far.

T:     I don't like this idea of your going to your room because it looks too much like brooding and sulking to people. If we can help you work out ways to do something else, would that help convince the social worker?

C:     I have no idea because I have no idea what my daughter has told them. They took her word for everything, and never asked me nothing, which seems awfully strange to me. I would never ever hurt those kids.

T:     I hear that powerful loyalty.

C:     My daughter is extremely hotheaded; if I ask her something, she blows up in my face, and I do it right back to her, and all the kids hear is yelling. And they are violent, because that is all they hear. And my daughter never controls them because my wife is there to do it for her. And after I get wound up ...

T:     So you are one of many hotheads in this family.

C:     It is passed down from generation to generation.

T:     This is not an easy problem to solve.

C:     I don't know if there is any way to solve it.

T:     Of course, you can. But if you do that, there is the danger they will feel bad about their temper. It may embarrass them to lose control when you don't. You are a pretty loyal guy, maybe you should go very slow on that so as to protect them. But just clarify for me. If they get mad and get in your face, and you stay calm, and even if they don't, if you are to change and feel calmness, would that be what you want from me?

C:     Yeah, but there is never an end, there's not an end to it. The only end is something I don't want to do. But if I was dead, I would be better off.

T:     Well, we don't know if you would or not. But as you pointed out, you want to help the grandchildren, and while it would possibly get you out of a bad situation ... we don't know ... the disadvantage is it would be a horrible blow to the grandchildren.

C:     Yes, that's right.

T:     So we are going to work on helping you to handle angry situations in a calm way.

C:     Yeah ...

T:     So let's imagine a miracle happens tonight after you leave my office, and while you are asleep, something happens, and when you wake up, you have become able to handle angry situations. Your daughter can say obnoxious things to you, your wife can say irritating things to you, and you listen to them. You don't blow up, you don't run to your room and hide; you don't blow up. Who is the first person who is going to notice that a miracle has happened?

C:  I am just thinking of my grandkids, the way they were yanked away.

T:  That was a horrible shock.

C:  The whole family says it is me.

T:  You are to blame, it's all on your head. You stay and tolerate it, you don't take the "easy" way out, and you get blamed because they are gone. Who is blaming you?

C:  My wife's side of the family. They say that's not the way to raise kids. I can't help the way I feel sometimes, so I go into my room so I don't do something I might regret. I know I shouldn't have done what I done. But they shouldn't have yanked them away like that.

T:  You know you shouldn't have been flashing guns around and talking about blowing your head off. But it was a spiteful thing to yank them away. Does you wife agree?

C:  She agrees with me. They are our kids, practically. And to have them yanked away.

T:  There's a lot of deep feeling there.

C:  I know I look like a hard-core person ...

T:  Yeah, you have all that Harley stuff, but you are really a more emotional guy than you look. You are really a very caring person.

C:  I have this image, being a biker and all that.

T:  It's image. (*Laughter.*)

C:  I carry that to work with me, and I snap back at everybody else. I need something to vent my frustrations. I've got holes in my walls and in my doors from punching them, so I don't hit someone.

T:  Yeah. What percent of your life do you think the anger controls?

C:  Oh, 75%.

T:  I hear you. Big piece. Tough deal, isn't it, to reclaim that much of your life. So what about the 25%? What about the moments that anger is not in charge of you?

C:  Oh ... I guess when I am by myself. It is strange ... I am going to be interrogated as soon as I get home, about being here so long. Was I really with you? She thinks I would be with a girl-friend, which I don't have. And have to account for every minute of every day or I must have been with a woman.

T:     And?

C:     Then she rants and raves and throws a fit. She sees secret messages on pieces of paper that doesn't have any writing on them. She sees things on my clothes; she's obsessed with thinking I have a girlfriend, and if I don't dash right home when I leave here, I must have been with a woman. And knowing that, when I get home, I am going to get interrogated, I can't handle that. And I am not doing anything wrong.

T:     This is good, this is a good situation you are in, because it seems to me you have a lifelong history of being hot tempered, even be-fore you married your wife, I would bet.

C:     Oh, yeah, she knew I was a hothead.

T:     So you have always been a hothead. If you were in some monas-tery where everyone treated you kindly, and you didn't have any temper problems, it wouldn't be much of an achievement. But if you can learn to control your temper in a situation like the one you have with your wife, you have really achieved something. If you say to me you are going to work hard, and really bust your butt to get the 75% of your life back, if you tell me, "Anger has jacked me around long enough, anger has made me its puppet. An-ger has controlled me, and I am going to fight to get my life back."

So if you work hard week by week to get your life back, even if your wife is still weird about your having a girlfriend, and you are less and less upset, if you kept that up, what would your fami-ly notice?

C:     I guess my Sheetrock wouldn't have holes in it. But the situation wouldn't change.

T:     You would change, even if they didn't; would that change the situation?

C:     I don't know. I don't think so.

T:     Well, there is a danger here, that if you work hard on throwing anger out of your life, and they don't work hard at anything, they are getting a free ride from you. And they are going to pick up on some of your changes and benefit without having to go through the hard work you are going through. They would benefit.

C: Why should I do all the work?

T: Good question, why should you?

C: It don't seem right. My wife don't do diddly-squat. I provide for her, I make the money, and I get ridiculed when I get home. I am not the one who should be here! (*Laughs.*)

T: I am not questioning that. I agree. But who is here?

C: Yeah.

T: Poor old Gordon. Got picked on again! (*Laughter.*)

C: Yeah, feeling sorry for myself. Seems like nobody else will, so I might as well.

T: That's wonderful.

C: I spend too much time thinking about it.

T: Yeah, you brood.

C: Mope around. A lot of people have told me that.

T: So I take this pen, which is a magic wand, and (*touches Gordon*) touch you and you go home, and tonight, during the night, your fairy godmother comes, and says, "Gordon, you've been a good boy, and I'm gonna give you a prize; you are peaceful, like a monk, even though you are living with crazy people." But if you can live with crazy people and not get angry, you have become strong.

Now that miracle happens in the middle of the night and tomorrow morning you wake up and you don't even remember the fairy godmother's visiting you. You get up, and you have been healed of anger. Your wife is still obsessed; your daughter comes around, and she is still a volcano; but you are healed. So what will those people notice about you that makes them think, "Gordon's different"?

C: They would think I was on drugs or something.

T: They might. What are they going to see that makes them think that?

C: I don't know. If I get this depression fixed, then I am an alky, or I am a drug addict, and I don't do either one. And that surprises people, like, "Oh, you're a biker, you have to do that." But I don't do that.

T: You must enjoy giving people that surprise. Now back to my question. I know you don't know the answer.

C:     My mind wanders and wanders and pretty soon I don't even remember the question you asked. (*Laughter.*)

T:     Well, let's struggle with it a bit. So here is this miracle that happens, and you feel peaceful, good, never felt this way. You wake up tomorrow morning, you start going about your business, but it is like this angry wound, this red open sore, is healed. Anger can't control you any more; the hurt is gone. You are a strong man now; people can touch you where the wound was, and it doesn't hurt. You are calm.

So what are they going to see that makes them think this miracle has happened?

C:     I would be more talkative, smile, which I never do.

T:     Let me write these down: be more talkative, smile, which I never do. You may have to practice. What else?

C:     I don't know, my reactions? The way I talk to her?

T:     Tell me about that.

C:     Talk in a more passive manner, instead of being apt to jump right back at them.

T:     So let's say you talk in a more peaceful manner. You talk more, but you are just peaceful. How will that help?

C:     It will help me up here (*points to head*). Because right now, I am scrambled. As long as I know I am OK, the rest of the world can have their problems.

T:     Help unscramble your thinking.

C:     I can't do anything to cure it; it is beyond my control.

T:     OK. I am going to take a brief break and then I'll return and we'll talk about this hard work you are going to do.

[*brief break*]

T:     OK, here is what I want you to do. First, you need to recognize that you are a person of deep love and commitment; you are a very caring and responsible person who wants to do the right thing, no matter how hard it is. You really love your grandkids, and you really love your wife, even when the going gets rough, you hang in there.

Because you have to do something to get your grandkids back in your home, I want you to carefully notice times when you are more peaceful and calm, when you smile, and when you talk, when you talk in a more talkative manner. It may only be 25% of the time, or even 15%.

You don't use alcohol or drugs, but you are addicted to anger. But I have never met an addict yet who didn't have some sober times, and just didn't give in to the alcohol or drugs. And the alcoholic only needs to be sober for one day. So I want you to notice carefully when you are free of anger. When you are smiling, talkative, and living in a peaceful manner. And it may only be once in a while, but tell me about that.

Now do you want me to write that down?

C:       Yeah, write it down.


In the second session, Gordon reported that there were times he felt angry, but he would go out to his shed and work on a go-cart engine for a friend's son, and the angry feeling would go away. He had not gone into his room to brood but had walked around the house looking for chores to do. He was instructed to keep up the good work. The social worker is convinced that he is no longer a danger and the grandchildren are back in the home.

At the third session, he brought his wife, and some marriage counseling addressed her jealousy. I asked about times when they didn't argue and what seemed to be different about those times. I suggested that when she was in a bad or upset mood, her brain was unlikely to be able to solve problems, so it might be better if she waited until she felt calmer before accusing him of being unfaithful. I asked her how she recovered from the bad feelings when she saw evidence that she thought meant he was unfaithful. She didn't have a method, so I suggested that when the feeling of suspiciousness tried to control her, she pay close attention to what she could do if she didn't give in to that temptation.

At the fourth session, he was feeling considerably better. He said that his wife was only slightly better about her suspicions, but they didn't seem to bother him so much. His Beck Depression Inventory Score was 17. I suggested that he continue until the Beck was lower, but he disagreed, saying he felt better than he had for years, and that was good enough.

## CONCLUSION

The use of solution-focused approaches to therapy will do less damage than will other therapeutic styles. A careful reading of the transcript will show several examples of the "one-down" position, of reframing, and of other "strategic" techniques. Yet, what did they contribute? The real turning point in the session seems to be when we began to think together about the outcomes Gordon would like to see, the answers to the Miracle Question.

Thus, it may be that strategic therapy empowered this client. But in retrospect, in examining my own transcript, I am left with the conclusion that a respectful attending to his goals, and ignoring the needs and desires of other people *for* Gordon, may be what helped us get on track and do some good.

Constructivist approaches to therapy are often criticized as ignoring values or as seeming to support the idea that all ideas are equal. My own experience with this was that strategic therapists are not value-free. I was supervised for three years by John Weakland, and when I posed such questions as Gordon's suicidality ("Is suicide an acceptable goal?"), John would shrug and remind me that the first rule of therapy is "CYA!— cover your assets."

So when Gordon talked of suicide as a potential outcome, I simply discussed the pros and cons in a fairly (apparently) evenhanded way. Yet my own desire to manipulate Gordon comes through in the transcript, when I use his position of love for his grandkids as leverage to bankrupt the idea of suicide:

C:     Yeah, but there is never an end, there's not an end to it. The only end is something I don't want to do. But if I was dead, I would be better off.

T:     Well, we don't know if you would or not. But as you pointed out, you want to help the grandchildren, and while it would possibly get you out of a bad situation ... we don't know ... the disadvantage is it would be a horrible blow to the grandchildren.

Strategic therapy borrows from Erickson the focus on determining the patient's position and using that therapeutically. In the present case, I tried to do that by enlisting Gordon to rebel against anger, suggesting that anger had "jacked him around" for a long time and was having its way with him. In subsequent sessions, this theme continued, with my asking whether anger had been able to screw around with his head or whether he had been able to outsmart anger. This is not particularly a "solution-focused" technique, but one that apparently was helpful in Gordon's case.

A student I was supervising once commented to me that I really seemed to believe in solution-focused therapy. I responded with an emphatic "No!" I do not believe in it, but I find it helpful and low in risk. With Gordon, it seems to me that Ericksonian skills of reframing, of using his position to promote positive change, were of some help.

I often find in doing supervision that students today are enthusiastic about learning about solution-focused therapy but are fairly ignorant of its foundation in Milton Erickson's understandings and concepts. There is a difference between an artist and a technician, and there is a difference between a counselor who uses rote scripts to promote change and the therapist who senses a variety of challenges and responds quickly to them. After many years, I am beginning to be that kind of therapist, responding flexibly and quickly to a variety of challenges.

### References

Berg, I. K., & Miller, S. D. (1992). *Working with the problem drinker.* New York: Norton.

De Shazer, S. (1988). *Clues: Investigating solutions in brief therapy.* New York: Norton.

De Shazer, S. (1991). *Putting difference to work.* New York: Norton.

Elkin, I., Shea, M. T., Watkins, J. T., Imber, S. D., Sotsky, S. M., Collins, J. F., Glass, D. R., Pilkonis, P. A., Leber, W. R., Docherty, J. P., Fiester, S. J., & Parloff, M. B. (1989). National Institute of Mental Health treatment of depression collaborative research program: General effectiveness of treatments. *Archives of General Psychiatry, 46,* 971–982.

Howard, K. I., Kopta, S. M., Krause, M. S., & Orlinsky, D. E. (1986). The dose-effect relationship in psychotherapy. *American Psychologist 41,* 159–164.

Johnson, L. D. (1995). *Psychotherapy in the age of accountability.* New York: Norton.

Johnson, L. D., & Miller, S. D. (1994). Modification of depression risk factors: A solution-focused approach. *Psychotherapy, 31,* 244–253.

Metalsky, G. I., & Joiner, T. E., Jr. (1992). Vulnerability to depressive symptomatology: A prospective test of the diathesis-stress and causal mediation components of the hopelessness theory of depression. *Journal of Personality and Social Psychology, 63,* 667–675.

Miller, S. D. (1994). The solution conspiracy. *Journal of Systemic Therapies, 13,* 16–37.

Pekarik, G., & Wierzbicki, M. (1986). The relationship between clients' expected and actual treatment duration. *Psychotherapy, 23,* 532–534.

Seligman, M. (1990). *Learned optimism.* New York: Knopf.

Shapiro, D. A., Rees, A., Barkham, M., Hardy, G., Reynolds, S., & Startup, M. (1995). Effects of treatment duration and severity of depression on the maintenance of gains after cognitive-behavioral and psychodynamic-interpersonal psychotherapy. *Journal of Consulting and Clinical Psychology, 63,* 378–387.

Steenburger, B. N. (1994). Duration and outcome in psychotherapy: An integrative review. *Professional Psychology: Research and Practice, 50,* 111–119.

Sweeney, P., Anderson, K., & Bailey, S. (1986). Attributional style in depression: A meta-analytic review. *Journal of Personality and Social Psychology, 50,* 974–991.

Talmon, M. (1990). *Single-session therapy: Maximizing the effect of the first (and often only) therapeutic encounter.* San Francisco: Jossey-Bass.

Wachtel, P. L. (1993). *Therapeutic communication: Principles and effective practice.* New York: Guilford.

Walter, J. L., & Peller, J. E. (1992). *Becoming solution focused in brief therapy.* New York: Brunner/Mazel.

Weiner-Davis, M., De Shazer, S., & Gingerich, W. J. (1987). Building on pretreatment change to construct the therapeutic solution: An exploratory study. *Journal of Marital and Family Therapy, 14*(4), 359–363.

White, M., & Epston, D. (1990). *Narrative means to therapeutic ends.* New York: Norton.

# 16

# Ericksonian Approaches to
# Pain Management

*Jeffrey K. Zeig & Brent B. Geary*

P ain management is a process of setting the patient on a train of activity that modifies the experience of pain as the patient carries it out. The job of the Ericksonian hypnotherapist is to create a series of constructive associations that will work in one of three directions: distraction, dissociation, or the alteration of sensation.

Milton Erickson added immensely to the literature on hypnotic pain control. The corpus of his work can be found in the *Collected Papers of Milton H. Erickson, M.D.* (Erickson, 1980a), edited by Ernest Rossi. The reader who is interested in additional information can go directly to the source.

## ASSUMPTIONS

Volumes have been written on pain management. But space allows only a cogent summary of hypnotic approaches that can be incorporated into treatments for pain. Several important areas will receive only brief attention; the authors encourage readers to study these topics further. This chapter assumes that the psychotherapist is working closely with the physicians attending the patient. Medical interventions should not be undertaken by nonmedical professionals. Family members often can—and should—be included in pain-management processes. Hypnosis should be integrated with other psychosocial methods to enhance their benefit to the patient. In sum, the treatment of pain should be comprehensive. Hypnosis affords great promise for a variety of patients and sources of pain. The following should be considered in a broad context, however, with ethics, collegiality, and other issues constantly borne in mind.

### The Assessment of Pain

Pain is a multifaceted experience. It must be properly assessed in order for it to be treated effectively. In the traditional diagnosis of pain, clinicians often focus on the organic causes and carefully gather information prior to providing treatment. In an Ericksonian assessment, the evaluative procedures in and of themselves effect pain control. In the process of evaluation, the therapist sets in motion a process of complementary assessment and intervention. There are five areas of assessment that are especially meaningful. An additional area, aspects of pain, will be covered as a separate category.

#### What Does the Pain Mean to the Patient?

The clinician can initially focus on subjective aspects of the pain. To discover what the pain means to the patient, the therapist needs to know whether the pain is a threatening pain, like angina; the intractable pain of cancer; or spasms of pain such as those experienced during labor. The therapist must understand whether the pain will be the patient's constant companion or will eventually recede.

As the therapist queries the patient about meanings of the pain, there might be evidence of pain relief, especially in the case of pain that is immediately experienced in the consulting room. As the therapist asks about the meaning of the pain, it subtly encourages the patient to "dissociate" from the actually experienced pain. Again, there are three primary hypnotic techniques for working with pain: dissociation, distraction, and alteration. These three principles should be kept in mind during the entire assessment procedure, because they often emerge as naturalistic examples of ways in which patients cope with discomfort.

#### Detailed Description

By procuring a detailed description of the pain, the therapist can effect experiential division in the gestalt of pain, thereby modifying the experience. This process builds on the "Farrah Fawcett principle."

A number of years ago, I (JKZ) worked at the Arizona State Hospital.

One day, while having lunch, other staff members and I mused over the cover of *People* magazine that displayed Farrah Fawcett, wearing a rather revealing bikini. One member of the staff looked at her ankles and commented that they were too fat. Another staff member pointed out that her calves were out of proportion to her thighs. Others opined that her waist was too small, her bust was not right, her neck was too long, her smile was crooked. By the time we had finished lunch, she no longer looked attractive.

The "Farrah Fawcett principle" illustrates that if you examine anything closely enough, it tends to lose its integrity. The clinician can use this principle by asking the patient about his or her pain in detail, even bordering on the absurd. For example, a therapist could ask about the size of the pain, the shape of the pain, the texture of the pain, the thickness of the pain, the duration of the pain, the weight of the pain, and so on. This microanalysis of the pain can effect both a desired division and a dissociation that can be utilized in treatment.

### Analogies

The use of analogies further helps the patient to distract and dissociate from pain. The therapist might ask simple analogical questions such as: "What is the pain like?" "What does the pain remind you of?" Analogies allow the patient to change the category of thinking about the experience of pain. The therapist can, moreover, prod analogies by asking the patient about dimensions of the pain. If the pain were a color, what color would it be? If the pain were a plant, what kind of a plant would it be? If the pain were a tool, what kind of a tool would it be? If the pain were a vessel to contain water, what kind of a vessel would it be? If the pain were a song, what kind of song would it be?

The use of analogies allows additional options for metaphorical interventions. For example, if the patient indicated, during trance, that the pain was like a tune, the therapist could change the tone and tempo. Such metaphoric interventions can directly affect the intensity of symptomatic experience.

### Expectations and Motivation

The patient's expectation of treatment needs to be thoroughly understood. Many patients seeking hypnosis have unrealistic expectations of what can be accomplished. For example, we have encountered patients who have had serious organic impairments, such as strokes, who believed that hypnosis can be used to restore prestroke functioning. Others hope that the hypnosis will take away all of their suffering. As understandable as they might be, unrealistic expectations must be clarified.

Patient motivation, a factor in all treatment situations, is especially important in pain control. Pain patients often have conflicting motivations. They suffer, but sometimes, owing to legal or disability issues, they must maintain the limitations imposed by pain. This predicament can defeat any gains that treatment might offer. The job of the therapist is to utilize the patient's expectations and motivation to the maximum extent possible. The therapist can incorporate positive expectations and motivations into the backbone of the treatment plan.

## Key Words

We have found it beneficial to take note of special words, phrases, and metaphors that patients use to describe pain. For example, if a patient describes pain as being "pressure," one might create an induction by reframing the concept of pressure. The patient can be instructed to attend to the "pressure" of his or her hand on his or her lap, noticing the variations in the experience of "pressure." Subsequently, that pressure can be modified, for example, through hand levitation. In such cases, the therapist works parallel to the symptom process. The idea of changing symptom words into solution words has been described by Zeig (1988).

### ASPECTS OF PAIN

Another assessment device involves understanding the aspects of pain.

## Learned Aspects

Again, pain is complex. It does not merely exist as sensation; some pain is learned. For example, dogs reared in isolation seem to experience pain differently from the way dogs reared in more normal surroundings do. Similarly, athletes who learn to ignore pain experience it differently from those who lack such training do.

## Cultural Aspects

People from different cultures differ in their report and expression of pain. For example, more phlegmatic individuals of northern European heritage often report less pain to the same amount of stimulation than do the more dramatic southern Europeans. The influence of modeling can be telling in the manner in which a patient presents pain. Those raised in expressive families may learn to amplify pain for attention. A stoic presentation is common among patients who grew up in quiet and contained households. Inquiring about family background often yields valuable information.

### Temporal Aspects

Some pain is composed of experienced pain, remembered pain, and anticipated pain. This is especially true for contractions of pain, in which there is a period of quiescence between spasms. Erickson reminded clinicians that if they could help the patient to feel only the experienced pain and to eliminate the remembered and anticipated pain, they could significantly change the amount of suffering.

### Pain and Suffering

Hilgard and Hilgard (1983) stressed that pain consists of both physical sensations and emotional suffering. They used two 10-point scales, asking patients to indicate the amount of pain and the amount of suffering. Most patients can readily distinguish between pain and the suffering that the pain causes. For example, a patient might rate the level of pain at four but the extent of suffering at eight. By demarcating pain and suffering, the therapist begins a process of dividing and conquering.

### Other Splits

We have used other splits in addition to that of pain and suffering in order to help patients. For example, we have asked patients to divide pain into harmful and harmless pain and needed and unneeded pain. Some pain is like an alarm. It serves a productive function, but, once the alarm goes off, the patient no longer needs the warning.

### Contextual and Relational Aspects

The context in which a sensation is experienced alters the way in which that sensation is interpreted. For example, Erickson reminded students that a woman seeing her husband off to war might say: "Squeeze me so hard you will break my ribs, kiss me so hard you will make me bleed, I want to remember that hug, I want to remember that kiss."

However, the most gentle touch of a rapist can cause searing, even indelible, pain.

By focusing on the aspects of pain, the therapist can realize a vital tenet for this type of work: pain *is* malleable. Pain is not a thing, it is a process. By thinking about the aspects of pain, the therapist absorbs an understanding that pain *can* be changed.

## PRINCIPLES OF WORKING WITH PAIN

There are five principles that we keep in mind that are important in the hypnotherapy of pain patients.

1. *You do not need an all-comprehensive trance.* In fact, all-comprehensive trances are usually unnecessary in therapy. A light trance may be enough to modify pain. Also, selective trances may be used; the patient does not need to have complete relaxation. Partial relaxation may be enough.

2. *Set the patient on a train of activity that modifies the experience of pain as the patient carries it out.* As the patient becomes experientially involved in patterns of behavior, thought, and action, the experience of pain decidedly changes.

3. *Patients have resources that make pain control possible.* The job of the therapist is to create an appeal to the experiential learnings and associations that exist inside the patient. We all have the experience of going to a movie with a tension headache and suddenly noticing that the headache has lessened or disappeared. Erickson reminded patients that they could go to a lecture hall and listen to an interesting lecture and not even realize the discomfort of the seat. On other occasions, they might sit in the same lecture hall listening to a boring lecture and experience considerable discomfort in the same chair.

4. *Pain is a process, not a thing.* The therapist must have faith in the patient's ability to modify experience. Often the patient thinks of a symptom as a static object, for example, "Here is *my* pain." Accepting the patient's definition might con the therapist. Rather, thinking about pain as a process might benefit both therapist and patient because processes can be modified, whereas it can be more difficult to modify things.

5.   *Reinforcement is often indicated.* It is rare to hit a "hypnotic home run" and in one fell swoop clear away a patient's pain or the misery that accompanies it. Instead, we have found that repeated hypnotic experiences are crucial in enlivening helpful associations, experiential learnings, memories, insights, and the other variables that are instrumental in pain management. It many cases, it is beneficial to provide patients with an audiotape of hypnotic sessions conducted in the therapist's office. This allows the patient to continue to experience the trance state and to derive benefits from it. Also, the therapist is thereby working with a more experienced subject who is versed in hypnotic potentials as tangible gains.

## TECHNIQUES

There are a number of techniques that are used both traditionally and by Ericksonian practitioners. We will describe seven of them.

### Glove Anesthesia

In traditional hypnosis, the therapist may suggest the experience of anesthesia in the hand. This method is called glove anesthesia. Subsequently, through arm levitation, the hand can be moved to other parts of the body where the anesthesia can be transferred into painful areas, thereby providing helpful sensations in the affected sites.

### Hypnotic Phenomena

In a classic paper, Erickson (1980b) posited that all hypnotic phenomena can be harnessed to modify pain. The essential part of the method is to discover which hypnotic phenomenon the patient can best elicit. For example, if the patient is good at dissociation, the patient can dissociate away from the pain. If the patient is good at amnesia, the patient can forget the pain. If the patient can effectively achieve hypermnesia, the patient can vividly remember a time that was more comfortable. If the patient is good at age regression, the patient can regress to bodily awareness in a time before the pain. If the patient is good at time distortion, the patient can increase the times of comfort and decrease the times of pain. Patients will provide clues regarding avenues to explore by the manner in which they talk about their pain, their goals for pain management, and methods they employ naturalistically to control discomfort.

*Displacement*

In a number of cases, Erickson worked to move pain. For example, he moved pain in one limb to another limb. This technique seems rather spectacular. Actually, displacement is a common human phenomenon. For instance, one can have a worry in mind that causes an acid stomach. Erickson liked to say that if a patient can have phantom pain, the patient can have phantom pleasure. In the same way, if a patient can displace negatively, he or she can displace positively.

*Modification*

The therapist can utilize particular strengths or associations of the patient. For example, if the patient is a musician, perhaps the pain could change in tempo. A woodworker might chisel a sharp pain into a duller pain. A student can learn something from the pain.

*Confusion*

Kay Thompson (1982) used word plays and ambiguities to help patients with pain. For example, she discussed the way in which pain can be experienced as a window. The window serves to keep unwanted elements outside, but still allows light and warmth inside. From the inside, one can look through the "pain" and experience the comfort on the other side of the pain. When one sees through the "pain," another perspective is available.

*Interspersal*

The interspersal technique is utilized to deliver messages on the social and psychological levels simultaneously. In a classic case, Erickson (1966) discussed the growth of a tomato plant on the social level, while, on the psychological level, he interspersed suggestions for pain control. The patient, Joe, was unresponsive to medical pain treatment. Erickson reminded him, "Joe, you are a florist and I am going to talk to you about tomato plants, but that is not what you really want to hear." Erickson continued by saying, "For example, you can imagine, Joe, how the little seed can, Joe, *rest in the bed*, and then there are the rains that can bring, Joe, *peace and comfort*." The purpose of the interspersal technique is not made obvious. Rather, the technique serves to "awaken" experiential learnings that were dormant. The therapist works to build a context in which unconscious processes are elicited indirectly.

*Amplification and Deviation*

Patients often present for therapy believing that they have no ability
to control pain. Sometimes the therapist can work to increase the experience of pain rather than diminish it. If patients are able to control experience by intensifying pain, then they might be able to decrease it.

## AN ERICKSON CASE EXAMPLE

Erickson was a credible clinician for pain patients because he was not
speaking hypothetically or hypocritically when he talked about pain control. Erickson himself was intimately familiar with the experience of pain.
When pain patients came to see him, they saw a man who was in constant chronic pain. However, Erickson's pain did not seem to substantially impair his enjoyment of life. In fact, he had ways of reframing his
own pain. He used to say, "I don't mind the pain. What I don't like is
the alternative." To Erickson, there was no acceptable alternative to pain;
as long as he had pain, he was alive.

The following case example of Erickson's (1980c) approach elucidates
some of the principles previously mentioned.

Erickson made a house call to a cancer patient. Kathy was at home because that is where she wished to do her dying. When Erickson came into
the room, she was lying on one side, in a fetal position, chanting, "Don't
hurt, don't scare me; don't hurt, don't scare me; don't hurt, don't scare
me; don't hurt, don't scare me." Rather than introduce himself in a more
traditional way, Erickson intervened by chanting with the patient, "I'm
going to hurt you, I'm going to scare you; I'm going to hurt you, I'm go-
ing to scare you; I'm going to hurt you, I'm going to scare you; I'm going
to hurt you, I'm going to scare you." Kathy asked, "Why?" Erickson
continued chanting, "I want to help you, I want to help you, but I'll scare
you, I'll scare you." Subsequently, he asked Kathy to "turn over mentally, not physically." He asked her to become absorbed in that activity.
Kathy replied by saying, "I think that I am on my left side."

This was an ingenious technique of distraction: rather than trying to
absorb the patient in relaxation, Erickson made a slight modification. He
absorbed the patient in the *memory* of a painful action. It was dissociated
from present *experience*. Erickson then said, "Kathy, I want you to feel a
mosquito bite on the sole of your right foot, biting, biting, it hurts, it
itches." Kathy tried to call up the experience that Erickson suggested, but

was unable to do so. She replied, "I am sorry, my foot is numb, I can't feel that mosquito bite." Utilizing that response, Erickson suggested that the numbness would spread throughout Kathy's entire body, except to where the surgical wound from the breast removal was located. "That place where the surgery was done will feel like a very bad, itchy, mosquito bite," he concluded.

Erickson utilized the patient's response, but left an area of pain. The purpose of this, Erickson explained, was recognition that patients sometimes have unacceptable feelings that they want to take out on themselves. Rather than modify all of the pain, he left one area of suffering. Erickson reported that Kathy was able to make a more satisfactory adjustment. She stopped her chanting and was able to better enjoy the rest of her days.

## CONCLUSIONS

Pain control is very much a matter of faith. There are three kinds of faith. First, the therapist must have faith in his or her own ability adequately to utilize the experiences that patients bring to the endeavor. Second, the therapist has to have faith in the ability of the patient. The therapist must realize that patients have within them resources that make pain control possible. Third, there must be faith that hypnosis, the relationship between the therapist and patient, can be successful in some way. This "article of faith" (i.e., the present chapter) has discussed some of the ways that pain can be modified and managed with hypnosis. Armed with faith—as well as knowledge, hope, experience, and other vital ingredients—the therapist and patient together can board that train of activity that modifies the experience of pain.

### References

Erickson, M. H. (1966). The interspersal hypnotic technique for symptom correction and pain control. *American Journal of Clinical Hypnosis, 8,* 198–209.

Erickson, M. H. (1980a). *The collected papers of Milton H. Erickson on hypnosis, Vols. I–IV,* E. L. Rossi (Ed.). New York: Irvington.

Erickson, M. H. (1980b). An introduction to the study and application of hypnosis for pain control. In E. L. Rossi (Ed.), *The collected papers of Milton H. Erickson on hypnosis, Vol. IV* (pp. 237–245). New York: Irvington.

Erickson, M. H. (1980c). *A teaching seminar with Milton H. Erickson*, J. K. Zeig (Ed.). New York: Brunner/Mazel.

Hilgard, E. R., & Hilgard, J. (1983). *Hypnosis in the relief of pain* (rev. ed.). Los Altos, CA: William Kaufman.

Thompson, K. (1982). The curiosity of Milton H. Erickson, M. D. In J. K. Zeig (Ed.), *Ericksonian approaches to hypnosis and psychotherapy* (pp. 413–421). New York: Brunner/Mazel.

Zeig, J. K. (1988). An Ericksonian phenomenological approach to therapeutic hypnotic induction and sympton utilization. In J. K. Zeig & S. R. Lankton (Eds.), *Developing Ericksonian therapy*. New York: Brunner/Mazel.

# 17

# A Warrior's Approach in Dealing with Chronic Illness

*Sandra M. Sylvester*
*(With a Contribution by Robert Nakashima)*

## OVERVIEW

WarriorHeart is a nonprofit organization that works with the chronically ill to help them reawaken a sense of purpose and well-being in their lives. At this time, WarriorHeart's work is focused on helping individuals who have multiple sclerosis (MS) to achieve maximum use of their bodies and minds through a program of neurological restructuring based on the work of Milton H. Erickson, M.D., and the ancient tai chi discipline of the martial arts.

## INTRODUCTION

In many instances, chronic illness (arthritis, cancer, diabetes, autoimmune diseases, neuromuscular diseases, chronic pain, etc.) takes the sufferer on a journey through successive stages. These stages may succeed each other rapidly or they may take years. At first, its onset may be so gradual that the illness is unnoticed or unrecognized for a time. To give one example: in the case of a neuromuscular disease, a fairly active woman may notice that she is lagging behind while hiking with friends, whereas, in the past, she would set the pace. She may notice that her hiking boots seem to be getting scuffed at the toes so that they begin to look much older than they are. Or that her feet seem to get numb after a short period of standing or walking; and wearing wider shoes does not seem to help. She may notice that she habitually sits down to dress or leans against a wall for balance. She finds that simple household tasks, like changing an overhead light bulb, have become something she dreads because being on a ladder and reaching causes her to lose her balance. She may make excuses about being clumsy as she spills things or breaks glasses or dishes more frequently. She may notice that her lifestyle is beginning to change, that she is not driving at night anymore, that she avoids being out when traffic is heavy because she has a feeling that her reaction time is not as quick or precise as it once was. She is plagued by fatigue and poor mental focus. Psychologically, she is losing her self-confidence. She begins to resist taking on additional responsibilities. Soon, she breaks through the denial and realizes that something is wrong.

Because her balance is impaired, this neurologically affected person begins to curtail her activities, becoming more sedentary and isolated. In time, with diminished movement, muscle atrophy occurs followed by stiffness and pain. This can result in a downward spiral of gradual and progressive mental and physical deterioration. Changing the direction of this downward spiral is imperative.

Many people who are chronically ill become experts on their illness by researching, reading, and consulting with others through word-of-mouth contacts. They try many or all of the traditional treatments, and alternative treatments as well. Eventually, the person with a chronic illness decides that it is time to get on with life, to make the best of a difficult situation. For some, this process of dealing with life's inevitable difficulties becomes an opportunity for growth, and the illness, even though unwelcome, is viewed as one of one's most precious teachers. This is the focus of the WarriorHeart program.

## THE EVOLUTION OF WARRIORHEART

The WarriorHeart program evolved through the collaboration of Robert Nakashima, a martial arts instructor, and the author, Sandra Sylvester, Ph.D., a psychologist trained by Milton Erickson in the power of the mind to effect physical and psychological changes. WarriorHeart began as a response to a request from the National Multiple Sclerosis Society to teach tai chi to people in wheelchairs. Through the process of teaching individuals with MS, the concept of WarriorHeart developed.

Now, three years later, WarriorHeart is a nonprofit organization whose purpose is to lift people with chronic illness out of their passive resignation to a level of feeling, being, and acting from which the uncertainties of the future can be faced with tranquillity, hope, and courage. At the present time, we are working exclusively with those with neurological impairments, although, as we grow, our program will expand to include persons with many chronic illnesses.

WarriorHeart is an interdisciplinary program coordinating meditation, stretching, range of motion, purposeful movement, and tai chi chuan. The program has been adapted and specialized to reach those whose mobility is impaired or who are in pain. A WarriorHeart student adheres to a code of honor, responsibility, and compassion while embracing the rigors of the program of daily meditation, exercise, and tai chi. This process is very demanding, requiring personal effort and commitment.

## THE WARRIOR IN WARRIORHEART

In facing a chronic illness, one of the first casualties is the loss of the sense of self. Thus, dealing successfully with a chronic illness involves redefining the sense of self, not by *what I can do* but by *who I am*. To be engaged in a daily battle with chronic illness is to take on the mantle of the warrior.

WarriorHeart opens the warrior path of self-mastery and greater fulfillment to those with chronic illness. Through mastering such skills as synchronizing mind and body, facing the world with openness and fearlessness, and finding the sacred dimension in everyday life, individuals learn to radiate goodness into the world. They acquire the sense of self-worth that comes from espousing the basic task of the warrior: to find a good and meaningful life that will also serve others.

Although chronic illness may compromise a student's physical ability, it does not in any way compromise the character of the student. Each component of the program is designed to help students realize the depth of their potential to enhance their quality of life, in spite of illness or disability. In fact, WarriorHeart students, although they may be recipients of social services, become empowered to help themselves.

The core of WarriorHeart is a blend of the philosophy and techniques of Milton Erickson with the ancient philosophy and techniques of the Chinese martial arts system of tai chi, both of which are grounded in the inseparability and inner connectedness of the mind and body working together seamlessly and fluidly. Both systems involve physical awareness and observation, and both systems rely on mental images to unlock hidden meanings and life lessons embodied in the daily experiences of unpredictability and change that come with facing a chronic illness.

WarriorHeart teaches that in facing life with a chronic illness, especially a progressive illness with no known treatment or cure, one is on a journey alone, facing unknown challenges. There will be times when anyone who is on this journey will want to quit because the obstacles are too great. Continuing the journey in spite of the difficulties creates within the individual a hero-warrior.

Erickson learned this as a teenager when he battled polio and taught himself how to stimulate movement and sensation in paralyzed limbs by inventing exercises using the everyday tools and landscapes of the yard and fields of his family's farm. He was realistic and pragmatic. He changed his plan to become a surgeon, which would have required long hours on his feet, and chose to become a psychiatrist, which allowed him to pursue his love of and fascination with the richness and complexity of the human mind and spirit. He learned the importance of his own daily practice to be able to maintain focused attention, economy of movement, and commitment to completing a task, no matter how long it took, with an intensity as if his life depended on it.

Based on the essence of Erickson's process of rehabilitation, we stimulate movement and sensation in individuals with MS by using classroom mirrors to augment impaired proprioception. In this way, students can utilize visual feedback to correct movements and body alignment. In time, with mindful repetition, movements that were once ataxic and spastic become fluid, graceful, and smooth.

We invent exercises using everyday activities, such as getting up from a chair, or standing at the sink to brush one's teeth, or turning over in bed, as opportunities to focus inward to a felt sense of physical grounding and balance. In these daily activities, students learn to move so that every part of the body participates in the action, with all parts working together. Our students learn how to stand with their weight balanced side to side, front to back, suspended from the ceiling, while grounded in the earth through various mental images that aid the nervous system.

Applying themselves to these and other exercises with a focused intensity—"as if your life depended on it"—day after day, whether they want to or not, is a commitment that demands the heart of a warrior. The repetition of the exercises helps establish new neurological pathways through a process known as neurological restructuring so that the body is better able to move in necessary and useful ways.

In teaching his residents and students, Erickson emphasized the importance of observing the patient. This process of keen observation was a lifelong practice, being of particular advantage to him as he gradually regained the use of his limbs and fine motor coordination after becoming a victim of polio at the age of 17. He was aided in his review and remembering of weight transfer by watching his toddler sister learn to walk. He experimented with his own body, relearning muscle function through observation and muscle memory.

In teaching neurologically impaired students how to coordinate movements, we model and demonstrate weight shift and movements involving all parts of the body working in synchrony. Thus, the students, after careful observation, imitation, and repetition, and after executing the movements in unison at a slow rhythm, are able to improve their balance, coordination, and sensitivity.

Erickson used natural images and concepts to teach life lessons: the constantly changing and interconnected life cycles of the seasons, plants, and animals; the relationships of the earth, the moon, and the stars. He drew on nature and natural development for examples in explaining complex psychophysiological relationships in very simple and easy-to-understand terms.

Often examples, stories, and visualizations help to capture the essence of an event by engaging the feelings, emotions, and past personal experiences, as well as the intellect. By using examples, stories, and visualizations, we can reframe an experience and uncover a hidden depth and meaning that greatly enriches it. As our most important example of reframing, WarriorHeart teaches that any person facing life with a chronic illness is called upon to take a hero's journey.

The common element of such journeys is that an ordinary person is called upon to do a very difficult task, a task that has great consequences for himself or herself. He or she travels alone, on an uncharted path, into unknown danger, where the forest is darkest. The person has no one to show the way, but only the purity of his or her intention and singleness of purpose as an internal guide. The process of persevering on the journey in spite of exhaustion, hunger, danger, and fear, forges the character of this person until a hero emerges. The process of continuing to walk one step after another in pursuit of the goal, rather than quit, creates the hero.

When chronic illness is approached as a hero's journey, tremendous empowerment ensues.

A second example of reframing can be found in the following story that encapsulates the essence of dealing with MS. An oyster attached to a cliff by the sea opened and closed its shell to feed by filtering nutrients out of the seawater. One day, the sea was unusually turbulent, and as the oyster was feeding, a grain of sand got caught under its very soft and delicate body. The sand had sharp and jagged edges. It felt very uncomfortable to the oyster. So the oyster did what all oysters would do in a similar situation, it tried to get the sand out. It tried every way it knew to dislodge that grain of sand. Finally, after many attempts to get rid of the sand, the oyster decided to learn everything it could about the grain of sand. It began to feel the shape of the sand, learn which edges were sharp, move the sand grain around to try to find a more comfortable position. As the oyster explored and examined the grain of sand, it left a very thin coating of its own mucus on the sand's surface. Day after day, the oyster moved this grain of sand around, continuously coating it with very thin layers of mucus. After many days and months, the oyster began to notice that the grain of sand did not hurt any more. After a much longer time, the grain of sand, which was once an irritant, became a pearl.

Such bursts of insight and empowerment are among the peak experiences of life. The way to reach them, however, is slow, methodical, daily practice: with noticing and respecting the smallest details of life, the natural ebb and flow of breathing, the rhythm of one season flowing seamlessly into the next, the warmth that comes when tension gives way to relaxation as we practice the WarriorHeart program; meditation, stretching, purposeful movement, and tai chi.

## THE WARRIORHEART PROGRAM

### Meditation

Meditation, which focuses the mind on breathing while grounding, aligning, and stilling the body, supports the flow of energy from the universe through the meditator. Students learn, in both sitting and standing meditation, the mental and physical relaxation that automatically reduces stress and balances the nervous system and brain. Meditation has become a standard prescribed treatment for cardiac care and cancer; it is the foundation of the WarriorHeart program. The concentrated mental focus of meditation is used during all of the other, following activities as well.

### Stretching

In an attitude of quiet concentration, WarriorHeart students learn about the flexibility, strength, and range of motion of their own bodies. They learn techniques to teach the weaker parts of their bodies to imitate the stronger parts. By stretching, students learn to separate MS from muscle atrophy. They can do something directly about the atrophy and indirectly about what is related to MS. Through practice, they can see and feel improvement in a matter of weeks. Our students report diminishment or abolition of pain, lessening of the frequency and severity of muscle spasms, and greater independence.

### Purposeful Movement

By aligning the body, centering the weight, and concentrating on rooting into the earth, students are gradually able to transfer their weight from one foot to the other while maintaining balance and relaxation throughout every moment. Changes and improvement in balance occur slowly, as new neurological pathways are developed through the process of neurological restructuring. It may take weeks and months of continued practice before changes are appreciated. Our students report falling less frequently and regaining balance more rapidly.

### Tai Chi Chuan[1]

Tai chi is an ancient Chinese system of health maintenance and self-defense that employs a series of slow relaxing movements in coordination with breathing, postural integration, and mental imagery.

On a purely physical level, the expressed goal of the tai chi practitioner is to gain a heightened sense of spatial awareness, and kinesthetic perception, or "body feel," as well as an all-around increase in strength, balance, and general well-being. The body gradually learns, through disci-

---

[1] By Robert Nakashima.

plined application of the principles of tai chi movements, to move with maximum efficiency and economy. For those with limited amounts of energy and stamina, this alone can have profound implications. For one, the conscious control of the body's energy system can mean a remarkable increase in the quality and meaning of a life lived in the shadow of a chronic, debilitating illness. Tai chi practice necessitates the absolute mindfulness of the body–mind relationship. In progressive stages, the modified tai chi forms taught by WarriorHeart lead the practitioner to new levels of insight and empowerment over physical being. For those whose illnesses have left them with a sense of alienation from their bodies, this is perhaps tai chi's greatest gift—a sense of reacquaintance with the best parts of themselves.

On emotional and spiritual levels, the practice of tai chi by those with chronic illnesses has produced equally encouraging effects, not the least of which is the fostering of a supportive spiritual community among those who have committed themselves to the tai chi principles. Tai chi is fundamentally a *relational* activity, although it can be practiced anywhere, at any time, alone or with groups. The student must build relationships to the teacher, to the other students, to his or her own sense of himself or herself, and, finally, to the universe. One of the most honored traditions in the martial arts community is the powerful, almost sacred relationship that binds teacher to student and the students with each other. Over the centuries, this set of relationships has been shown to accelerate learning, to help ward off the boredom and depression that invariably accompany any difficult journey, and to enrich whatever lifestyle one has chosen.

Ultimately, tai chi constitutes a wholesome discipline that systematically addresses areas that no other single modality of therapy or treatment can claim. An ancient sage once observed, "Walk with the disease, keep company with it, for that is the way to be rid of it." The implicit lesson of tai chi practice is that *there is no opponent.* The "enemy" (i.e., the disease), therefore, must be blended with and redirected, rather than fought to an exhausting stalemate. The martial arts contain a wonderful metaphor for resolving conflict by *dissolving* it. Tai chi, above all, stresses the virtue of yielding and neutralization rather than head-on confrontation. In this way, the person suffering from a chronic illness can learn to apply these timeless principles to the most difficult issues of day-to-day living.

## CONCLUSION

The WarriorHeart program seeks to reawaken the sense of purpose or reason for being that often gets clouded in people affected by MS or other chronic illnesses. Based on the work of Milton Erickson, and the principles of tai chi, WarriorHeart students are taught techniques that allow them to form a different relationship with their bodies. As a result, they often demonstrate more fluidity and grace in their movements, an overall calmness that comes from getting their minds and bodies to work together, and an acceptance that MS is simply a part of their lives, something with which they will deal as each moment unfolds.

The principles of building energy, causing energy to flow, and rebuilding the patterns in the nervous system are illusive. To make these illusive principles tangible, WarriorHeart uses pictures, or mind scenes, to reframe problems and engage the body/mind/spirit in concentrated focused attention. These mind scenes, together with the physical techniques provided by the various components of the WarriorHeart program, afford a context for establishing new neurological memories and pathways in WarriorHeart students.

# 18

# Ericksonian Approaches to
# Psychosomatic Conditions

*Harriet E. Hollander*

Psychosomatic illness refers to chronic conditions with identifiable physiological pathology in which anxiety, stress, beliefs, and expections play a significant role in precipitating symptoms or influencing their severity. Although psychosomatic conditions require medical diagnosis and treatment, they frequently improve with nonmedical interventions, such as psychotherapy, including hypnosis.

Among the psychosomatic conditions that involve both physiological and psychological factors are asthma, arthritis, fibromyalgia, migraine, and irritable bowel syndrome. Ulcers, once considered a psychosomatic disorder, are now understood to be the result of heliobacter invasion and require antibiotics. However, as one gastroenterologist observed when referring a patient for hypnosis, "Stress increases stomach acidity in this client, reddening and inflaming the gut, leaving him vulnerable to heliobacter infection. I have noted ulcer flare-ups in him in the absence of heliobacter bacteria." Ulcers, for some individuals, constitute a mind–body illness requiring both medical and nonmedical approaches.

Psychosomatic illnesses are diagnostically distinct from conversion reactions. Psychological factors play a significant, although unconscious, role in conversion reactions, but physiological pathology is absent. There is a gray area in which clearly psychological events or maladaptive habits lead to physical pathology. Bruxism in adults in an example, causing tooth breakage, temperomandibular jaw pain, or headache.

In children, chronic gagging following a single traumatic event in which there was choking during the intake of solid food may result in a phobic fear of food and of vomiting in a public place, such as at school. Food refusal attributable to a fear of gagging may be accompanied by complaints of nausea, stomach upset, and constipation due to altered food habits, with a long-term risk of irritable bowel syndrome.

## ERICKSON'S CONTRIBUTIONS TO THE TREATMENT OF PSYCHOSOMATIC ILLNESS

Among Erickson's most notable contributions are those concerning the treatment of mind–body illnesses, with a focus on the pain and anxiety associated with these conditions. Although his treatment was individualized for each patient according to the problem presented, Erickson held certain basic assumptions about the treatment of pain and psychosomatic illness.

Erickson (1985b) did not believe that there was much point in telling someone who was sick or in pain that the hurt was in some way "unreal," since contradicting the reality of suffering would make no sense to the patient. He accepted organic pathophysiology as "real," while directing his therapy to the person's reaction to the illness.

Erickson engaged the patient in utilizing personal resources for therapy and hypnosis. Personal resources were defined as the wealth of past experience and mastery, as well as hypnotic ability. He emphasized the importance of utilizing the subject's contribution in every possible way, firmly believing that hypnosis belongs to the subject and is not an illustration of a therapist's power.

Rapport in hypnosis, Erickson wrote (1985d), "exists well beyond the relationship between the subject and hypnotist." Rapport exists in relation to the patient's goal and self processes in the therapy situation. The effectiveness of treatment, particularly with such complex conditions as psychosomatic illness, will depend less on what therapists plan or intend than on their willingness to enable the patient's personality to play a significant role in achieveing a therapeutic goal.

## ADDRESSING BELIEFS AND EXPECTATIONS

Erickson (1985a) was perfectly willing to provide direct instruction to clients, in or out of trance, about the nature of the unconscious. For example, to alleviate pain, which is often facilitated by trance deepening, Erickson might explain, as a client experimented with different levels of hypnotic awareness, the reality of unconscious experience. He would tell clients that the unconscious mind deals with ideas and memories and understandings. These ideas, memories, and understandings are facts. They are "concrete." As an example, he would suggest that patients could have their "unconscious" develop a state of numbness even if they held the *belief* that such a condition could not exist. He would address their uncertain *expectations* of hypnosis by suggesting that they didn't need to "manacle" their unconscious processes in the name of reality. He would reframe negative beliefs and expectations by suggesting, "Your unconscious can be as creative as it needs to be" (1985d), while also advising (and further discharging negative beliefs and expectations) that you can't dictate to your unconscious (1985b).

## ERICKSON'S APPROACH TO PAIN

Pain can be dealt with by anesthesia, analgesia, or distraction. Distraction involves a shift, not necessarily in hypnosis, from awareness of pain to memory of comfort (Erickson, 1985a). Erickson (1985d) recognized that clients already knew that they could manipulate their body responses without having a hypnotic experience. He pointed out that clients came to him who were able to inhibit the knee-jerk response, increase blood flow in one hand and decrease it in the other, raise and lower blood pressure, or dilate the pupil of only one eye without going into hypnosis. He advised therapists that in order to carry out a hypnotic intervention, they needed to know what was possible physiologically, what the client could achieve physiologically, and what the client wanted to accomplish.

### Treatment of Symptoms

Erickson (1985e) strongly held that hypnotic interventions are about altering and transforming pain and altering and transforming symptoms, not about getting rid of them. People report pain imagery. A headache can be splitting, a gut can feel as though it were burning. A client can visually or kinesthetically displace the splitting sensations of the headache to a different part of the head or to a different place in the body. The burning sensation in the gut can be altered so that the level of burning heat diminishes to a strong warmth.

## Utilization of Client Resources

Erickson (1985f) saw hypnosis as an opportunity to elicit and then utilize a broad range of response possibilities in the client. His creative hypnotic suggestions were probes into these response potentials. They included providing clients with the experience of autohypnosis, in which the client would hypnotize an imaginary "friend," producing a hand levitation (1985b). Clients learned trance deepening, with its beneficial reduction of pain awareness through relaxation, arithmetic progression, hand levitation, trance without awareness, willingness to wait in hypnosis for symptom change, ideomotor responses, posthypnotic suggestion, and hypnotic amnesia (1985b).

## Post-Erickson Approaches

Ericksonian approaches to healing continue their evolution. Rossi (1996) employs ideomotor hand levitation or hand opening and closure to put clients in touch with their own self-healing experiences. Clients discover that their hands levitate or open or close when they are ready to utilize their own resources in healing. Hands return to rest when adequate understanding or resolution of the psychological aspects of the psychosomatic condition has been attained.

More recently, Lankton (1998) demonstrated how one can suggest to clients who *believe* that their real physical pain cannot be diminished because it has a physiological basis that they can relieve their *anxiety* about *expecting* to be burdened with a chronic condition. He shows how a wide and encompassing utilization of multiple Ericksonian approaches and hypnotic phenomena can bring about a distinctive and client-verifiable reduction in pain level.

## PRINCIPLES OF TREATMENT

The following key Ericksonian approaches were utilized in the case examples cited.

1. To gain *rapport*, establish your full acceptance of the seriousness and reality of the physical "body" illness. Then explore the client's view of the mind–body connection by listening to how the client assesses the contributing role of stress and anxiety.

2. As you listen and watch, assess the client's beliefs, expectations, and typical pattern of description of the illness in order to *utilize* them in the healing intervention.

3. *Induce* trance by explaining hypnosis and the role of the unconscious, as an *induction* to a hypnotic experience.

4. *Suggest* hypnotic phenomena—anesthesia, analgesia, distraction, displacement, hand levitation—that the client can *utilize* during problem exploration and for deepening.

5. Give the client time to *rest and consolidate* the hypnotic experience. Provide *posthypnotic* suggestions that make use of self-awareness and autonomy.

## Case Examples

### Karen: Accepting Client's Choice of Goals

Karen, age 14, was first brought to treatment in the aftermath of a choking episode that left her so traumatized that she even feared to drink the prescribed fortified liquids that would prevent her from becoming malnourished. She complained of a feeling that there was an obstruction in her windpipe. This sensation, globus hystericus, is diagnosed as a conversion reaction and has no physiological basis.

Karen had seen, over a 10-week period, a behaviorist, a child analyst, and several medical specialists. The physicians were concerned when she began to complain of nausea, constipation, painful stools, and stomach pain, resulting in a further reduction in her food intake. Karen recognized that her anxiety prevented her from eating. However, she believed the obstruction in her throat to be a reality.

The therapist acknowledged the reality of the experience of "globus hystericus." Karen was told that hypnosis would help her reduce her fear of the obstruction by enabling her to numb it. She could then bypass the obstruction, and eventually it would shrink. Hypnotherapy over several sessions was utilized to reduce the globus hystericus, which made it possible for her to "nibble" during the session. However, she was unable to eat at home, which is consistent with the resistance typical of conversion reaction.

The therapist became aware that Karen needed to master her trauma through "self-help," or through experiences that reflected an internal locus of control. She was, therefore, informed that she had been given the best of available treatments. Now, the therapist suggested, it was up to her to cure her problem by watching videotapes of herself in hypnotic trance. She had to be "willing to wait" to alter her symptoms on her own timetable. The girl seemed pleased with this therapeutic suggestion and diligently watched her tapes, without parental prompting, until, after two and a half weeks, her normal eating behavior was restored. She remarked that she "just had to do it herself." The more physiologically based symptoms of constipation and stomach pain went into remission.

Like many adult clients, this teenager experienced a common paradox of treatment. She saw her symptom as "non-self." The therapist was asked "to just treat my symptom" as if it were outside her "self," so she could get on with her life. She resisted the therapeutic help she wanted as a threat to the integrity of her wish for self-mastery, which was restored as she paced her own learning experience in hypnosis.

### Matthew: Psychosomatic Treatment of Irritable Bowel Syndrome

Matthew, a highly functioning executive in his early 50s, had lost a battle to retain control of his manufacturing company. He received a substantial financial severance package but was unemployed and so had to reduce his standard of living. His wife, by a second marriage, had expected more and began to criticize his entrepreneurial ability, his parenting skills with their new baby, and his sexual functioning. After several years of unemployment, he became ill and was diagnosed with irritable bowel syndrome. Despite medical treatment, together with cognitive and then psychodynamic therapy, his condition worsened, and he sought hypnotic help.

Addressing Beliefs and Expectations

As the first session began, Matthew informed the therapist that any suggestions to relax invariably made him extremely tense. He was only able to sustain a willingness to "do nothing," his idea of relaxation, when he treated himself to a shave and had to wait with hot towels on his face during a skin treatment. He also relaxed while he waited on the massage table for the masseuse to enter or when instructed to rest at the end of the massage. He feared that his worsening condition would require surgery.

As his therapist, I told Matthew that his case was indeed challenging, and that traditional hypnosis would not work because the experience would be contrary to his habitual patterns. However, I assured him that an appropriate, highly individualized hypnotic intervention could be formulated that would result in symptom relief.

In the first session, because he wanted hypnosis, I suggested that he resurrect those images that led to "doing nothing," or his so-called relaxation. As he initiated a trance on his own, I remarked that I would make a tape of the session that he could use to practice an approximation of hypnosis for stress reduction. Continuing to address him conversationally, while pacing his breathing, I encouraged him to take charge of his hypnotic experience. He could imagine in hypnosis how he would respond to criticism if he could react as he wished. Or he could let himself concentrate on his own version of "doing nothing" and rehearse that.

While he was in trance, I informed him that some gastroenterologists considered surgery a poor choice of treatment for irritable bowel syndrome. During hypnosis, I had him identify gaseous distress and experiment with its *displacement*. He was given a posthypnotic suggestion to notice in the future what situations were connected with pain relief.

Utilizing Client Resources

At the next session, Matthew reported noticeable improvement in his comfort level. He informed me that he had begun to recognize how he reacted to the stress of his marital situation. He became anxious and tense and his symptoms intensified. Interestingly, I observed that he became more relaxed, particularly in the abdominal region, as his indignation rose.

To make use of this observation, I invited him to continue describing his reaction more fully. I asked him to hold a biofeedback card registering changes in skin temperature as he spoke so that he could ratify the calming effect on his gut of venting his anger.

He began to describe his abuse at home, but appeared to be in a light hypnotic state, although his eyes were open. At my suggestion, he looked briefly at the card and observed that, despite his external agitation, the card registered a change indicating greater calm. He continued speaking of his abuse with eyes closed in a deepened hypnotic state. He was then able to rest, retrieving his previous image of "doing nothing" with considerable ease. He was given a posthypnotic suggestion to make good sense of his hypnotic experience and to act on his learning.

Over the next several sessions, the client concluded that he could use hypnosis during the sessions to access his thoughts and feelings. He learned, to his surprise, that for him the overt expression of anger brought inner calm, and he began to confront his stresses at home. He now believed that his condition would improve, and he experienced a reduction in pain symptoms.

## SUMMARY AND CONCLUSION

Psychosomatic illnesses involve belief, expectations, anxiety, and stress that affect physiological pathology. The use of hypnotic interventions to address these psychological factors often results in attendant changes in pain and the remission of symptoms. The client's personality and goals become a full part of the therapist's intervention, undertaken with the cooperation of the client, who creatively carries out the hypnotic work.

---

**The Erickson Approach**

- Validate physiological symptoms.
- Identify and utilize beliefs, expectations, fears, stresses, and pain descriptions.
- Induce hypnosis by explaining it.
- Suggest hypnotic phenomena that match the client's abilities as a multilevel intervention leading to symptom alteration.
- Give posthypnotic suggestions for self-awareness and autonomous activity.

---

### References

Erickson, M. H. (1985a). An introduction to the study and application of hypnosis in pain control. In E. L. Rossi & M. O. Ryan (Eds.), *Mind–body communication in hypnosis: Healing in hypnosis* (pp. 217–279). New York: Irvington.

Erickson, M. H. (1985b). Utilizing natural life experience for creative problem solving. In E. L. Rossi & M. O. Ryan (Eds.), *Mind–body communication in hypnosis: Life reframing in hypnosis* (pp. 1–133). New York: Irvington.

Erickson, M. H. (1985c). Reframing problems into constructive activity. In E. L.

Rossi & M. O. Ryan (Eds.), *Mind–body communication in hypnosis: Life reframing in hypnosis* (pp. 133–188). New York: Irvington.

Erickson, M. H. (1985d). Hypnotic alterations of physiological functions. In E. L. Rossi & M. O. Ryan (Eds.), *Mind–body communication in hypnosis: The seminars, workshops and lectures of Milton H. Erickson* (pp. 1–65). New York: Irvington.

Erickson, M. H. (1985e). Symptom-based approaches in mind–body problems. In E. L. Rossi & M. O. Ryan (Eds.), *Mind–body communication in hypnosis: The seminars, workshops and lectures of Milton H. Erickson* (pp. 65–201). New York: Irvington.

Erickson, M. H. (1985f). Special states of awareness and receptivity. In E. L. Rossi & M. O. Ryan (Eds.), *Mind–body communication in hypnosis: Life reframing in hypnosis* (pp. 223–266). New York: Irvington.

Lankton, S. (1998). *Examining the resolution of anxiety and pain problems using hypnosis* (videotape). Milton H. Erickson Foundation, Brief Therapy Conference: Lasting Impressions, New York.

Rossi, E. L. (1996). *The symptom path to enlightenment*. Pacific Palisades, CA: Palisades Gateway.

### Suggested Readings

Erickson, M. H. (1985). *Mind–body communication in hypnosis* (vols. 1–3), E. L. Rossi & O. Ryan (Eds.). New York: Irvington.

# 19

# Hypnosis: Adjunct to
# Medical Maneuvers

*Norma Barretta & Philip F. Barretta*

When patients manage "intractable" pain, recover or heal more quickly than is "normal," are "cured" of incurable illness, or go "into remission" instead of dying, we who have done hypnotic work with such patients are often confronted with the "Semmelweis phenomenon" (A. Freedman, personal communication, September 1998).

"How do you know it was the hypnosis?" the doctor asked.

"Maybe it was something else," or "Well, this is an unusual case," or "Perhaps it was misdiagnosed."

The cynics are certainly certain it was *not* the hypnotic work the patient did.

In the late eighteenth century, Ignaz Philipp Semmelweis concluded that young mothers were dying of puerperal fever because attending physicians did not wash their hands between seeing patients and thus were infecting the postpartum women who delivered in hospitals. Women who had their babies at home rarely suffered the same fate.

Even when Semmelweis demonstrated that the death rate from puerperal fever was practically zero with midwives (who washed their hands between deliveries) and staggering with physicians (who did *not* wash their hands) doing the deliveries, his critics still laughed at him.

It took almost a century to prove that Semmelweis was right.

"He who is certain is not open to learning."
— Confucius

In 1924, at the University of Wisconsin, Milton Erickson described himself as "too naive about medical problems and too eager to experiment to
exercise reasonable caution in a medical situation" (Erickson, 1967, p.
166), and so he hypnotized a young athlete who had bitten through his
tongue and could not speak (and who really *should* have had sutures), and
reported: "Within four hours the young athlete was free of swelling, pain
and the handicap" (p. 166).

Almost every collection of Erickson's work includes examples of his
considerable success with pain management, anesthesia, and the reduction
of or need for medication. Obviously, Erickson made extensive use of
hypnosis in many, many such cases, as well as with himself. On one of
our visits to Phoenix, Phil asked Dr. Erickson how he managed his own
battles with pain.

His response clearly indicated that he noticed Phil's left hand, which
at that time showed minor signs of arthritis.

Gazing quite obviously at Phil's hand and then looking directly at
him, Dr. Erickson said, "I *take an hour* when I first wake up to *get all the
pain out*" (personal communication, October 1978).

Upon our return to California, Phil began to take very long hot
showers every morning. Twenty years later, he continues this pattern and
has full use of his hands. He experiences pain only when he doesn't remember to "take an hour."

In *The Nature of Hypnosis and Suggestion* (Rossi, 1980, Vol. I), Erickson
states: "An intense memory rather than imagination" will provide an
associative pathway. Bandler and Grinder (1981, pp. 61–63) made use of
this concept in many of the techniques of neuro-linguistic programming
(NLP), especially in "anchoring" and "anchor collapsing," where anchoring refers to creating and reinforcing a posthypnotic suggestion, and
anchor collapsing means removing a previous posthypnotic suggestion.

Distraction, displacement, and reinterpretation, together with the utilization of early memories to replace current pain, were Erickson's tools
in managing pain (Rossi, 1980, Vol. I).

Kay Thompson played with ambiguity in her approach to pain. She spoke of "panes of glass," which could be easily shattered and disposed of (personal communication, 1985).

Deborah Ross (1992) describes several cases in which patients maintained pain as a protective measure. Ross used metaphor to guide patients into more useful ecological and comfortable ways of protecting themselves. She recommends that such cases be followed up, perhaps twice a year, to pace the wellness.

There have been many reports throughout history of the use of hypnosis to relieve pain; as early as 1847, Esdaile discussed its application in surgery and medicine in his book on *Mesmerism in India.*

Beyond this, hypnosis can bring about healing as well as relief. Erickson reported many terminal cases of pain control. In June 1997, Harold Crasilneck described the case of Janelle at the 14th ISH Congress on Hypnosis in San Diego. An infiltrating carcinoma with metastases to the bone caused constant pain after a radical mastectomy, radiation, and chemotherapy. Her prognosis was limited and there was a "hot spot" on her bone scan when she consuled Dr. Crasilneck. After three days (53 hours) of long repetitive sessions, she reported a "religious" experience while in deep trance. Repeated radiological studies showed no sign of cancer.

Dr. Crasilneck calls his approach "bombardment," which, together with the autoimmune system's positive response, acted as a catalytic agent in destroying the cancer.

## CASE REPORTS

### Judy and Marilyn

In our own work with medically referred patients, we have had two cases of uterine fibroid tumors. Judy, then 35, came to us in 1977, upset because a hysterectomy had been prescribed to stop the heavy bleeding caused by several fibroid tumors. She had just remarried and thought she might want to have another child. She did not want to undergo the surgery. When asked what she thought might work, she said, "Heat. I can burn them out." Hypnosis was used to create a "million-candlepower" flame (in her mind's eye), which she moved down into her uterus. During our third session, she asked that we hold our hands above her abdomen during the trance. We did so and felt an intense heat in the area. After six sessions, Judy returned to her gynecologist to be reexamined. He found no evidence of fibroid tumors. He called it "an unusual case," dismissing her hypnotic work as irrelevant.

Almost 20 years later, Marilyn came in for presurgical preparation for a myomectomy, the removal of fibroids, in lieu of a hysterectomy. We audiotaped her hypnotic session, which she was to repeat by listening to the tape for the month or so preceding the scheduled surgery.

She seemed to be obsessed by the thought that she could die. The metaphor we used was the familiar Erickson "dog story" of Roger Drassett, the basset, who lived to a very old age by changing his lifestyle (moving to Arizona). We also reminded her of how easy it is to delete things on a computer. She was very familiar with computers and so she deleted the thought of dying during the surgery.

Fifty-three tumors were removed from Marilyn's uterus. She was told it would be six weeks before she would recover. She was back at work full-time three weeks later.

### Tom's Story

Two years later, Marilyn's husband, Tom, was to have a kidney transplant. Since he is a columnist and author and sometimes a medical writer, Tom reports his own experience:

A persistent skeptic, I had no great faith in the power of hypnosis, but since it had apparently worked so well for Mar, I was willing to give it a try. During our session, I told Dr. Barretta everything I feared about my then-putative transplant operation. It was a laundry list that included everything from rejection and pain to discomfort from the catheter I knew the surgeon would insert in my bladder and keep there for a few days after the transplant.

After I'd explained all this to Norma during our first half-hour together, she told me to relax, close my eyes, lean back in her office recliner, and simply listen to her. I did, as her tape machine silently recorded her talking to me about all the issues I had raised. Afterward, I listened to that tape every day until surgery. Sometimes I fell asleep while listening. Other times, I'd feel nervous and edgy while listening. In the end, my own mood or physical state didn't seem to matter.

I think my buoyant mood just before surgery was, at least in part, the product of all that listening to comforting, positive suggestions. No one can ever quantify how much the hypnosis contributed to my state of mind, but I have no doubt that it was a factor. In all my 53 years, I'd never been so calm and happy heading into a critical event as I was then. Hypnosis was the only difference I could see between my lead-up to this occasion and how I'd prepared for everything from college exams to key business meetings, and even my wedding ...

... With my throat burning from the anesthetic tube used during the surgery and the sense that I was sneaking something every time I took a sip of water, the first night after the operation was pretty miserable, the worst night I was to have for many months after the transplant. Nurses woke me every hour or so to draw blood and check my vital signs and I found myself arguing with one nurse over the frequency of the interruptions. Finally, at 4 A.M., with the sense that I wouldn't be allowed to sleep very long anyway, I decided to get out of bed. I did it gingerly at first. But soon I was able to walk quite well, even dragging around my heavily laden IV pole and catheter. By 6 A.M., I felt a huge surge of energy, more vitality than I'd felt in many years. "Is this what I've been missing?" I asked myself. "It's incredible!" I took a hike around the hospital's postsurgery floor. Months earlier, I had asked Tanya Heinen of the Polycystic Kidney Research Foundation how far transplant patients usually walk during the first day after surgery. She told me about Ed Farmer, a former major league pitcher and a radio announcer for the Chicago White Sox, who she said had set the record by walking to the nurses' station near his room within less than a day of his transplant. That was one reason I was grinning broadly when I walked right past the nurses' station, and then on to Tammy's [his donor] room to check on her. She was out cold, with Hannah [the donor's mother] sleeping on a chair beside her bed.

I walked on, to the amazement and bemusement of the nurses watching me. Next, I encountered one of the doctors on the surgical team, who reacted with a crooked grin when I told him I was ready to go home right then. Of course, I knew I couldn't. Being in a hospital is a bit like being in a prison. Just as a prisoner needs the warden's signature before walking out, a patient needs the written say-so of a doctor. And none of them was about to sign me out just yet, even if I already felt well enough to leave (about 15 hours posttransplant).

Blood-test results showed exactly why I felt so chipper and energetic. When the night nurse, Kazu, took my blood at midnight, the creatinine reading—which is the best measure of kidney function—was 7.9, meaning the poisons in my blood were at the same level as if my kidney function were about one-eighth of normal. When it was taken again just before 6 A.M., it was 2.6, the lowest it had been in more than seven years. The readings would get steadily lower, too, until they stabilized between 1.1 and 1.3, well within the range of normal kidney function. This meant my new kidney was taking hold quickly, cleaning out the poisons that had sapped my energy as they circulated for many years in my body. As I walked, I began to understand that I had not realized for years how crummy I'd really felt.

I spent the rest of that day prowling the halls with my IV and catheter whenever I didn't have guests—which wasn't often. Oh yes, the catheter . . . People told me in advance that it would not be uncomfortable. But I felt from the start that it made me feel continually that I had to urinate urgently. It was worse in some sitting and lying positions than in others. This was the single least comfortable thing I experienced in the days immediately following transplant. But while I listened to Dr. Barretta's tape on the second night after the operation, I decided to try something new. Whenever the urge would become strong or frustrating, I would stand up and simulate urinating, even though anything emerging could only run down the catheter tube. This was in keeping with the tape's suggestion of trying a "different approach" whenever something difficult or inconvenient occurred. Within hours, I became much more comfortable with the catheter.

Besides the sudden energy I felt, there were two other remarkable developments on my first day posttransplant: One was that I became aware that I had felt virtually no pain. The other was the disappearance of my dialysis fistula, a good sign.

While the disappearing fistula was no big surprise to anyone but me, my lack of pain astonished every doctor who came to see me on rounds. I had so little discomfort from the six-inch incision on my abdomen that I never took so much as a Tylenol pill, let alone the morphine drip that was readily available. I attribute this partly to the pain tolerance I had built up over years of occasional kidney pain episodes: Next to them, what I felt from the new slit was like a mosquito bite. Partly, also, I credit Dr. Barretta's tape, which suggested daily that the way to handle pain was simply to equate it to a tiger residing under my bed, whose nose I could push back down whenever it became rambunctious. I listened to that tape every night in the hospital and called that image to mind whenever I'd twist or bend in a way that brought a sudden stab of pain. Again, it will never be possible to measure precisely how much effect the hypnosis had, but I'm utterly certain it played a major role.

Similarly, Dr. Barretta stressed in our session that my body would not react against the new organ and reject it as a foreign object, but instead would welcome it as a productive and permanent resident. Was it a coincidence that my immunosuppressant doses were reduced much more quickly than normal, to the point where I was taking the usual lifetime maintenance dose of several medications less than three weeks after transplant? No one can say. "All we can say is that hypnosis certainly can't hurt," observed the attending physician.

What a difference 20 years can make!

On September 26, 1998, we attended a first anniversary celebration of Tom's kidney transplant and wished the "new kidney" on the block our best.

### Deborah and Carol

Another presurgical preparation was a transanal excision of a villous adenoma (removal of a colon polyp). Deborah, a vibrant, active, and busy career woman with a family to care for, was concerned about being "out of it" for a long time following surgery. She was also an avowed "coward" about pain. Her tapes included several metaphoric instructions to displace the pain from kinesthetic to visual so that she could watch the pain drift out to sea (she lives near the Pacific Ocean) until she could no longer see it.

Another tape included many healing messages; one she particularly liked was about dogs who went to obedience school (she was very disciplined in her approach to life), where they learned to stay at rest when necessary, and they learned, quite quickly, to heel rapidly. (Thank goodness, the unconscious mind can't spell—unless properly instructed, of course!)

Deborah, our patient, told us:

> I was awake and conversing with Dr. B., the anesthesiologist, during the entire surgery, telling jokes, laughing. Although I'd planned to use your tape during the procedure, I didn't because I was so calm and completely at ease; no anxiety at all.
>
> After the surgery, I was experiencing an extreme "spinal headache." I listened to the postsurgery tape and the headache disappeared. I'm sure the hypnosis kept the anxiety at bay and assisted in the healing process.

Our latest patient (September 1998), Carol, 32 years old, had been diagnosed with a stage 4 melanoma originating above the knee some 20 months earlier, and now metastatic to the abdominal and chest lymph nodes. She came in emaciated, despondent, discouraged, but with a strong belief she would survive.

It is our opinion, as well as our experience, that being able to elicit metaphoric symbols from a patient is more useful than imposing symbols or creating them. Erickson concurred: "Leading the patient to 'see what I, the patient, can do' is much more effective than letting the patient see what things the therapist can do with or to the patient" (Haley, 1967).

We encouraged Carol to assign a symbol to her immune system, strong, invincible, powerful.

She selected an army, somewhat similar to the Roman legions who were victorious for several centuries, to represent her T cells, ever vigilant and on constant patrol, seeking out and destroying anomalous invasive, unwelcome cells. The macrophage cells would be symbolized by a professional maid service to clean up and dispose of the debris. Repairs would be done by a "Mr. Fixit," capable of fixing any and all things.

She was to undergo several biochemotherapy treatments during the month of October. She was hypnotically instructed to greet the chemotherapy as a welcome ally in her battle. Together with her invincible army, now armed with state-of-the-art chemotherapy, the cancer would be destroyed. She would be ever so slightly hungry after each treatment.

She missed her next appointment because she was so weak from the chemotherapy treatment. However, she was eating! At her next appointment, on November 3, she had gained weight, about 20 pounds, and her latest radiological study showed that she was in remission.

## CONCLUSIONS

There is no doubt that hypnotically prepared patients learn to manage pain, and to undergo surgery, chemotherapy, and radiation with far less discomfort and fewer side effects. They have less blood loss, less swelling, less fever. They are subjected to less anesthesia; there is little or no post-surgical nausea. They recover more quickly.

Patients for whom the prognosis was poor often survive, and some are even freed of the condition they had been entertaining: The party is over!

We remain uncertain as to why hypnosis works as well and as often as it does. But that uncertainty keeps us open to a new learning.

---

**Remember to:**

1. Think of hypnosis as a useful adjunct to medical treatment (traditional or alternative) and tune up your belief in "miracles."
2. Emphasize each person's own responsibility for self-care and well-being. Hypnosis enhances personal power.
3. Tap into the person's resources and use his or her symbols in your metaphors.
4. Use the greatest pharmacy on the planet: It exists between the patient's ears.
5. Select your language carefully: Words can have a powerful ameliorative effect when they are woven into a tapestry of the patient's own selection.

---

### References

Bandler, R. (1975). *Patterns of the hypnotic techniques of Milton H. Erickson, Vol. I.* Cupertino, CA: Meta.

Bandler, R., & Grinder, J. (1981). *TRANCE-formations.* Moab, UT: Real People Press.

Bergman, B. R. (1993). Major surgery under hypnosis. *Hypnos, 20*(1).

Enquist, B. (1997). Pre-surgical hypnosis and suggestions in anesthesia. *Hypnos, 24*(4).

Freedman, A. (1998, September). Uncertainty and institutional change: The Semmel-weis phenomenon. Unpublished paper and personal communication.

Haley, J. (Ed). (1967). *Advanced techniques of hypnosis and therapy: Selected papers of Milton H. Erickson, M.D.* Orlando, FL: Grune and Stratton.

Justice, B. (1987). *Who gets sick: Thinking and health.* Houston, TX: Peak Press.

Kroger, W. (1979). Personal communication.

Lankton, S., & Lankton, C. (1983). *The answer within.* New York: Bruner/Mazel.

Ross, D. (1992). Symbolic pain: Metaphors of dis-ease. *Hypnos, 19*(4).

Rossi, E. L. (Ed.). (1980). *The collected papers of Milton H. Erickson on hypnosis (Vols. I–IV).* New York: Irvington.

Rossi, E. L., Ryan, M. O., & Sharp, F. A. (1983). *Healing in hypnosis.* New York: Irvington.

Roud, P. C. (1990). *Making miracles.* New York: Warner Books.

Schmidt, C. (1992). Hypnotic suggestions and imaginations in the treatment of colitis ulcerosa. *Hypnos, 19*(4).

Simonton, C., Simonton, S., & Creighton, J. (1978). *Getting well again.* Los Angeles: Tarcher.

Yapko, M. (1990). *Trancework.* New York: Brunner/Mazel.

Zeig, J. K. (1980). *A teaching seminar with Milton H. Erickson.* New York: Brunner/Mazel.

## 20

# Facilitating Generativity and Ego Integrity: Applying Ericksonian Methods to the Aging Population

*Helen Erickson*

There are more elderly persons alive today than at any other time in the history of the world (*Healthy People 2000*). The fastest growing sector of our society are those 85 and older, followed by those 65 and older. Those most vulnerable to the onset of new health problems are people 55 years of age and above (*Healthy People 2000*). While traditional health care is designed to treat sickness and disease, these data suggest that the cost of such care might create a major social problem in the new millennium. And yet, little has been done to explore possibilities that might cut costs by promoting health and healing rather than merely treating sickness and disease.

Perhaps this is so because many in our society perceive aging persons as being on a decline—a decline in physical, mental, emotional, and social health—and feel that little can be done to alter their trajectory. They associate normal age-related changes with sickness and believe that "getting older" is synonymous with "being old." They often assume that turning 60 means that "the body and mind are past their peak"; turning 70 means that "chronic disease and dementia are just around the corner."

Although it is true that some age-related changes result in a decline, age-related changes can also result in growth. Whether decline or growth occurs is dictated by the individual's perception of the events themselves. That is, how one sees such changes influences the outcome. Perceptions of change without meaning or purpose produce negative outcomes; negative outcomes produce a further decline in the aging person. On the other hand, attributing positive meaning and purpose to normal life changes results in growth; growth enhances our sense of well-being and increases our ability to contribute to the well-being of others. Some of our greatest humanitarians, scientists, and philosophers created their best work in their later years—take Franklin Delano Roosevelt and Viktor Frankl.

Another of these exemplar seniors was Milton Erickson, M.D., who practiced his profession until his death at the age of 79. He founded the American Society for Clinical Hypnosis, launched the Society's journal, wrote 150 articles, coauthored numerous books after his 55th birthday, and was actively involved in life until his final illness. Few people who knew him thought of him as an invalid or an "old man"; instead, he was viewed as a dynamic person, a brilliant scientist, a wise teacher and mentor, a father, husband, grandfather, and friend. Although he certainly had numerous physical ailments that interfered with his mobility, he maintained multiple roles and was alive emotionally, socially, mentally, and spiritually until his last breath. He set an example for those who followed; he showed us that we can continue to grow and explore, to be curious and productive, and to live a full and happy life until the last breath is taken. His life and his life work afforded an incentive and direction for health-care providers concerned with the well-being of aging adults.

This chapter presents a model derived from my exposure to Erickson's teachings that has been used to enhance the lives of persons of all ages (Erickson, Tomlin, & Swain, 1983; H. Erickson, 1988, 1990a, 1990b). In this chapter, it has been customized specifically for the aging population. Two purposes here are to present basic philosophical/conceptual considerations and to discuss their implications for practice.

## PHILOSOPHICAL/CONCEPTUAL CONSIDERATIONS

### Mind–Body–Spirit Dynamics

There are continuous interactions among the multiple components of the mind, body, and spirit so that stimuli in any one part of the person produce multiple responses in the other parts (Ader, 1981; Benson & Stark, 1996; Dienstfrey, 1991; Friedman & VandenBos, 1992; Gallager, 1993; Goleman & Gurin, 1993; Klivington, 1997; Miller, 1998; Savva, 1998; Watkins, 1997). These responses depend on the individual's conscious and/or unconscious perception of the stimuli (Dafter, 1996; Morris, 1998; Moskowitz, 1992; Moyers, 1993), the state and trait resources available to contend with the stimuli (Erickson, Tomlin, & Swain, 1983; Erickson, 1988, 1990b), the cultural context (Morris, 1998; Shafer, 1998), and other simultaneous or time-related stimuli (M. Erickson, 1983; H. Erickson, 1990; Rossi, 1986). The outcomes of these responses will determine one's overall health (Dafter, 1996; Erickson, Tomlin, & Swain, 1983; H. Erickson, 1988, 1990b; Wickramasekera, 1998).

## Health

Humans have a natural drive toward holistic health. Health is not a physical or mental absence of disease, but an ability to live a quality life and to maintain meaningful roles in society. That is, although sickness and disease will influence our physical capabilities, happy humans are able to grow, maintain meaningful roles, experience well-being, transcend daily hassles, and live quality lives in spite of sickness and disease. This is holistic health.

Facilitating holistic health is contingent upon understanding basic human nature—understanding what facilitates our inherent drives and what interferes with our natural processes. Relevant factors include (1) needs, growth, mutuality, and self-fulfillment; (2) attachment, loss, and grief; (3) developmental processes; and (4) linkages.

## Needs, Growth, Mutuality, Self-fulfillment

All humans have an innate drive to achieve growth, mutuality, and self-fulfillment (M. Erickson, 1983; Erickson, Tomlin, & Swain, 1983). The degree to which one's needs are met determines one's potential for growth at any given point in life. Need satisfaction produces assets and unmet needs produce deficits. Need assets facilitate growth whereas need deficits impede growth.

There are five types of needs: biophysical, affiliation, individuation, affiliated individuation, and spiritual needs (H. Erickson, 1992). The first two are lower-level needs, whereas the need for affiliated individuation and spiritual well-being are higher-level types. Mutuality depends on affiliated individuation (Erickson, Tomlin, & Swain, 1983); self-fulfillment is contingent on relationships that facilitate the satisfaction of higher-level human needs.

## Lower-Level Needs

### Biophysical Needs

The human body consists of multiple, interactive subsystems, such as the immune, hypothalamus–pituitary–adrenal, respiratory, cardiovascular, and urinary tract systems. Biophysical needs are related to the dynamic interactions among these multiple subsystems. The degree to which these needs are met determines the degree to which the body will work efficiently and effectively. Most biophysical needs are obvious, for example, the need for oxygen, food, and movement. Others, although less obvious, sometimes are more important, such as chemicals necessary for the functioning of the Krebs cycle. Minimal satisfaction of biophysical needs is necessary to physical life.

### Affiliation and Individuation Needs

Affiliation needs are those that are met when one person feels linked to another in such a way that he or she experiences a sense of connectedness with some degree of safety, security, and a sense of being valued with minimal conditions. Individuation needs are related to feelings of individuality, self-esteem, personal worth, and pride in uniqueness. Satisfaction of affiliation and individuation needs depends on past life experiences and one's current view of interactions and relationships with other humans, with animals, and/or with a higher power, such as God.

Many adults assume that it is inappropriate to have affiliation needs because these feelings imply dependency on another. They have difficulty distinguishing between dependency and an affiliated linkage. They perceive that there is a dichotomy between dependency and independence, and that it is necessary to sacrifice one in order to have the other: we are either dependent or independent. Such individuals often seek independence at the expense of the satisfaction of their affiliation needs. Because aging mandates increased dependence on others, a distinction between dependency and affiliation needs becomes paramount for the older person.

## Higher-Level Needs

### Affiliated-Individuation

An intrapsychic phenomenon, this takes place when a person perceives himself or herself as simultaneously connected to and separate from a significant other (Erickson et al., 1983; H. Erickson, 1990a) and perceives permission from the other member of the dyad for both affiliation and individuation. The balance between affiliation and individuation need satisfaction will determine the degree to which affiliated-individuation occurs. Satisfaction of the need for affiliated-individuation affects the degree to which one can attain a sense of healthy, growth-producing mutuality. Mutuality involves a reciprocal relationship between two people wherein affiliated-individuation is experienced by each member of the couple. When people achieve a sense of affiliated-individuation, they have an inherent drive toward satisfaction of spiritual needs.

Spiritual Needs

These needs are met when we find meaning and purpose in our lives that transcend lower-level needs. It is possible to have spiritual needs met when others are not. The pursuit of meaning and purpose is dependent on a healthy balance between affiliated-individuation and mutuality. Finding meaning and purpose in life, an essential aspect of the healing process, helps the individual discover the essence of his or her being and leads to self-fulfillment.

Although spiritual needs exist across the life span, they tend to be more important for the aging adult. Thus, affiliated-individuation, mutuality, and self-fulfillment are of major concern for those working on the developmental stages of generativity or ego integrity as described in the following.

*Need Satisfaction, Assets and Deficits*

When needs are met repeatedly, need assets are produced. Need assets become resources that can be used to maintain holistic health, respond to acute stressors, or contend with ongoing stress states (Erickson, Tomlin, & Swain, 1983). When needs are not met, need deficits result. The balance between need assets and deficits *at any given time* will determine the nature of one's *state* resources, which are needed to cope or contend with immediate life experiences. The continuous production of need assets results in growth, whereas continuous need deficits result in deprivation. Need deprivation impedes growth (Erickson et al., 1983; H. Erickson 1990a, 1990b).

**Attachment, Loss, and Grief**

When a phenomenon or object meets one's needs repeatedly, attachment to that phenomenon or object results. Attachment phenomena/ objects can be concrete or abstract and vary across the life span. Whenever there is a real, threatened, or perceived loss of the attached phenomenon/object, the grief process occurs. The exact nature of the process depends on the meaning of the lost object to the individual. Some objects are significant in that they represent a loss of self, whereas others represent the loss of factors that support the self. The first are of greater significance and are more difficult to resolve.

In all cases, there are several emotional responses, including feelings of denial, anger, and sadness. An individual's ability to work through the grief process depends on the availability of a new phenomenon or object that meets his or her needs repeatedly. When one exists, bonding to the phenomenon or object ensues, followed by attachment. The new phenomenon or object takes on significance, the old object is "let go," and the grieving process is resolved (Erickson et al., 1983; H. Erickson, 1990a, 1990b; Kinney & Erickson, 1990).

When the individual perceives that there are no phenomena or objects available that can and will meet his or her needs, he or she will either hang on to the memory of the old phenomenon/object or "give up" on its availability. In either case, the grieving process is unresolved, and morbid grief sets in and lingers until a new attachment occurs.

### Developmental Processes

Because development is inherent, sequential, and epigenetic (E. Erickson, 1963; Erickson, Tomlin, & Swain, 1983; H. Erickson, 1990b), all humans are in a continuous developmental process. The balance between need assets and deficits over a prolonged period will determine the nature of one's developmental residual. While developmental processes are common to all humans, the nature of one's developmental residual is unique. Continuous growth produces health-facilitating developmental residuals, including strengths and virtues related to each stage of development.

Interference with growth has the alternate effect: health-impeding developmental residual. The balance between positive and negative developmental residuals at any given time will determine the nature of one's trait resources; these are also needed in coping or contending with immediate life experiences. Trait resources influence how people view and experience life events and how they respond to them (Erickson, Tomlin, & Swain, 1983; H. Erickson, 1990a).

## Linkages

As indicated above, humans have an inherent drive to satisfy their needs. The phenomenon that repeatedly meets one's needs becomes an attachment phenomenon. Attachment phenomena may be concrete or abstract in nature, and they vary throughout life. The real, threatened, or perceived loss of an attachment phenomenon results in a grieving process. One's ability to find alternative attachment phenomena that fulfill one's needs will determine the degree to which the grieving process is resolved. The effect of unmet needs is to diminish the resources needed to work through the grieving process. The result can be unresolved grief or morbid grief.

Resolution of the grief process requires that alternative need-satisfaction phenomena or objects be identified—phenomena or objects that can meet the person's needs repeatedly so that he or she can let go of the previously attached-to phenomenon or object. Because need satisfaction is necessary for continuous growth, and continuous growth is necessary to produce healthy developmental residuals, these relationships are important for the aging person.

Everyone has an innate tendency to seek healthy developmental outcomes, but developmental processes can be stagnated by unresolved losses and morbid grief. The nature of the developmental residual produced at each stage of life provides a base for future growth and development. Thus, a strong trust residual (stage 1) provides a healthy base for the development of a strong autonomy residual (stage 2), which, in turn, provides a healthy base for a strong initiative residual (stage 3), and so forth. On the other hand, a strong mistrust residual (stage 1) will predispose one to a sense of shame and/or doubt (stage 2), which predisposes one to a sense of guilt (stage 3), and so forth. Because developmental residuals from previous life stages will determine how one perceives one's current life and how one interprets and copes with new life events, each person's approach to these tasks is unique. However, a person's behavior and attitudes can be assessed and interpreted within the context of the developmental process as it is affected by need satisfaction, loss, grief resolution, and attachment to new objects.

## IMPLICATIONS FOR PRACTICE

### Focus of Care

Clearly, the therapist's orientation to health care will determine the phenomenon on which he or she focuses. Those who use a traditional medical model will be concerned primarily with the treatment of sickness and disease or the prevention of physical or mental deterioration. They are likely to focus on signs and symptoms and to interpret their observations within the context of a curing model. Those who use the model described above will be concerned primarily with facilitating healthy processes and promoting well-being.[1] They are more likely to view signs and symptoms as symbolic and will interpret their observations within a healing model. Professionals who follow a traditional model will assess what's wrong with the body and/or mind and plan treatment to address these problems. Their goals will be to control or cure the sickness or disease and/or to make the person suffering from such conditions as comfortable as possible. The second type of therapist will assess need assets, losses, grieving processes, and developmental residual. The treatment goals will be to help clients attain affiliated-individuation, mutuality, and self-fulfillment.

### The Aging Adult

Aging adults are often confronted with an increase in losses and challenges not previously experienced. Their bodies and minds start to change, they slow down physically, and they have diminished sensory input capability. They are faced with changing roles, the losses of loved ones, and shifting responsibilities and relationships. They often experience social stigmas, which are usually unintended, but exist nevertheless. Whereas aging adults sometimes struggle to maintain control over their lives, professionals often imply that they should expect physical and mental deterioration and that they might be better off if they retired or gave up activities that seem to tire them. The professionals suggest that it is time for them to do "what they want." The unspoken implications are that they no longer have much to offer and that time is limited. Although there may be truth to the latter assumption, aging adults need to be valued for their accrued knowledge, life experiences, and general wisdom. They want to be able to share their lives with the younger generation in ways that are meaningful to them and to the recipients of that wisdom.

---

[1] For these practitioners, physical problems are also addressed. The difference is that the person is the focus of care, not the disease. Disease processes are viewed as factors that interfere with well-being and the quality of life. Signs and symptoms of disease are perceived as symbolic and are treated from both a physical and a psychosocial standpoint.

They want to believe that life continues until the last breath (and perhaps beyond that), and that life continues to provide an opportunity to make contributions and to be the most that they are capable of being. They don't want to admit that it is time to step aside, go into retreat, or withdraw from life, and simply fill their hours with meaningless motions or wait for time to pass.

However, as with all human beings, the aging adults' developmental residuals will determine how they approach the later part of their lives, their behaviors and their attitudes. Thus, to understand the clinical implications of using Ericksonian techniques with the aging adult to facilitate uniqueness, it is necessary also to understand commonalities.

## Life-Stage Tasks

Aging adults focus on the developmental tasks of generativity and ego integrity respectively. The stage of generativity is preceded by intimacy. During intimacy, adults gain a sense of being connected to significant others and emerge from this stage with either a love for humankind or a sense of isolation and disconnectedness. The first results in positive developmental residual and the second in negative residual. Their developmental residual influences how they approach the next stage of life and the type of resources they are able to mobilize as they work on related life tasks, and that will be demonstrated through their behaviors and attitudes.

### Positive Residual

During the stage of generativity, the emphasis shifts to a concern for society with a focus on one's personal contributions. At this stage of life, people question themselves about the meaning and purpose of their lives. They seek an understanding of the meaning of their contributions to society and of what legacy they will leave behind. They move into the stage of ego integrity with a wisdom about life in general, a sense of completion, and a knowledge that because they have lived, others will be happier, safer, and more content, and will enjoy a better future. These adults do not perceive an end to their lives (although they recognize that physical decline will occur), but instead they perceive a continuation of the essence of their being across time.

### Negative Residual

When adults have difficulty negotiating the stage of intimacy, a sense of isolation evolves, leaving a developmental residual that predisposes them during the stage of generativity. Rather than moving into generativity with feelings of being connected and a concern for humankind, they feel isolated and turn inward. During the stage of generativity, they become more self-absorbed and less concerned with others, and drift toward a sense of despair. They struggle to find meaning in life, but have difficulty. As they merge into the stage of ego integrity, they come to believe that life has no meaning and that their lives in particular were futile. They begin to look toward the end, often with fear and trepidation.

No human is truly a paradigm of all positive or all negative residuals. Instead, we are all a combination of the two. The degree to which one's needs are met, losses are grieved for, grief processes are resolved, and new attachment objects are found will determine the balance. Herein lies the challenge for the therapist working with this population. To understand better the personal orientation of aging clients, therapists need to be able to model their world, to understand their uniqueness. Modeling is the natural precursor of role-modeling. Modeling and role-modeling[2] evolve as a pattern of communication between the two people (therapist and client) develops.

## Modeling and Role Modeling

At some level, all humans know what has interfered with their well-being, what they need to do to get well, and what will help them grow. This is called self-care knowledge (Erickson, Tomlin, & Swain, 1983; H. Erickson, 1990a). Self-care knowledge is both conscious and unconscious information. The clinician's job is to facilitate the client's ability to (1) articulate what is known consciously, (2) bypass resistances to discovering what is known unconsciously, (3) integrate conscious and unconscious knowledge, and (4) use what is known.

*Modeling* (Erickson, 1975; Erickson, Tomlin, & Swain, 1983; H. Erickson, 1990b; Kinney & Erickson, 1990) is the technique used to initiate a working relationship so that the therapist can understand the person's unique view of the world, including resistances, lifetime patterns, losses, and therapeutic needs. Modeling enhances intercommunication between

---

[2] The concept of "modeling" and "role-modeling" were first proposed to this author by Milton Erickson. It took about 15 years of study before their importance was understood and appreciated.

the therapist and client, as well as intracommunication (within the multiple parts of the client). It requires that the therapist *step into the world of the client*, build a mirror image (as much as possible), and interpret that world within a conceptual model. Modeling includes the interpretation of both verbal and nonverbal cues in order to understand (to the extent possible) the uniqueness of the client. This includes an understanding of the multiple roles and relationships that are important to him or her in experiencing mutuality and self-fulfillment.

While modeling can be accomplished by observation and interpretation of nonverbal cues only, the therapist's understanding can be enhanced by a brief dialog with the client. Information that is useful includes a description of the situation, the factors related to this situation, what is expected to happen, what can be done about it, and the client's goals. Observation of verbal and nonverbal responses not only provides information about the client's conscious and unconscious concerns, but it also enhances the therapist's understanding of the client's perceived safety in the current situation. Safety in the relationship and safety in disclosure are very important for all people, but more important for the aging. This information provides a starting point for the therapist to utilize the client's world view in therapy.

*Role modeling* is the process used to plan strategies that will help clients grow and become more fully themselves, to move toward a higher level of self-fulfillment, and to gain a healthy sense of mutuality. Because many therapists are younger than their clients, they sometimes become confused about the older client's orientation to the world. When a therapist is dealing with the life task of intimacy, it may seem that all of life is about developing happy, healthy relationships wherein one feels connected and loved and can reciprocate with love. However, for healthy older adults working on the task of generativity, feelings of being connected, loving, and being loved are no longer of paramount interest; these feelings are assumed and a basic part of the person's life. Instead, they are concerned with finding ways to experience a continued affiliation with loved ones and loved ideas as they pursue their own uniqueness and gain an understanding of their contributions to society.

Persons who have a preponderance of negative developmental residual are searching for ways to be connected and to make meaning of their lives. Although they may state that they want to be left alone, don't trust, have learned not to love, and don't believe in life after death, they, too, are searching for a sense of mutuality and self-fulfillment. Their despair (often presented as clinical depression or overt hostility) is a clue for the therapist that there are unmet needs, unresolved losses, and the resulting morbid grief.

### Building Rapport

*Communication* between therapist and client starts as we model the client's world and as we role-model. It begins with the first interaction, which may be as subtle as an exchanged glance, a handshake, or even a motion toward a chair, or as overt as a direct statement (Klivington, 1997; Watzlawick, 1967). Thus, it is important to remember that one "cannot not communicate" (Watzlawick, 1967) when the other member of the dyad realizes that communication is occurring. Cues that are sent from one to the other set the stage for the following messages. Messages send both content and contextual information and are interpreted within the framework of the receiver. Because all messages are based on perceptions of either the equality or inequality of the two communicating members (Watzlawick, 1967), the therapist's attitudes toward aging are important when working with older clients. Sometimes what we say is therapeutic, not because of what we say, but of how we say it (Watzlawick, Weakland, & Fisch, 1988).

People come to a therapist because they have exhausted their own conscious resources; they do not know how to help themselves to be happier and healthier. They come learning from past experiences that affect their current expectations, hopes, and resistances. The aging adult needs to have a deep sense of the "I" and "we" states of being, as well as the "you-and-me" state of being. The person also needs to see freedom and acceptance in all three states. Because happy humans are never static (Erickson, Rossi, & Rossi, 1976), the therapist's job is to facilitate growth within the context of normal developmental processes so that clients can live their lives to the maximum of their abilities (Erickson, Tomlin, & Swain, 1983).

*Expectancy* is a basic concept in Ericksonian work. When clients come for help, they expect *something* to happen; either they will get help or they won't. The older adult often holds back to assess the safety in disclosing. The therapist might interpret this *waiting* as evidence of resistance, however, it should be remembered that "you can't wait for something to happen without knowing it is going to happen" (Erickson, Rossi, & Rossi, 1976, p. 88). The therapist's ability to take advantage of the client's expectation is basic in Ericksonian work. The way we build on this natural state—a state of expecting that something is going to happen—depends on how we communicate with our clients and what we communicate. They are able to receive our messages because they have a natural drive toward mutuality and inherent suggestibility.

*Suggestibility* "is (also) basic in (Ericksonian) hypnosis. Many attempts have been made to define hypnosis, both in terms of the phenomena involved and in terms of possible causal mechanisms, but no definition has yet satisfactorily answered all the questions raised ... Bernheim advanced the concept that a suggestion is the basic factor in producing and utilizing hypnosis. Suggestions need not be of a verbal nature only. They can occur at any sensory level. These include, of course, the olfactory, the gustatory, the auditory, the tactile, the visual, and many others. Suggestion and hypnotizability are very highly correlated" (Erickson, Hershman, & Secter, 1981, p. 20). Because people inherently strive for growth and mutuality, they are also highly receptive to suggestions that fit into the context of their world orientation.

## Bypassing Resistance

Since the aging adult comes to the therapist expecting that something is going to happen and is highly suggestible, bypassing resistance to trance induction is just a matter of applying basic Ericksonian philosophy and techniques. Key considerations are induction and trance work techniques.

### Induction Techniques

Given that most older adults have concerns about relinquishing a sense of control, many are resistant to traditional induction techniques. They are, however, very receptive to a naturalistic or conversational induction: incorporating and interspersing[3] (M. Erickson, 1983; Erickson, Rossi, & Rossi, 1976; Rossi & Ryan, 1992; Zeig, 1980), self-disclosure,[4] sensory ori-

---

[3] Interspersing is the random inclusion of purposeful comments intended to induce trance or facilitate trance work.

[4] Self-disclosure in this situation refers to the therapist's sharing his or her philosophy about self-care knowledge described above and how it relates to the therapist's belief about people. This can be accomplished by stating something to the effect that all people know what it is that interferes with their health and well-being, what they need to be happier, and what will help them grow. I often add that I believe that people want to be the most that they can be and that life circumstances sometimes interfere. I also indicate that there are no rights or wrongs, only learnings about how to be more effective and how to get our needs met more efficiently.

entation,[5] early learning sets[6] common to most people, truisms,[7] client storytelling,[8] and client integration.[9] Each technique assists the aging adult to gain a sense of comfort with the therapist and a sense of control over his or her current experience, and to develop a yes-set.[10]

Confusion techniques (Erickson, Hershman, & Secter, 1981; Erickson, Rossi, & Rossi, 1976) also work with the older adult. Generally, adults have had many experiences with the health-care system, and thus have an expectation of how the provider will behave, what the provider will ask, and what he or she will expect. Usually, they anticipate the typical handshake and the questioning; they perceive that the therapist will expect cooperation and compliance. When the therapist does not respond in the expected ways,[11] the client becomes confused and is then open to conversational techniques.

## Trance Work

Whereas several techniques are useful in working with aging adults, some are more useful when working with someone with high levels of positive developmental residual and others are more effective with those who have high levels of negative developmental residual. Some work well

---

[5] Orientation to external stimuli, such as sound, sight, and smell with a gradual refocus to internal stimuli, such as the rhythm of the heartbeat, feeling the chest go in and out as we breathe deeply.

[6] Most people can remember when they first learned their ABCs, first started to learn how to ride a bike, first learned to add 1 and 1. When invited, most can also remember how difficult each task seemed before it was completed, and how simple it was after accomplished (Erickson, Rossi, & Rossi, 1976).

[7] Truisms build on early learning sets. For example, to state that it was very difficult to tell an "m" from an "n" and sometimes even to tell an "m" from a "3" is to state something that is true for most people. The more we know about the client's world, the easier it is to use truisms to bypass resistance (Erickson, Rossi, & Rossi, 1976).

[8] Client storytelling is initiated by asking the client to tell you a story, any story that pops into his or her mind. You can expand by saying that it might be a story from recent life experience or something from a much earlier time in life. The important thing is that it just seems to come to the client's (conscious) mind.

[9] This is achieved by asking the client to find pleasure in remembering and suggesting that at some time in the future, he or she might be curious as to why this story came to mind.

[10] The yes-set is developed by creating a set of experiences that the client can recognize and with which he or she can resonate, resulting in feelings of safety and a willingness to proceed. The yes-set is necessary to bypass resistances designed (unconsciously) to protect the self from others (Erickson, Rossi, & Rossi, 1976).

[11] For example, rather than a quick and clean handshake, when the therapist lingers and applies slight upward pressure to the under side of the wrist, followed by a slight downward pressure to the top side of the wrist, a handshake induction occurs. When this is followed by other "surprises," such as the therapist's sitting in what is obviously the client's chair or starting with an unexpected story, further confusion leads to deepening of the trance.

with both types of persons. For example, storytelling can be used with nearly all individuals. When there is high positive residual and minimal negative residual, the goals are to help the person draw on his or her own strengths, to recognize those strengths, and to learn to use resources in new ways. In this situation, the client either has the resources but doesn't know that he or she has them, or has easy access to resources and simply needs some assistance. Often such persons have had long stretches of time when they were comparatively happy and well. They present themselves with new physical problems (often associated with major losses), feelings of sadness, and a sense of life being turned upside down. They need help in finding new ways to meet their need for affiliated-individuation, a sense of purpose for their recent life experiences, a meaning in their lives, and self-projection. Reframing (M. Erickson, 1983; Rosen, 1982; Rossi & Ryan, 1992; Zeig, 1980), indirect suggestions, reintegration, displacement, visual imagery (Erickson, Hershman, & Secter, 1981), use of analogies and time distortion are easily applied techniques that work well.

On the other hand, when there is high negative residual, the therapist will be challenged by symptoms that reflect both the negative residual and the client's natural drive toward growth. Often the client's behaviors and attitudes reflect lack of trust[12] and/or mistrust, self-doubt,[13] shame,[14] guilt,[15] inferiority,[16] identity confusion,[17] and isolation.[18] Simultaneously, because there is also the propensity for growth, their behaviors

---

[12] Lack of trust differs from mistrust. The first indicates that the client has minimal affiliation needs met without conditions; the second indicates that the client has learned that it is not safe to be affiliated. People who lack trust often talk about feelings of abandonment.

[13] Self-doubt sometimes presents itself by behaviors that suggest self-assurance. However, those with self-doubt who demonstrate the attitude that they are always right and don't make mistakes are generally people who are not sure enough about themselves to allow scrutiny by self or others.

[14] Shame differs from modesty. The first is founded in a sense of diminished worth, the latter in a sense of self-respect. People who have negative residual related to this stage in life often talk about being rejected.

[15] Guilt differs from assumption of responsibility. The first is founded in a sense of being discovered as guilty of wrongdoing, the latter is the willingness to recognize human vulnerability and freedom of choice. Some will project responsibility for their life situation onto others with extreme hostility. Hostility is a sign of morbid grief related to this stage in life or earlier.

[16] Inferiority differs from humility. Inferiority sometimes presents itself in behaviors that seem to demonstrate the opposite, that is, self-importance. Humility is the healthy recognition of one's worth within the context of the larger scheme of life.

[17] While many older adults appear to have adequate support systems, many others feel alone and isolated within those support systems. They have a sense of emptiness, and often futility, in their relationships. However, they may continue such relationships because of the fear of being truly alone.

[18] Two interesting case examples are provided in H. Erickson, 1990b.

will indicate that they wish to have healthier relationships and to find new ways of coping.

They often present themselves in conflict. They indicate that they want to "get rid" of old habits, "stop" destructive behaviors, and be happier. However, when a traditional therapist suggests ways to achieve these goals, the client will sabotage each possibility. This happens because the therapist's suggestions are focused on building positive residual without consideration of undoing negative residual at the same time. The therapist must do a dance with this type of client, moving back and forth between the two types of residual.

Strategies that are particularly useful include reframing (M. Erickson, 1983; Rosen, 1982; Rossi & Ryan, 1992; Zeig,1980), seeding (Zeig, 1980), anecdotes (Zeig, 1980), embedded commands (Zeig, 1980), and storytelling. Analogies or metaphors (Rossi & Ryan, 1992) are not very useful for negative residual below developmental stage 3 (i.e., initiative and guilt), since metaphors require abstract cognition. Developmental residuals related to developmental stages 1 and 2 have incorporated preconceptual thinking and require communication within that context. Although segmentation (Erickson, Rossi, & Rossi, 1976) is extremely helpful for this type of client, it is always necessary to integrate learning as the client progresses.

## SUMMARY

This chapter describes relationships among developmental processes, need satisfaction, attachment, loss, and grief, and the relevance of applying Ericksonian techniques to the aging population. The intent was to provide the reader with a general overview, not an in-depth description, of this model. The aim was to help the reader better understand how to facilitate healing in this population with consideration for affiliated-individuation, mutuality, and self-fulfillment.

### Case Example

Mrs. S.'s daughter had volunteered her mother for a study of persons with Alzheimer's disease and their caregivers. Mrs. S., 85 years of age, had lost her second husband two years earlier and had recently moved from another state so that she could live with her daughter. Mrs. S.'s physician diagnosed her as having clinical depression and early-stage Alzheimer's disease. Her daughter stated that her mother did nothing all day but sit on the sofa and tear up tissues. She refused to participate in family activities, seemed unable to recognize her daughter, and called her son-in-law by her deceased husband's name. The daughter told me that Mrs. S. might not respond to me, and that she refused to leave the house, so I would have to go to her for the first visit, which I agreed to do. When I arrived, Mrs. S. was sitting on the sofa, apparently unaware that I had entered the room. As I approached her, I introduced myself, and told her that I was a nurse and was interested in finding people who would be willing to take part in a study. I briefly described the study and then invited her to participate. She responded with the comment, "Oh no, dearie, I'm too old. I don't have anything to offer anyone any more. I just want to die." Using a surprise technique to induce trance, I responded, "Well, it seems to me that you don't understand the problem. The truth is not that you are too old, but that you are too young!!" I then asked her if she wanted to know how I knew that. For the first time, she looked at me. I explained that I knew that she was too young because the matron of honor at my wedding was 86, and then stated, "So, you see, you are not too old, but too young. But I might just let you participate anyway because you remind me of her. She was a wonderful woman and my husband's grandmother."

Mrs. S. looked surprised, began to smile, and invited me to sit down and let her sign the consent form. I asked her if she would like to tell me a little about herself, anything that came to mind, and encouraged her to feel the sofa on which she was sitting, to get as comfortable as possible, perhaps to feel the back of the sofa against her back and her feet on the floor. I then encouraged her to notice how quietly she was breathing and to feel the delightful rhythm of her strong heartbeat. As she visibly relaxed, I suggested that she might want to be curious about what she would remember and what she would choose to talk about.

She immediately started to talk about a time that she remembered when she was 3 years old. Her voice changed, and she sounded much younger. She said that she felt frightened and alone, that she had been abandoned and a part of her was missing. I reminded her that I was with her, and even as she continued to be curious and explore, my voice would go with her. I again suggested that she might want to feel the comfort of her back against the sofa and her feet on the floor and to remember that her back and feet were connected to the rest of her so that she might be able to let that gentle comfort settle throughout her body.

Again, her voice changed, this time sounding a little older; she was on a ship, running everywhere and looking for someone. She again stated that she was frightened and felt alone; she said that she thought that she was about 3 years old and that she was going to America. I reminded her that my voice would go with her on her journey and that she would remember that the problem was that she was too young, but that she would soon learn that she was safe and that she would grow, and as she grew, she would know new ways to explore and be curious without being afraid. She told me that I was exactly right and that she would be happy to see me again. I suggested that she might be able to remember what she'd learned and to use her information to help herself find ways to be happy. She agreed.

While we were setting a date for our next meeting, her son-in-law and daughter entered the room. She immediately stood up, hugged her daughter, called her by name, and greeted her son-in-law by his name. When I left her, she was standing at the door waving goodbye with a big smile on her face.

The following week, Mrs. S. arrived for the first group session. She sat down and immediately started talking about her family. She stated that she was born in Lithuania, that her father had left her mother and herself when she was a newborn; he'd come to the United States to start a new life. When she was 18 months old, her mother joined her father and she stayed behind with an aunt. When she was about 3 years of age, she and her aunt came to America. She showed us pictures of herself in Lithuania and on Ellis Island. She commented that she had completely forgotten that she wasn't born in this country and found it curious that she should be thinking about it now. She said that she seemed to be on a journey to find herself, and then laughed with pleasure at her own "joke."

In later sessions, Mrs. S. described her fears when she was sent to boarding school and when her first husband died, and her inability to cope when her second husband died. She talked about learning not to trust that someone would be there to help her, about her shame concerning her background, about her feelings of guilt and betrayal (since her parents had worked so hard to make a better life for her). She confessed that she wasn't sure that she had wanted to be a mother, that she hadn't really been able to find a satisfying role for herself in life (although she taught school for nearly 45 years), and that she never felt really close to anyone (even though she needed to be married), always felt isolated from others, and was feeling hopeless when I first met her.

Throughout the sessions, I continued to reframe, to seed ideas, and occasionally to use embedded commands. For example, at one point, she talked about being a real dummy when she was little because she felt lost and ran all over the ship looking for someone (most likely her mother), even though her aunt had warned her that she might get lost. I suggested that she was a very *smart* little girl, she knew what she *needed* and what she wanted, and that this is generally how it is—*we know more about ourselves than anyone else does* no matter who they are—although we don't always know what we know! And wasn't it nice to know that she was no longer such a little girl and that now she could get what she needed and wanted, and that probably there were a lot of commonalities between the little girl and young 85-year-old woman talking with me. I also told her that it would be interesting for her to learn more about what she knows, but doesn't know she knows and that her learning would help her really *know* herself.

Although Mrs. S. occasionally showed signs of disorientation and confusion, her MMSI score and her Memory and Behavior score (measured by the Zarit and Zarit Memory and Behavior Checklist) improved, she was able to participate in family activities, and she enjoyed life for several more years. Her daughter summarized it all in a simple statement: "Thank you for giving me back my mother."

## CONCLUSIONS

Ericksonian philosophy suggests that all humans have the desire to live healthy, happy lives; to find meaning and purpose in their lives; and to become the best that they can be. This holds true even as the body and mind are declining owing to the natural passing of time. When we use strategies that focus on the strengths of our clients, and help them to become more fully alive (even as they approach physical death) and to live their lives to the fullest, we are truly helping them heal and transcend.

When Marc Ian Barasch, a middle-aged journalist, was diagnosed with throat cancer, he tried both traditional and nontraditional treatment modalities. As he describes in his resulting book (Barasch, 1995), he described that there is a universal pattern, which he calls the healing path. According to Barasch, the healing path is analogous to a life transformation. He concluded that the "point of getting well is not necessarily to go back to normal, but to reclaim the soul." This chapter was written in an effort to help practitioners find new ways to help their clients discover the essence of their being, to reclaim their souls.

## References

Ader, R. (Ed.). (1981). *Psychoneuroimmunology*. New York: Academic.

Barasch, M. (1995). *A soul approach to illness: A healing path*. New York: Penguin Books.

Barnfather, J., & Erickson, H. (1989). Construct validity of an aspect of the coping process: Potential adaptation to stress. *Issues in Mental Health Nursing, 10*, 23–40.

Benson, H., & Stark, M. (1996). *Timeless healing: The power and biology of belief*. New York: Scribner's.

Consumers Union (1995). Working out chronic illness. *Consumer Reports on Health, 7*(10), 113–120.

Dafter, R. (1996). Why negative emotions can sometimes be positive. *Advances: The Journal of Mind-Body Health, 12*(2), 6–18.

Dienstfrey, H. (1991). *Where the mind meets the body*. New York: Harper Collins.

Dossey, L. (1993). *Healing words*. San Francisco: Harper Collins.

Erickson, E. (1963). *Childhood and society*. New York: Norton.

Erickson, H. (1975). Personal communication with M. Erickson.

Erickson, H. (1988). Modeling and role-modeling: Ericksonian techniques applied to physiological problems. In J. Zeig & S. Lankton (Eds.), *Developing Ericksonian therapy: State of the art*. New York: Brunner/Mazel.

Erickson, H. (1990a). Self-care knowledge: An exploratory study. *Modeling and role-modeling: Theory, practice and research*, vol. 1, pp. 178–202.

Erickson, H. (1990b). Modeling and role-modeling with psychophysiological problems. In J. Zeig & S. Gilligan (Eds.), *Brief therapy: Myths, methods and metaphors*. New York: Brunner/Mazel.

Erickson, H. (1992). Lower and higher level needs: Affiliation, individuation, and affiliated-individuation. Unpublished manuscript.

Erickson, H., Tomlin, E., & Swaim, M. (1983). *Modeling and role-modeling: A theory and paradigm for nursing*. Englewood Cliffs, NJ: Prentice-Hall.

Erickson, M. (1983). *Healing in hypnosis*. In E. Rossi, M. Ryan, & F. Sharp (Eds.). New York: Irvington.

Erickson, M., Hershman, S., & Secter, I. (1981). *The practical application of medical and dental hypnosis* (first published in 1961). Chicago: Seminars on Hypnosis Publishing.

Erickson, M. H., Rossi, E. L., & Rossi, S. I. (1976). *Hypnotic realities.* New York: Irvington.

Frankl, V. (1984). *Man's search for meaning* (3rd ed.). New York: Simon & Schuster.

Friedman, H., & VandenBos, G. (1992). Disease-prone and self-healing personalities. *Hospital and Community Psychiatry 43*(12), 1177–1179.

Gallager, W. (1993). *The power of place: How our surroundings shape our thoughts, emotions and actions.* New York: Poseidon.

Goleman, D., & Gurin, I. (Eds.). (1993). *Mind-body medicine.* New York: Consumer Books.

*Healthy People 2000: National Health Promotion and Disease Prevention Objectives 1991.* Washington, DC: U.S. Department of Health and Human Services.

Justice, B. (1998). Being well inside the self: A different measure of health. *Advances in Mind-Body Medicine, 14*(1), 61–68.

Kinney, C., & Erickson, H. (1990). Modeling the client's world: A way to holistic care. *Issues in Mental Health Nursing, 11,* 93–108.

Klivington, K. (Ed.). (1997). Information, energy, and mind-body medicine. *Advances: The Journal of Mind-Body Health, 13*(4), 3–36.

Klivington, K. (1998). Information, energy and healing: Challenges to biology and medicine. *Advances: The Journal of Mind-Body Health, 13*(4), 36–42.

Miller, D. (1998). More on "information, energy, and mind-body medicine." *Advances in Mind-Body Medicine, 14*(4), 287–292.

Morris, D. (1998). Illness and health in the postmodern age. *Advances in Mind-Body Medicine, 14*(4), 237–250.

Moskowitz, R. (1992). *Your healing mind.* New York: Morrow.

Moyers, B. (1993). *Healing and the mind.* New York: Doubleday.

Rosen, S. (1982). *My voice will go with you: The teaching tales of Milton H. Erickson.* New York: Norton.

Rossi, E. (1986). *The psychobiology of mind-body healing: New concepts of therapeutic hypnosis.* New York: Norton

Rossi, E., & Ryan, M. (Eds.). (1986). *Mind-body communication in hypnosis: The seminars, workshops, and lectures of Milton H. Erickson* (Vol. 3). New York: Irvington.

Rossi, E., & Ryan, M. (Eds.). (1992). *Creative choice in hypnosis: Milton H. Erickson.* New York: Irvington.

Savva, S. (1998). Toward a cybernetic model of the organism. *Advances in Mind-Body Medicine, 14*(4), 292–301.

Shafer, W. (1998). Incorporating social factors into the mind-body and wellness fields. *Advances in Mind-Body Medicine, 14*(1), 43–60.

Watkins, A. (Ed.). (1997). *Mind-body medicine: A clinician's guide to psychoneuroimmunology.* Edinburgh: Churchill Livingston.

Watzlawick, P. (1967). *Pragmatics of human communication: A study of interactional patterns, pathologies and paradoxes.* New York: Norton.

Watzlawick, P., Weakland, J. & Fisch, R. (1988). *Change: Principles of problem formation and problem resolution.* New York: Norton.

Wickramasekera, I. (1998). Secrets kept from the mind but not the body or behaviors: The unsolved problems of identifying and treating somatization and psychophysiological disease. *Advances in Mind-Body Medicine, 14*(2), 81–98.

Zarit, S., & Zarit, J. (1990). *The memory and behavior problems checklist and the burden interview.* Unpublished manuscript. Pennsylvania State University.

Zeig, J. (Ed.). (1980). *A teaching seminar with Milton H. Erickson.* New York: Brunner/Mazel.

Zeig, J. (1990). Seeding. In J. Zeig & S. Gilligan (Eds.), *Brief therapy: Myths, methods and metaphors,* New York: Brunner/Mazel.

# 21

# Ericksonian Approaches to
# Dissociative Disorders

*Maggie Phillips*

E rickson's collected papers and other publications offer numerous accounts of his study of dissociative phenomena. Yet he rarely wrote about what he called "unusual" dissociation (Erickson, circa 1940/1980), which contributes to such conditions as posttraumatic stress disorder (PTSD), psychogenic amnesia, depersonalization, derealization, and multiple personality disorder (MPD), now called dissociative identity disorder (DID).

Long before it became popular as a topic for discussion, however, Erickson was very interested in the multiple personalities as an opportunity to study alterations in consciousness, along with the development and organization of personality structure and functioning. He wrote several articles (Erickson, circa 1940; Erickson & Kubie, 1939; Erickson & Rapaport, circa 1940/1980) exploring the phenomenon he called "dual personality." In these cases, his identification of secondary, alternative personalities surfaced spontaneously during hypnotic exploration of various neurotic symptoms in patients referred for his consultation.

One of Erickson's more colorful cases was that of "Miss Damon" (Erickson & Kubie, 1939), a 20-year-old psychology student who volunteered for a series of hypnosis experiments, and who suffered from obsessive phobias involving unlocked doors and an inexplicable hatred of cats. During lengthy sessions of automatic writing, she revealed unknowingly, through her written responses to Erickson's questions, that another personality, "Jane Brown," was present and knew the source of Miss Damon's fears. Erickson employed a mirror to stimulate visual hallucination, and through this and other means, "Brownie" helped in retrieving childhood memories related to a traumatic encounter with her grandfather at around the age of 3 years. She brought them to Miss Damon's conscious awareness and assisted in the emotional processing of the traumatic material, which resulted in the permanent resolution of the phobias.

## ERICKSON'S POSITION ON
## DISSOCIATIVE DISORDERS AND MULTIPLICITY

Erickon's diagnosis and understanding of multiplicity differed from the views of current researchers in several ways (Richeport, 1994, pp. 416–417).

1.  He did not find abuse a major etiology; in fact, he never discussed abuse.
2.  He believed that there were only two or three main personalities in most multiples, with additional split-off personality fragments.
3.  He rejected the concept of Hilgard's "hidden observer" and other explanations of subpersonalities, offering instead the principle of multiple unconscious awarenesses of self that occur, much as hypnotic trance has diverse expressions in a given individual.
4.  His clinical data refuted the commonly held belief of an underlying hysterical dynamic and instead suggested a broader psychodynamic basis, including an obsessive-compulsive structure.
5.  He did not involve family members in treatment or inform them of the patient's diagnosis, believing that the family system would adjust to the patient's therapeutic changes.
6.  He did not agree that hypnosis created iatrogenic multiplicity because he did not believe that hypnosis could produce an enduring personality.

Although Erickson did not define dissociative disorders as such, he recognized that the human personality was not "a simple limited unitary organization" and that its structure would reflect the complexity of an individual's experiential background (Erickson, circa 1940/1980, p. 262).

From this perspective, Erickson viewed the existence of separate subpersonalities as a common personality characteristic. This conceptualization is quite compatible with those of his predecessors (Janet, 1887; Prince, 1906/1969) and with those of his contemporaries (Alexander, 1930), as well as with current theories of dissociative personality functioning (Spiegel, 1993), especially the model of the dissociative continuum and ego-state functioning (Phillips & Frederick, 1995; Watkins & Watkins, 1997).

Experts in the field of dissociation agree that resolving dissociation helps to facilitate more integrative functioning (Kluft, 1993; Putnam, 1989; Ross, 1989; Van der Kolk, van der Hart, & Marmar, 1996; Watkins, 1992). Ahead of his time, Erickson had as his goal not to fuse or blend the subpersonalities, or even initially to reduce dissociation, but instead to utilize the secondary personalities as aids to the therapy process (Richeport, 1994). In most cases, he left the amnesia intact until the primary personality could benefit from the important information, skills, and attitudes the alternative ones presented. Then he helped to break down the dissociative barriers to allow the separate personalities and fragments to confront each other.

In practice, Erickson's methodology parallels that of John and Helen Watkins (Watkins & Watkins, 1979, 1991, 1997), who developed ego-state therapy, a hypnotic model designed to identify, activate, and work therapeutically with the aspects of self that are differentiated by the nature of the dissociative barriers that separate them. In normal, highly functioning individuals, the dissociative barriers are minimal and highly flexible, allowing for fluid, integrative functioning. In those with more fragmented, dissociated personalities, the degree of dissociation is greater, and in MPD (DID), the ego states are completely separated from the primary personality. Bur regardless of the degree of dissociation separating the ego states, therapy goals are the same: to resolve internal conflicts that are largely unconscious in order to achieve more cooperative and integrative personality functioning (Watkins & Watkins, 1997).

Like John and Helen Watkins, Erickson (circa 1940/1980; Erickson & Kubie, 1939) believed it was important to contact the subpersonalities, once identified; to communicate with and to accept them; and to form a collaboration or alliance in order to teach them how to help the main personality with its problems. In the case of Ellen (Erickson, circa 1940/ 1980), a 24-year-old married woman who worked as his secretary, Erickson made contact with Mary, the subpersonality, taught her to talk, and motivated her to help Ellen recall several dissociated traumatic memories. This work helped to facilitate the resolution of Ellen's sexual problems with her husband and other behavioral difficulties related to internal fragmentation.

In Erickson's other published case of multiple personality (Erickson & Kubie, 1939), he recognized the protective function of Jane Brown, the alter ego of Miss Damon, and helped the two to recall the painful traumatic incident that appeared to underly her phobic symptoms. In these two instances, he was able to help his patients break down amnestic barriers so that they could share co-consciousness and shift their functioning from alternating personalities to coexisting, cooperative ones.

In an unpublished case, that of Vicky (Haley & Richeport, 1991), Erickson was able to achieve co-consciousness but not integrative functioning. Because one of the secondary personalities was heterosexual and the primary personality was homosexual, with neither wanting to give up control of the self, Erickson suggested that they direct personality functioning during alternate weeks.

Although Erickson did not detail his work with other cases of "unusual" dissociative functioning that did not fit the criteria for MPD, it is likely that he followed his general principles of therapy. These methods involved accepting dissociative and amnestic symptoms as he would any other type of symptoms, utilizing them as assets to therapy, and directing their purpose into more acceptable areas of functioning.

## FOLLOWERS OF ERICKSON AND THEIR APPROACHES

Several students of Erickson's work who participated in his teaching seminars have applied Ericksonian approaches to their work with MPD and dissociative-disorder clients. Jay Haley, for example, followed Erickson's principles when supervising other therapists, and in his own work with a few clients diagnosed with MPD in the 1980s (Grove & Haley, 1993; Richeport, 1994). In one reported case, Haley worked with the supervisor of a therapist who was having difficulty believing the authenticity of his client's multiplicity and who insisted on fusing the subpersonalities who appeared. With Haley's help, the supervisor was able to convince the therapist to accept a secondary personality, utilize its abilities and characteristics as important resources, negotiate communication and collaborative agreements between the personalities, eliminate amnestic episodes, and facilitate co-consciousness (Richeport, 1994).

John Beahrs (1982a, 1982b), another of Erickson's students, has been working more extensively with dissociative and MPD clients in recent years, specializing in work with combat veterans. He includes using an Ericksonian perspective to view the disturbed behavior of his more intractable clients as a type of spontaneous hypnosis. For example, in the case of a severely psychotic woman who was being treated with large doses of antipsychotic medications, Beahrs talked with her as he would with any patient who had entered an altered state as part of a planned hypnotic session. Within one meeting, she had accepted his suggestions that her hypnotic abilities were skills that she would be able to use to greater benefit under her conscious control, and remained virtually free of psychotic symptoms thereafter.

Beahrs (1982a) described using a similar approach with other clients who had disorders of self-identity, including those with MPD. In each case, validating the positive aspects of their symptoms and instructing them to perform them even more functionally led to significant improvements. He wrote extensively about hypnosis as multiplicity (Beahrs, 1982b), basing his views on Hilgard's (1977) work with the "hidden observer" and the Watkinses' study of ego states (Watkins & Watkins, 1979, 1998) or "latent alter-personalities" (Beahrs, 1982b, p. 35). Beahrs' work builds on these views, along with those of Erickson, to suggest that dissociated aspects of the self in a hypnotic state function very similarly to the secondary personalities found in severe dissociative disorders. Since this is the case, their dissociative skills can be utilized, much as hypnotic abilities can.

A third among Erickson's students, Michele Richeport (1994), has written an interesting chapter exploring his methodology as a cross-cultural approach to multiple personality. She points out that Erickson's interest in spirit mediums may have influenced his abilities to diagnose and treat clients with this type of dissociative condition. This is illustrated by the fact that his astute powers of observation and unparalleled understanding of hypnosis and spirit states allowed him to distinguish between shifts in personality functioning and altered states of consciousness. His detection in natural settings of "conflicting responses, reactions, and patterns of behavior" helped him to become acutely alert to unusual behavioral expressions and their alterations (Richeport, 1994, p. 418).

Richeport notes several similarities between Erickson's therapy with multiplicity and the practice of spiritism. Within both perspectives, individuals are encouraged to identify and develop unusual behaviors, such as hallucinations, visions, and spontaneous hypnotic states. They are encouraged to identify and express "other selves" through automatic writing. Secondary personalities are contacted and encouraged to collaborate with the therapist in order to help the main personality with its difficulties, just as spirit guides and entities are employed for similar purposes.

Erickson's views of multiplicity and dissociation now have been extended in Steve Gilligan's self-relations model (Gilligan, 1997). Gilligan's premise is that individuals dissociate from the center core of their beings when it is violated or neglected. They develop a persona in order to protect against the overwhelming pain of these core injuries, which, for some people, becomes their whole identity. According to his view, denial of the central core produces suffering, which, in turn, necessitates the use of further defenses and precipitates further dissociation from the authentic center. This kind of dissociation results in a separation of the cognitive self from the somatic self. Gilligan's solution is to help an individual respond to dissociative symptoms that are alienating by viewing the symptoms as a "call" to return to the original core through development of an integrated, relational self. This integrated self connects the "sponsorship capacities of the cognitive self with the life-giving 'fressen energies' of the somatic self" (Gilligan, 1997, p. 27). Gilligan's self-relations model is true to Erickson's belief that the "other selves" created by dissociation are to be used as resources to accomplish the goal of therapy, which, in this case, is the resolution of symptoms through relationship with these disconnected selves to create a less fragmented, more authentic self.

Other Ericksonians have contributed to a solution-oriented approach to the problems resulting from disruptive dissociation. Yvonne Dolan (1991, 1994) has examined extensively the treatment of the dissociative difficulties related to PTSD from childhood sexual abuse. She (Dolan, 1994) strongly endorses Erickson's approach of discovery, contact, and collaboration by reminding readers that eliciting traumatic memory without simultaneously eliciting the resources needed to provide a corrective experience for the client amounts to a "rape of the unconscious" (Erickson & Rossi, 1989).

Like Erickson, she perceives dissociation as a separation from important self-resources that must be repaired by creating new associational bridges. In part, this is accomplished by inviting the client to consider questions focused on identifying solutions in the present and future rather than focusing on associational links to past trauma. Examples are, "What will be the first (smallest) sign that things are getting better, that sexual abuse is having less of an effect on your current life?" and "What will you be doing differently when the sexual abuse is less of a current problem in your life?" (Dolan, 1994, p. 407).

Dolan suggests that solution-focused therapy and related techniques help traumatized clients gain more control of symptoms, while providing relief and stabilization. Additionally, she proposes that methods that focus on present resources and future goals will help restabilize clients long enough for them to complete developmental tasks, help establish the inner resources needed for psychological survival of the retrieval and processing of traumatic events, and hasten the integration and resolution of trauma. Her techniques (Dolan, 1991), based on solution-oriented approaches developed by other Ericksonians (De Shazer, 1985, 1988; O'Hanlon & Weiner-Davis, 1989), include the utilization of associational cues to promote comfort and safety; rituals and therapeutic directives for containment, self-nurturing, and self-expression; and experiential bridges that help to heal dissociative splits.

Although Dolan primarily addresses PTSD rather than dissociative disorders, there is general agreement that the dissociative responses that contribute to the formation of MPD also contribute to PTSD, although they tend to result in less complete inner fragmentation and personality division (Phillips & Frederick, 1995; Spiegel, 1993; Watkins & Watkins, 1997). Other Ericksonians have contributed to the literature on the application of Erickson's principles to posttraumatic and dissociative difficulties. They include various positive utilizations of posttraumatic/dissociative symptoms (Phillips, 1993, 1995b; Phillips & Frederick, 1995) and trauma-related transferences (Phillips, 1997b); the use of multilevel messages, homework assignments, and therapeutic metaphors to motivate clients to deal with symptoms and various aspects of trauma (Alon, 1985); the employment of therapeutic ritual to resolve traumatic experiences and facilitate new identity (Gilligan, 1993); the utilization of multilevel metaphors to change affect, attitude, behavior, self-image, and identity (Lankton & Lankton, 1989); and applications of indirect suggestion and metaphor to encourage strengths and the integration of rape trauma, and to revive a sense of mastery (Brown, 1985).

## AN INTEGRATIVE ERICKSONIAN APPROACH TO
## DISSOCIATIVE CONDITIONS

Recently, drawing on my Ericksonian training, as well as my background in more classical hypnosis, I developed a model for the treatment of the dissociative range of clinical conditions, including PTSD, MPD/DID, and the dissociative disorders. This four-stage model, as described by my coauthor and me (Phillips & Frederick, 1995), is called the SARI model. This is an acronym for the following tasks of therapy: (1) *Safety* and *Stabilization*; (2) *Accessing* and *Activation*; (3) *Resolution* and *Renegotiation*; (4) *Integration* and new *Identity*. The SARI model closely parallels the basic sequence of recovery from trauma identified by numerous experts in the trauma/dissociation field, even though slightly different terms are used (Courtois, 1991; Herman, 1992; Kluft, 1993).

During the first stage of work, the therapeutic focus is on the use of direct and indirect hypnosis for mastery and ego strengthening. Strategies range from indirect techniques, such as metaphor, seeding, calibration, and utilization of posttraumatic symptoms, to formal hypnotic techniques, such as ideomotor/ideosensory signaling, age progression, and positive regression.

Once the client has achieved a reasonable degree of *safety* and *stabilization* within the therapy situation, as well as in everyday functioning, the next task is to *access* the origins of dissociative conditions while *activating* inner resources to provide corrective experiences. Indirect approaches, such as "safe remembering" (Dolan, 1991), are used, along with more formal techniques, such as direct and indirect ego-state therapy. The ego-state perspective is especially important in cases where there is serious internal fragmentation that results in self-identity problems. During this stage, "other selves" or subpersonalities are identified and activated. The therapist forms alliances with these ego states, which are always presumed to be helpful resources (Erickson, circa 1940/1980; Watkins & Watkins, 1979).

The "R" stage, which is often interwoven with the tasks of the previous stage, involves *reassociating* dissociated experiences and parts of the self with the client's mainstream consciousness. Within this process, the client connects with split-off subselves, and secondary personalities are also reconnected with each other. Conflicts between ego states that drive trauma-related symptoms and contribute to continued dissociation are *resolved*, while aspects of past traumatic events are *renegotiated*.

In the final stage, the client is helped to *integrate* therapy experiences, as well as to achieve more integrated personality functioning. During this time, the need for dissociation is reduced, more complete co-consciousness is attained, and a more cooperative coexistence of conflicting ego states and alternative personalities is accomplished. As this occurs, the client is helped to expand identity and integrate positive future orientation more fully.

SARI is an integrative model because, although it is based on Ericksonian principles and concepts, it integrates powerful aspects of other therapy traditions, including hypnoanalysis, to provide comprehensive treatment that can promote fuller, more integrative functioning of the self.

## CLINICAL CASE EXAMPLE

Jennifer, as reported elsewhere (Phillips & Frederick, 1995; Phillips, 1997b), a 45-year-old professional woman, was transferred to me by her previous therapist because both Jennifer and the therapist felt that they were at an impasse in her therapy. Jennifer had been given a diagnosis of DID/MPD, which was supported by her current clinical presentation and past history. On disability compensation and unable to work because of her numerous symptoms, she was interested in using hypnosis to explore internal aspects of herself and to resolve experiences of physical and emotional abuse that had begun as early in childhood as she could remember. Jennifer believed that these abuse experiences had contributed to her sense of internal fragmentation, her amnesia for long periods of time in the past, and her tendency to "lose time" in the present.

Although Jennifer was anxious to begin using hypnosis to explore intrusive flashbacks and "body memories" that were clearly contributing to her current difficulties in functioning, she was at high risk for destabilization. She reported frequent suicidal thoughts and depressive feelings even though on medication, mutilated herself several times per week, and engaged in daily bingeing and purging cycles.

I explained the SARI model to Jennifer and clarified that our first priority was to help her to achieve a sense of mastery over her symptoms during therapy sessions, as well as in her everyday life. I expressed my concern that the use of formal hypnosis at that time might worsen her situation, especially since she and her referring therapist had told me that previous inner exploration of alter personalities seemed to result in confusion and the escalation of self-destructive behaviors.

As we discussed what our plan would be, I said to her, "Jennifer, you are a highly intelligent woman. I would insult you if I told you that I was going to repeat the techniques your previous therapist used, ones that didn't work then, and would likely do nothing more now than retraumatize you." Jennifer replied, "Well, since you put it that way, of course, we can't do that. But what *can* we do? I feel like I'm spinning out of control." I immediately reassured her that whatever we did would be designed to help her gain control, and that the control might come subtly and gradually, or it might come dramatically, but she would be sure that she was finding control because her symptoms would let us know by subsiding. My carefully worded assertions of certainty against the backdrop of her chronic uncertainty had a significant impact, and I had both her attention and her cooperation.

I told her that we would be trying a new type of hypnosis to work with the inner parts of her personality initially that would approach this contact more scientifically with less chance of risk. When she agreed to this, I began to "talk through" to generic "other selves" that might be connected to the suicidal thoughts and cutting behaviors. I told them how important I believed they were; that only they, and they alone, could help Jennifer move past her impasse; and that we needed their help. I further explained to them that they could demonstrate their considerable power by decreasing her symptoms, and that I realized that without their participation, we would not be able to accomplish this. I established ideosensory signals (Phillips, 1995a), suggesting that the alters connected with these symptoms could demonstrate their control by increasing or decreasing sensations of severe pain in her hips, which Jennifer had been complaining about, in response to the questions I asked. To her surprise, Jennifer reported the desired decrease in discomfort as a "yes" signal. I continued in this manner until I had established a positive connection with several inner states and negotiated agreements to control the suicidal thoughts and cutting behavior. The terms of the contract were designed to benefit the as yet unknown secondary personalities, as well as the primary personality.

Within four sessions, cutting had ceased and other self-destructive behavior had diminished. We continued to work on various self-care and health issues for several more sessions until she was more stabilized. At that point, Jennifer commented that she felt curious about what more we could achieve with direct access to the parts that had been helping us so far. As we began our second-stage work, Jennifer was more grounded and comfortable in contrast to her earlier demeanor of anxiety and desperation.

We then began an informal assessment of her hypnotic responses. Jennifer told me she had never really felt comfortable in her body during previous hypnosis sessions. I reassured her that we would help her to find out how she could relax her body automatically without learning anything new. Although she was intrigued by this idea, as we began progressive relaxation, she complained that she could not experience her body's relaxing because whenever she tried, she floated away from her body. I congratulated her on having an excellent hypnotic response and suggested that she enjoy that "floating far away" feeling for a while and then find out whether she could come back into her body for a few seconds to enjoy the contrast. After a pause, she told me that she found going back and forth interesting, and then easier and easier. I invited her to continue practicing bridging between the dissociated state and reconnection with her body.

After a few sessions, dissociative responses were no longer distracting and she could choose to connect for longer periods with various body sensations, utilizing them to identify several parts of her inner system that appeared to be related to these somatic expressions. We then began a period of formal ego-state therapy, activating several subpersonalities that could communicate either verbally or through ideomotor or ideosensory signals. Altogether, we worked with about six child alters, ranging in age from 4 to 17, and also with four or five adult alters, including two main helpers and several secondary personalities apparently connected to self-destructive behaviors. Numerous traumatic events were accessed through the revelations of these ego states, and the more mature secondary personalities were encouraged to provide nurturing, corrective experiences. For example, two young adolescent subpersonalities longed to look more attractive by losing weight and giving more attention to grooming. Although this was not a need of the other ego states, an adult state agreed to spend some part of every morning supervising the "adolescents" in reading women's magazines for ideas about finding a new hairstyle, brushing her hair, and riding an exercise bicycle. More cooperative relationships were established among all the alters as they successfully helped with self-care, developed more positive eating behaviors, and contributed to healthier interpersonal relationships. When a friend offered Jennifer a free airline ticket to Spain, she was eager to test the gains she had made.

When Jennifer returned, she shared many positive experiences with me. For the first time in her life, she said, she had felt like a "normal person," interacting well with others and feeling little anxiety or depression.

It appeared that she had been able to sustain the previous changes we had made and that we were in the "resolution" phase of therapy. Within a few weeks, however, her functioning began to decline. She reported a return of self-punishing thoughts and inner voices, along with suicidal thoughts and the urge to hurt herself. Formal hypnosis sessions that had once been helpful seemed to trigger further fragmentations. The subpersonalities, previously cooperative and expressive, now reported panic and exhaustion.

During our sessions, Jennifer became quiet and more passive. When I commented on this change, Jennifer replied that she didn't see much sense in talking, and that I needed to put her into hypnosis, talk to the parts inside, and tell them what to do. Recognizing this as a regressive reaction even though I did not fully understand what had precipitated it, I decided to utilize her recent healthy experiences in Spain as a model for a new kind of partnership. I told her that I believed we needed to evaluate what we had been doing in light of her recent difficulties, and that during this reevaluation, we would not be using hypnosis, ego-state therapy, or any other techniques until we had a solid understanding of where we were and where we were going together.

Although Jennifer was alarmed, I told her that I felt that our work was not supportive of the experiences she had had in Spain. Instead, we were treating her as someone depressed, someone whose pathology needed "fixing," rather than as the carefree woman who had had a fabulous vacation. I clarified that I did not feel we had a joint partnership and that we needed to create an environment where we could be equal partners, supporting the ways in which she had felt equal to people with whom she had interacted in Spain and equal to the various adventures she had had. During the next few weeks, Jennifer made several changes. She began to come prepared with a list of goals for every session. She remembered and shared dreams, which she had never done before in therapy, since her dreams up until then were highly fragmented nightmares that had little continuity.

Afterward, I initiated very little direct internal work. Instead, we focused on tasks that appeared to be more integrative, such as discussing weekly solution-oriented plans for herself based on therapy homework assignments. As her functioning improved and restabilized, material about infancy and early childhood experiences surfaced through dreams, inner awarenesses, and journal writing. We speculated that her prior regressive episode might have been related to her first four years of shuttling back and forth between a loving, nurturing grandmother and her unstable, sadistically abusive mother. The time in Spain seemed to symbolize her grandmother's care, while her unsuccessful transition to her relatively isolated, empty daily life appeared to represent abandonment to her mother's misuse and neglect.

With this recognition, we were able to process information related to Jennifer's early years of life and to complete many related developmental tasks that were needed to sustain a constant level of good self-care. These included negative affect regulation, work on self and object permanence and constancy, and the development of more consistent, yet flexible, interpersonal boundaries. Utilizing her positive, loving relationships with her three nephews, she learned to transfer much of the healthy caretaking she demonstrates with them to nurture the more immature and primitive parts of herself. As she began to feel less overwhelmed by negative affect and somatic sensations, Jennifer was also able to participate in network chiropractic care, which allowed her to resolve many somatic symptoms, form a more positive body image, and initiate gradual weight reduction.

A week before the completion of this chapter, Jennifer left for a two-month retreat in Mexico. She commented that she was amazed by all the changes we had made. She felt a more solid integration of therapy work than ever before and told me she was filled with hope about "finally growing up." As we closed the session, she told me she was looking forward to examining the possibility of returning to work, which she had postponed until she felt strong enough to sustain a consistently positive future orientation, a milestone she believed she had finally reached.

## ADDITIONAL CONSIDERATIONS

Although dissociative-disorder clients present some of the most fascinating challenges to clinicians, they are also some of the most difficult to treat. Even the most experienced practitioners can find themselves overwhelmed by the multiplicity of problems and depleted by the complexity of demands. Ericksonian approaches can ease the treatment process in several important ways for both client and therapist, but as Erickson himself said, "Hypnosis is not a miracle worker" (Erickson, circa 1940/1980, p. 264).

Ericksonian techniques are not presented here as a substitute for solid training and supervision in the diagnosis and treatment of trauma and dysfunctional dissociative conditions. However, when used within a therapy framework that is grounded in principles of what makes any psychotherapy effective, including secure boundaries, clear roles, and well-formed, ethical treatment plans, they can be invaluable interventions.

## SUMMARY AND CONCLUSIONS

Several important principles have been presented in this chapter. First, Erickson did not perceive multiple personality and unusual forms of dissociation as forms of pathology, but rather as unique phenomena that cause difficulty because of the amnesia and disconnection they generate. This premise leads to his principle of utilization, which I view as the cornerstone of treatment with this difficult, yet rewarding, population.

Erickson's utilization approach is an indirect form of hypnosis that works well with people who may be unresponsive to more direct techniques. Through utilization, the therapist accepts and cooperates with all the client's attitudes, behaviors, and symptoms, no matter how obstructive to the therapy process they may appear to be. From this point of view, negative characteristics and symptoms are construed as assets rather than as resistances to be overcome. Alon (1985) has pointed out that this approach of acceptance may be particularly helpful with traumatized individuals because it does not require initial change, which can threaten their need for control.

When applying the utilization principle to therapy with dissociative populations, positive utilizations are particularly effective with the presenting personality style; beliefs about trauma, abuse, dissociation, and recovery; posttraumatic and dissociative symptoms; and ego states and secondary personalities as resources. With more complex chronic dissociative problems, it is also essential to utilize the psychological defenses and transference issues that inevitably arise as unique opportunities to understand the creative adaptive maneuvers that have developed in an attempt to protect what Gilligan (1997) has called the "central core" of the self.

In the case of Jennifer, utilization was used at crucial times throughout the four stages of therapy. During the initial stage, I employed her obvious intelligence and her need for control to form and strengthen our alliance. Some of her dissociative symptoms were also utilized to achieve safety and stabilization through indirect contact with internal parts of her personality system. During the second stage of work, I used her dissociative responses to formal hypnosis to teach her how to achieve mastery over the dissociative process so that she could achieve a more complete body connection and mental focus. From there, we were able to activate and work with fragmented aspects of her personality to resolve conflicts that contributed to symptoms and originated from terrifying abuse experiences in childhood. During the third stage of work, we weathered a debilitating regression by utilizing a growth-enhancing vacation experience and negative transference reactions to form a more mature, mutual partnership. Now, as we prepare to enter the fourth stage of treatment, we continue to take advantage of various challenges in her everyday life to identify developmental tasks that require completion and contribute to her new identity as a more cohesive, competent adult who can finally look forward to a satisfying future.

A second principle is the use of methods that, from the beginning of therapy, emphasize the importance of strengthening clients and helping them to gain a positive sense of control that stimulates changes in desirable directions (Beahrs, 1982b). I have found that focusing more on strengths than on pathology, and more on solutions than on causality, is integral to achieving consistent progress in therapy.

Third, it is essential to address internal fragmentation and self-identity issues both directly and indirectly. As Beahrs (1982b) has pointed out, "The first dilemma posed by dissociative disorder to the clinician is the question of whether it is meaningful and useful for him to perceive alter-personalities and their ego state equivalents within a given patient as having a unique sense of identity of their own" (p. 111). Ultimately, because every client is a whole that is composed of many parts, the issue of whether to address interventions to the whole personality or to the component parts of the client's internal system can be answered only by assessing which approach will be the most beneficial for the client and most likely to facilitate cohesion at a given time.

The degree of permeability of the boundaries that separate personality states from each other and from the main personality must also be considered in decisions about working with secondary personalities versus the personality as a whole. Erickson perceived that "no matter how rigid the boundaries, they are not absolute ... and will shift from time to time" (Beahrs, 1982b, p. 86). This is in agreement with the Watkinses' (Watkins & Watkins, 1979) observation that the major distinction between common ego-state problems and more severe dissociative disorders relates to poor information exchange between alternative personalities, which is governed by dissociative and amnestic barriers. Treatment methods, therefore, should be designed to maximize the internal flow of information.

In my work with Jennifer and other clients like her, I've found that when incomplete early developmental issues take precedence, there may be significant impairment to the formation of a cohesive self-constellation. Direct work with ego states may under these circumstances evoke more fragmented, archaic functioning. This can be corrected by addressing specific developmental tasks for the whole personality, or in more indirect ways with individual ego states that need this type of intervention. In other cases, dissociative clients with strong fears of loss of control or significant trust issues related to past trauma or prior, unsuccessful therapy may oppose direct access to inner personality states. These and other situations lend themselves to the use of indirect ego-state therapy techniques (Phillips & Frederick, 1995). Thus, the Ericksonian principle of indirection can be invaluable in navigating the tumultuous waters of dissociated personality structures.

Fourth, in working with dissociative conditions, it is paramount that the roles of the therapist and client be clearly identified and the therapeutic boundaries carefully drawn. Results of research (Phillips, 1998) recently conducted to study individuals who have achieved exceptional recovery from childhood abuse and trauma indicate that a strong working relationship between the client and therapist is highly correlated with ratings of a successful individual therapy experience. Unlike traditional approaches, Erickson advocated the cooperation principle, which suggests that therapy experiences "unfold from an experiential, interpersonal encounter in which therapist aligns with client, thereby enabling both parties to become increasingly receptive to each other" (Gilligan, 1987, p. 11). This kind of cooperative alignment seems to fit the criteria for the neutral therapeutic stance called for in working with traumatic memory issues (Phillips, 1997a), where the therapist must not harm the client by either disbelieving or encouraging belief in recollections of childhood trauma and abuse that may or may not have occurred. In Erickson's reported work with "unusual" dissociation, emphasis was always placed on reconnecting dissociated personality states and helping them to do the work that was necessary to strengthen personality functioning, rather than on authenticating retrieved memory experiences. He was not afraid to take strong positions with the client or with secondary personalities to achieve these important functional goals (Richeport, 1994).

### Ericksonian Principles and the
### Treatment of Dissociative Disorders

- A four-stage sequential framework called the SARI model has been suggested for the integration of Ericksonian with other hypnotic and nonhypnotic approaches to deliver comprehensive treatment to this challenging population.
- The principle of utilization is the foundation for helping dissociative clients to achieve more integrative functioning. This includes positive utilization of the client's unique personality style, presenting values, attitudes, and beliefs, as well as of posttraumatic symptoms, defenses, and transference reactions.
- It is essential to emphasize strengthening more than pathology, and solutions more than causality, to sustain consistent therapeutic progress.
- When addressing internal fragmentation and self-identity issues, indirect approaches can be helpful in making the initial contact with secondary personalities, using them as important therapeutic resources, orchestrating collaboration between personality states and the total personality, and addressing necessary developmental issues, especially when control and trust are overriding concerns.
- Erickson's emphasis on mutual cooperation is a helpful paradigm for clarifying the roles of client and therapist, and the boundaries between the client and therapist and between secondary and primary personalities. His focus on functional goals, rather than on memory issues, has stood the test of time and remains an important therapeutic legacy.

### References

Alexander, F. (1930). The psychoanalysis of the total personality. Nervous and Mental Disease Monographs, no. 52.

Alon, N. (1985). An Ericksonian approach to the treatment of chronic posttraumatic stress disorder patients. In J. Zeig (Ed.), *Ericksonian psychotherapy, Vol. II: Clinical applications* (pp. 307–326). New York: Brunner/Mazel.

Beahrs, J. (1971). The hypnotic psychotherapy of Milton H. Erickson. *American Journal of Clinical Hypnosis, 14,* 73–90.

Beahrs., J. (1982a). Understanding Erickson's approach. In J. Zeig (Ed.), *Ericksonian approaches to hypnosis and psychotherapy* (pp. 58–84). New York: Brunner/Mazel.

Beahrs, J. (1982b). *Unity and multiplicity.* New York: Brunner/Mazel.

Brown, R. (1985). The treatment of two cases of rape using Ericksonian hypnosis. In J. Zeig (Ed.), *Ericksonian psychotherapy, Vol. II: Clinical applications* (pp. 307–326). New York: Brunner/Mazel.

Courtois, C. (1991). Theory, sequencing, and strategy in treating adult survivors. *New Directions for Mental Health Services, 51,* 47–60.

De Shazer, S. (1985). *Keys to solution in brief therapy.* New York: Norton.

De Shazer, S. (1988). *Clues: Investigating solutions in brief therapy.* New York: Norton.

Dolan, Y. (1991). *Resolving sexual abuse.* New York: Norton.

Dolan, Y. (1994). An Ericksonian perspective on the treatment of sexual abuse. In J. Zeig (Ed.), *Ericksonian methods: The essence of the story* (pp. 395–414). New York: Brunner/Mazel.

Erickson, M. H. (circa 1940/1980). The clinical discovery of a dual personality. In E. Rossi (Ed.), *The collected papers of Milton H. Erickson on hypnosis, Vol. III* (pp. 261–270). New York: Irvington.

Erickson, M. H., & Kubie, L. (1939/1980). Permanent relief of an obsessional phobia by means of commmunication with an unsuspected dual personality. In E. Rossi (Ed.), *The collected papers of Milton H. Erickson, Vol. III* (pp. 231–260). New York: Irvington.

Erickson, M. H., & Rapaport, D. (circa 1940). Findings on the nature of the personality structures in two different dual personalities by means of projective and psychometric tests. In E. Rossi (Ed.), *The collected papers of Milton H. Erickson, Vol. III* (pp. 271–286). New York: Irvington.

Erickson, M. H., & Rossi, E. L. (1989). *The February man: Evolving consciousness and identity in hypnotherapy.* New York: Brunner/Mazel.

Gilligan, S. (1987). *Therapeutic trances: The cooperation principle in Ericksonian hypnotherapy.* New York: Norton.

Gilligan, S. (1993). Therapeutic rituals: Passages into new identities. In S. Gilligan & R. Price (Eds.), *Therapeutic conversations.* New York: Norton.

Gilligan, S. (1997). *The courage to love: Principles and practices of self-relations psychotherapy.* New York: Norton.

Grove, D., & Haley, J. (1993). *Conversation in therapy: Popular problems and uncommon solutions.* New York: Norton.

Haley, J., & Richeport, M. (Eds.). (1991). *Erickson on multiple personality* (audiotaped conversation). New York: Norton.

Herman, J. (1992). *Trauma and recovery*. New York: Basic Books.

Hilgard, E. (1977). *Divided consciousness: Multiple controls in human thought and action*. New York: Wiley.

Janet, P. (1887). L'anesthésie systematisée et la dissociation des phénomènes psycho-logiques. *Revue philosophique, 23*, 449–472.

Kluft, R. (1993). Clinical approaches to the integration of multiple personalities. In R. P. Kluft & C. Fine (Eds.), *Clinical perspectives on multiple personality disorder* (pp. 101–133). Washington, DC: American Psychiatric Press.

Lankton, C., & Lankton, S. (1989). *Tales of enchantment: Goal-oriented metaphors for adults and children in therapy*. New York: Brunner/Mazel.

O'Hanlon, W., & Weiner-Davis, M. (1989). *In search of solutions*. New York: Norton.

Phillips, M. (1993). Turning symptoms into allies: Utilization approaches with post-traumatic symptoms. *American Journal of Clinical Hypnosis, 35*(3), 241–249.

Phillips, M. (1995a). Our bodies, our selves: Treating the somatic expressions of trauma with ego-state therapy. *American Journal of Clinical Hypnosis, 38*(2), 109–121.

Phillips, M. (1995b). "The face": From post-traumatic symptom to therapeutic ally. *Hypnos, 22*(1), 6–11.

Phillips, M. (1997a). The importance of role integrity for therapists working with traumatic memory issues. Paper presented at the 1997 Fall Meeting of the International Society for the Study of Dissociation, San Francisco.

Phillips, M. (1997b). Spinning straw into gold: Utilization of transferential resources to strengthen the hypnotic relationship. *American Journal of Clinical Hypnosis, 40*(2), 118–129.

Phillips, M., & Frederick, C. (1995). *Healing the divided self: Clinical and Ericksonian hypnotherapy for post-traumatic and dissociative conditions*. New York: Norton.

Prince, M. (1906/1969). *The dissociation of a personality*. Westport, CT: Greenwood.

Putnam, F. (1989). *Diagnosis and treatment of multiple personality disorder*. New York: Guilford.

Richeport, M. (1994). Erickson's approach to multiple personality: A cross-cultural perspective. In J. Zeig (Ed.), *Ericksonian methods: The essence of the story* (pp. 413–442). New York: Brunner/Mazel.

Ross, C. (1989). *Multiple personality disorder*. New York: Wiley.

Spiegel, D. (1993). Dissociation and trauma. In D. Spiegel (Ed.), *Dissociative disorders: A clinical review* (pp. 117–129). Lutherville, MD: Sidran.

Van der Kolk, B., van der Hart, O., & Marmar, C. (1996). Dissociation and information processing in posttraumatic stress disorder. In B. van der Kolk, A. McFarlane, & L. Weisaeth (Eds.), *Traumatic stress: The effects of overwhelming experience on mind, body, and society* (pp. 303–325). New York: Guilford.

Watkins, J. (1992). *The practice of clinical hypnosis, Vol. II: Hypnoanalytic techniques.* New York: Irvington.

Watkins, J., & Watkins, H. (1979). The theory and practice of ego-state therapy. In H. Grayson (Ed.), *Short term approaches to psychotherapy* (pp. 176–220). New York: Wiley.

Watkins, J., & Watkins, H. (1991). Hypnosis and ego-state therapy. In P. A. Keller & S. R. Heyman (Eds.), *Innovations in clinical practice, Vol. 10* (pp. 23–37). Sarasota, FL: Professional Resources Exchange.

Watkins, J., & Watkins, H. (1997). *Ego states: Theory and therapy.* New York: Norton.

## Suggested Readings

Dolan, Y. (1991). *Resolving sexual abuse.* New York: Norton.

Erickson, M. H. (circa 1940/1980). The clinical discovery of a dual personality. In E. Rossi (Ed.), *The collected papers of Milton H. Erickson on hypnosis, Vol. III* (pp. 261–270). New York: Irvington.

Erickson, M. H., & Kubie, L. (1939/1980). Permanent relief of an obsessional phobia by means of commmunication with an unsuspected dual personality. In E. Rossi (Ed.), *The collected papers of Milton H. Erickson, Vol. III* (pp. 231–260). New York: Irvington.

Herman, J. (1992). *Trauma and recovery.* New York: Basic Books.

Phillips, M., & Frederick, C. (1995). *Healing the divided self: Clinical and Ericksonian hypnotherapy for post-traumatic and dissociative conditions.* New York: Norton.

Richeport, M. (1994). Erickson's approach to multiple personality: A cross-cultural perspective. In J. Zeig (Ed.), *Ericksonian methods: The essence of the story* (pp. 413–442). New York: Brunner/Mazel.

Spiegel, D. (Ed.). (1993). *Dissociative disorders: A clinical review.* Lutherville, MD: Sidran.

Van der Kolk, B., McFarlane, A., & Weisaeth, L. (Eds.). (1996). *Traumatic stress: The effects of overwhelming experience on mind, body, and society.* New York: Guilford.

Watkins, J., & Watkins, H. (1997). *Ego states: Theory and therapy.* New York: Norton.

# 22

# Mandatory Counseling: Helping Those Who Do Not Want to Be Helped

*Dan Short*

T here are two types of clients, those who want assistance and those who have been told to get help. Correspondingly, dysfunction can come in the form of a chronic inward struggle or as a chronic struggle with social forces. The latter is an externalized disturbance that results in troubled relationships or criminal activity (e.g., acts of violence, sexual abuse, neglect, or drug abuse). Thus, the suffering caused by the disorder is felt more by society than by the individual. When the individual does feel pain, his or her attention is cast outward so the person does not blame himself or herself but blames others for the misery. This type of behavior is described in the fourth edition of the *Diagnostic and Statistical Manual of Mental Disorders* (*DSM*-IV) under a variety of personality disorders. In contrast, voluntary clientele typically suffer from neuroticism, an inner conflict that is most bothersome to the person who has internalized the problem.

The difference between these two patterns of response is of such significance that a clinical intervention that works with one may only increase the level of dysfunction in the other. That is not to say that the goals of therapy must differ, but rather that the manners in which clients respond to the influence of the therapist can radically differ. The following information is intended to supplement the training of professionals who provide mental health services to persons who have externalized disturbances. The skills outlined in this chapter are not meant to stand alone as an independent treatment modality; instead, the following is a set of guidelines that distinguish the manner in which therapy is delivered.


## BEGIN WITH A COMMITMENT TO CHANGE

It is a mistake to assume that the client automatically will be receptive to information presented during therapy.[1] By definition, this type of client is not interested in self-improvement. He or she may perceive therapy as a waste of time or as a threat to his or her identity. Therefore, it is necessary to instill a belief in the importance of treatment, and thus a willingness to change. Change is more likely to occur when the therapist begins by securing the client's commitment to change *his or her* behavior (Zanna & Cooper, 1974).

C:      (*Sarcastic tone of voice.*) I'll just listen and you can tell me whatever I need to know.

T:      If you have a problem you want to tell me about and work on, then I will meet with you. If you cannot tell me about a specific problem related to your behavior, then there is no reason for us to meet.

C:      (*Angry.*) I have to be here. The courts are making me come!

T:      If you have legal problems, I will give you the number of a lawyer. I only work with counseling problems.

C:      (*Long silence.*) Well ... maybe I do have a problem with my temper ...

Declining to work with a person who refuses treatment is perhaps the simplest way to evoke a commitment to change. As stated by Milton Erickson (Haley, 1985), "Whenever you start depriving people of anything, they are going to insist that you give it to them" (p. 123). Another

---

[1] For a discussion of Erickson's view on this issue, see J. K. Zeig, 1985, pp. 110–111.

option is to continue to meet but refuse to begin therapy until a commitment to change is made (i.e., pretherapy meetings are not counted toward court requirements). Once a verbal commitment is obtained, it can be further ratified through the signing of a contract, prepayment for future sessions, or some other effortful activity. Motivation is crucial to the success of mandatory counseling, and, as research has shown, the more energy a person invests in an activity, the more likely it is that the person will view it as important (Aronson & Mills, 1959; Bem, 1967; Deutsch & Gerard, 1959).

## REQUIRE A CONFESSION

This type of client spends a lot of time and energy hiding the reality of the disturbance from others and himself or herself. The client is reluctant to admit his or her own shortcomings and instead blames the behavior on others. As long as someone else can be identified as the "bad guy," the client does not feel the need to examine his or her own inadequacies (Carver & Scheier, 1981). With this façade intact, the client is not motivated to change anything about himself or herself, and is likely to dismiss or ignore therapeutic interventions. A confession is important because such clients need to focus on their problematic behaviors (Petty & Cacioppo, 1986), rather than on the idealized images they have of themselves.

It should be recognized that the client has not yet admitted to having a problem, if the problematic behavior is framed in a past tense. A description of that which one "used to do" carries little emotional significance and is, therefore, an empty confession.

C:   It has been six months since I pushed her. I know that was wrong and now I'm here to learn *whatever* I can. (*Smiles.*)

T:   I need to find out how aware you are of the damage caused by your original act of violence. What problems would you guess still exist after that single act of violence, over six months ago?

C:   Well ... she still ducks her head whenever I move my hand real quickly. That really bothers me.

T:   So she does not feel safe with you?

C:   I guess not.

As the client tells the therapist about the problems caused by the behavior, there is an increased willingness to accept new ideas, much more so than if the client had been lectured by the therapist.

When the client is too quick to elaborate on or share insights regarding a "special" problem, then you may be dealing with a decoy. As a rule, the most serious problems are withheld from the therapist rather than described so freely. For a person who spends most of his or her time hiding thoughts and feelings, self-exposure is not simple.

C:     I've never told anyone this before, but I think I might have been abducted by a UFO. I think my memory may have been washed out so that I would not remember the event. Do you know anything about these kinds of problems?

T:     UFOs are a fascinating topic, and I'm sure I could talk with you about it for hours, but that is not why we are here. Are you willing to discuss with me the problems caused by your behavior?

This client never again expressed a concern about UFOs. Less important problems tend to disappear when they no longer serve a purpose.

A plea of insanity is a fairly useless confession and, therefore, unacceptable. When an individual is convinced that he or she has no control over his or her behavior, that person is excusing himself or herself from any attempt to use good judgment or moral reasoning. The client should not be given the opportunity to label the behavior as uncontrollable. Once this belief is stated, the client becomes less amenable to change. Instead, the client is asked to admit to mistakes. A bad decision, rather than some nonvoluntary force, is always easier to change.

## ADHERE TO PREDETERMINED
## RULES AND PROCEDURES

A true expert has the ability to make a difficult and complicated task seem simple because of the ability to "troubleshoot." In other words, he or she acts to prevent bad situations from occurring. This skill is essential when helping individuals who have a problem with respecting others. A useful method for preventing unnecessary problems is to make a list of rules and procedures that are read to the client, signed by the client, and sent home with the client. For example, when no one is allowed into a group without bringing payment, then clients are less likely to "forget" their money. A good set of rules and procedures evolves over time. Whenever the therapist is caught off guard with a difficult situation, a new rule is added so that the situation is less likely to arise again.

Ironically, those with externalized disturbances are often masters of the victim role. Not only does victimization prevent therapeutic progress, but it also allows the client to gain some control over the therapist and the interview process. Bad luck and a troubled life enable the client gradually to claim more and more privileges (e.g., coming late, coming without money, asking for appointments at special times). However, the effective therapist does not cater to the passing fancy of the client. Like a hole in a dam, a small infraction should be dealt with as quickly as possible. It is not helpful for the therapist to stretch his or her limits. This type of client is likely to dominate or take advantage of a do-gooder therapist. Instead, the client should be able to trust that the therapist is strong enough to uphold the boundaries. It is wise for a therapist to set and maintain boundaries that are stricter than they need be so that the therapist is not emotionally affected when the boundaries are tested or breached.

## MAINTAIN THERAPEUTIC AUTHORITY

When working with individuals who have externalized disturbances, it is essential for the therapist to trust his or her own decisions, values, and intentions. It is counterproductive for the therapist to question himself or herself during therapy. According to Harry Boyd (1993), "This work forces you to set your own values in order, and to establish and maintain your own priorities. If you do not develop a clear and consistent sense of who you are and what you want, personality-disordered patients will eat you alive." In some instances, such a client will brag about the ability to find another person's weak spot and use it against that person. That is why a therapist should not answer very personal questions. Although the client is entitled to information about one's training and theoretical background, it is not helpful to share emotionally loaded information, such as times when you have felt inadequate. This information might benefit someone with an internalized disturbance, but it only creates problems when dealing with clients who are looking for reasons to discount authority figures. For this reason, the therapist would be wise to have a consultant who will provide a healthy environment in which to question one's decisions or areas of concern.

At the beginning of therapy, the client will want to ascertain, "Can I manipulate or control the therapist?" If the answer to this question is Yes, the therapist becomes another pawn in the game. Although the therapist may want to talk to the client as a human with equal rights, he or she should keep in mind the powerful influence of a role-conferred advantage. Persons in positions of authority can influence others (Hofling, Brotzman, Dalrymple, et al., 1966). Therefore, if the client walks away from a session having achieved a leadership position, then the words and actions of the therapist are less influential.

An important means for maintaining therapeutic authority is to base one's opinions on facts that the client cannot easily dispute. For example, "Most of those I have seen succeed in therapy first learn how to admit to their mistakes. Only then are they able to make progress." This statement is very difficult for the client to deny because it is based on the therapist's experience.

With regard to "choosing one's battles," it is a bad idea to become preoccupied with whether or not the client is telling the "truth" about circumstances outside of the office. The client will always win this type of debate because he or she can easily bend the facts to fit his or her purposes. However, when your statements are based on behavior that occurs in the office, you are no longer dependent on the client's self-report. While making a point, the effective therapist always returns to concrete realities of which there is sound evidence or proof. This evidence is collected during the course of therapy through video tapes or a log of calls and conversations. When a client is told something important, it should be written down so that the client can see that a record has been made. This makes it more difficult for the client to undermine the therapist's self-confidence by making such statements as, "You never told me that!" or "It's not my fault I wasn't here, you told me the wrong appointment time!"

Clients often use intimidation to undermine the personal authority of the therapist. The most effective type of intimidation is delivered via indirect messages.

C:    Whenever someone crosses me, I am one crazy son-of-a-bitch. I once killed a man using my bare hands. That son-of-a-bitch made the mistake of crossing me.

T:    I will not work with someone who is too unstable to do counseling work. Are you currently dangerous?

C:      That depends on what you mean.

T:      I mean that I will not work with you if you are a threat to my well-being.

C:      (*Different tone of voice.*) That was a long time ago. I'm different now.

Intimidation tactics need to be confronted in a careful but direct manner. When a threat is made using an indirect means, then the therapist needs to make the content of the message or gesture overt by asking if the behavior is intended to be a threat. When a client backs down and describes himself or herself as safe, then the client is committing to more positive behaviors. Although some threats may be ignored, it is unwise to discount any serious threat. This would only encourage the client to prove himself or herself. Instead, the therapist should remain calm and confident, while clearly defining unquestionable boundaries.

When working with any person, whether the suffering is primarily internalized or externalized, one needs to recognize that the client's most unreasonable actions seem justified in his or her own mind. It is what the client understands to be the correct thing to do. That is why during therapy, the client must temporarily relinquish his or her command. In some ways, it is as though the client has once again become a child and is now looking for a type of parenting that may not have been available during childhood. In this position, the client may experience both terror and security. The terror lies in having no means of guarding or defending oneself. The security is in the possibility of being rescued from one's own chronic mismanagement of social and personal resources.

## BE SPECIFIC AND THOROUGH

By definition, an individual with an internalized disorder has a pathological self-view. Therefore, the stigma of a formal diagnosis can be counterproductive. But this is not true for individuals with an externalized disturbance. When working with this type of client, a formal diagnosis of the problem is just as crucial to treatment as is any intervention that follows. The failure of an expert to identify the dysfunctional nature of the client's behavior could be interpreted by the client as a sanction of his or her actions.

C:     (*Describes all of his frustrations with his partner.*)

T:     Sounds like you have been experiencing some difficult times at home.

The following week:

C:     I told my girlfriend that you agreed with me, that it was really her who needs the help, and not me.

In this example, the therapist's mistake was that it was not specifically stated to the client that he had a serious problem. Similarly, verbal reinforcement needs to be very specific so that it is not used by the client as blanket approval of all of his or her actions.

Often, vague answers are no answer at all. A vague response means that, for whatever reason, the person is not being forthright. He or she may be uninterested in the topic, or it may be hitting too close to home, making it difficult to respond.

T:     How was your week?

C:     Went great. Really not much to talk about.

T:     Did you have any disagreements with your girlfriend?

C:     Well, we had a little misunderstanding, but it wasn't any big deal.

T:     What was the biggest mistake you made during the disagreement?

C:     Well, after she pushed me and called me a "bastard," I just left because I don't have to put up with that kind of abuse.

T:     What mistake did you make?

C:     Well, I'd been out drinking, so I might have gotten louder than I should.

T:     You screamed at her. What else did you do?

C:     I called her a bitch.

T:     Why was it a mistake to yell at her and call her a bitch?

It is important to ask very direct questions because the client may never volunteer the most important information.

After teaching a new skill, the client should be given an opportunity to verify his or her accurate understanding through practice. This allows the therapist to test the client's knowledge.

T:    Do you understand all of what I just told you?

C:    Yeah, I got it. I kind of do this already, anyway.

T:    For this to work right you have to use all three steps in the correct manner. Are you sure that you don't have any questions?

C:    No. I got it just fine.

T:    Great. Now we will do a role-play. I will role-play your partner and you role-play yourself using a time-out.

C:    What do you mean?

T:    We are going to practice what you have just learned.

C:    I'm not sure I'm ready for that.

T:    It is all right if you do not do it perfectly the first time. Almost everyone has to practice this more than once.

When the therapist does not take the time to be specific and thorough, therapeutic effectiveness is greatly diminished. The only assumption that the therapist should make is that he or she will need to investigate carefully what he or she is told. According to Erickson, "Too many people listen to the problem and they don't hear what the patient isn't saying ..." (Zeig, 1985, p. 126).

## CREATE AN ATMOSPHERE OF SAFETY

One should remember that for any client, honest self-disclosure can be difficult (Jourard, 1971). For those who initially perceive the therapist as "the enemy," the vulnerability associated with honest self-disclosure can be very disconcerting. At first, this type of client may spend a lot of energy trying to convince others that he or she does not need help. However, behind that façade lies a fragile ego. Later in therapy, the client may admit, "I am scared of my own actions ... I don't know what I may do next." The client may have been thinking about this problem for months or even years, but when he or she reached the therapist's office the role of "client" felt too threatening, so a wall of denial was constructed. The phrase "psychological nudity" describes some of the awkwardness and fear experienced when asked to relinquish familiar defenses. The client dreads being officially labeled "a living failure." Ego protection is important because when people lose all hope in their own goodness, there is no longer reason to live or to promote the survival of others. Some clients come to therapy already teetering at the very edge of an existential crisis.

During therapy, the client must learn how to endure extended periods of uncomfortable self-examination. As a child, the client may have been severely criticized for the smallest of errors. Therefore, he or she does not appreciate the difference between being a complete failure and having made a mistake. In the case of the former, there is no reason to continue living. In the case of the latter, the individual still has reason for hope. Therefore, the client is taught to see his or her mistakes, and, at the same time, to maintain healthy self-respect. It is useful to confront self-abuse just as sternly as abuse against others. This helps the client to deal constructively with shame and to refocus on his or her responsibility for the behavior.

C:     Now that I've straightened myself out, or at least more so than I was ... I don't think I am finished yet ... but anyway, I sometimes think about things and how I have treated others and I realize what an asshole I really was. It literally makes me sick to my stomach to think about all that I did.

T:     It would be easy to start abusing yourself right now. But I think that it would be the wrong thing to do. In fact, it might only make you more likely to abuse others in the future. We can only treat others as well as we treat ourselves. You can't go back in time to change the things that happened, so what can you do right now? What is something that would be beneficial to everyone?

C:     I have already begun trying to do an equal good for every bad I ever did.

T:     That is a really great idea ... a good way to use the energy created by these memories.

C:     Yeah, but my daughter is the one who I have hurt the worst and I am not allowed to see her.

T:     Right. Going to visit your daughter might only cause more damage, so how can you do an equal amount of good for some other child? Have you ever donated money to an orphanage?

C:     Actually, I've been thinking about doing something like that.

Another means of protecting the client is to maintain a strong group alliance. A difficult confession can be responded to with acceptance, "We all make mistakes. That is why group is so helpful. We can learn from each other." The use of the pronoun "we" allies the entire group with the client. However, sometimes a client may come under attack from another group member, in which case it is the therapist's responsibility to protect the attackee by inviting the attacker to engage in a moment of self-examination.

One of the most important aspects of survival is the search for safety. This is something the client should be able to find in therapy. When you provide adequate protection, it enables the client to relinquish defense mechanisms, such as denial and blame. Therapeutic safety should not be used as an excuse to ignore difficult problems or to avoid uncomfortable confrontations. The effective therapist is safe and powerful simultaneously.

## DO NOT ACCEPT RESPONSIBILITY FOR THE CLIENT'S CHOICES

Although the therapist is responsible for the quality of his or her work, it is a mistake to assume responsibility for the client's dysfunctional behavior. Therefore, one should not base one's personal pride or sense of worth on whether or not the client changes dysfunctional behavior. Accepting credit for the client's success is also troublesome because, by implication, the therapist must also accept responsibility for the client's failures. When this boundary is tested, the focus of attention should be shifted back to the client.

C:    I did what you told me to do, and it worked great!

T:    Good for you! And what other goals would *you* like to accomplish?

The most effective therapist is careful not to become too invested in an endeavor that should belong to the client.

To avoid internal conflict created by feelings of ambivalence, this type of client is likely to delegate the role of superego to an outside authority figure. While working with alcoholics, Milton Erickson suggested that hypnosis can be counterproductive because it places a dependency "of the wrong sort" on the therapist (Rossi & Ryan, 1992, p. 61). Before these expectations have time to develop, the therapist should refuse to accept, as a liability, the client's future behavior.

C:    Don't worry, I'm going to keep to every appointment from now on!

T:     Actually, I am not worried about your coming to every appointment from now on, because if you get yourself expelled from the program, it will not affect me or my life in any manner. Things will go on just as if I had never met you.

C:     Don't you care what happens to me?

T:     If you decide to sabotage yourself, there is absolutely nothing I can do. However, if you want to try and make something more of your life, then I might be able to help. Do you want help?

C:     Yeah ... hell, yeah!

T:     Then tell me all of the different ways in which you can sabotage yourself in counseling, if you choose to do so.

In other instances, to appreciate fully the ability to make decisions, the client will need to have his or her choices outlined.

T:     The purpose of this orientation meeting is for you to decide whether or not you want to attend counseling. ...

C:     (Interrupts.) I already know I don't want to be here, but I have to, because some goddamn caseworker came to my home and stuck her nose where it doesn't belong!

T:     You are free to leave at any time. You can go straight down the hallway. The door at the end will open up into the parking lot.

C:     You are not listening to me. I said that I don't have any choice but to be here!

T:     Everything you do is by choice. There are six other men who were also court-ordered to counseling and they chose not to attend this meeting tonight ...

C:     (Interrupts.) Yeah, but I'm not going to jail and being here is the only way to keep out.

T:     It's not my job to keep you out of jail. I am here to help those who sincerely want help for themselves.

C:     (Stands up and begins to pace.) God damn it! What I am trying to tell you is that I don't need to be here. Have you ever had someone sent here who really didn't need it? Just tell me that, is it possible that someone could not need this counseling!

T:     (Calm but firm tone of voice.) You are interrupting the meeting and making it impossible for others, who want to be here, to get the information they need. Therefore, you can either sit down and listen to what I have to say or you can leave the room right now.

C:     (*Sits down. Does not speak again until after the meeting has ended.*)

This is an example of an important shift in awareness, from the actions to the therapist to choices that are available to the client. As may be true for all types of therapy, "leading the patient to 'see what [he] can do,' is much more effective than letting the patient see what things the therapist can do with or to the patient" (Erickson, 1963, p. 291).

### DEMONSTRATE CALMNESS AND STABILITY

The more disturbed the client, the more critical it is for the therapist to model calm, respectful behavior. This interaction alone is therapeutic and will help stabilize the client. When speaking with clients, it is helpful to use a smooth, soft voice, with the rest of one's body in an utterly relaxed and comfortable position. It does not matter whether the client is suffering from an internalized or externalized disturbance, as either would benefit from the experience of therapeutic intimacy and safety.

The therapist must not be too sensitive to personal attack, but must be able to deflect acts of aggression and hostility while remaining calm and focused on the task at hand. Just as a good parent does not rely on spanking to teach a child not to hit others, the therapist must always remain aware of the behavior he or she is modeling. The client who is harshly confronted or demoralized by the therapist will leave therapy ready to displace those negative feelings onto someone else.

Conversely, the therapist should avoid efforts to impress or win the favor of the client. Content seduction is sometimes a problem while speaking with a client who has learned to use others' ego needs. To remain effective, the therapist should get his or her ego needs met by someone other than clients.

T:     I don't think you have admitted to yourself how serious this problem really is.

C:     You really are pretty sharp. I don't think I've ever had a therapist as good as you. Those guys at that other counseling place were a joke. I don't think it does any good just to gang up on a client and yell. Do you?

T:      What is it that you are afraid of?

Without stopping for explanation, the expert therapist will return the client's attention to the original topic.

Providing therapy for clients who have severe behavioral problems can be very challenging. If you find yourself confronted by behavior so disturbing that you must depersonalize the client, then you have been excessively affected. Under these conditions, referral is necessary. To continue to work with such an individual is unethical and hazardous to your mental health.

## MAKE IT EASY FOR THE CLIENT TO
## GIVE IN AND WIN

Most individuals want to feel good about who they are. This is especially true of someone who has not yet learned how to take pride in his or her actions. The therapist should recognize this fact and use it therapeutically. When a client becomes vulnerable by confessing to a bad mistake and sincerely wants help, then it is the role of the therapist to frame the confession as successful behavior.

C:      I feel pretty stupid about the whole thing, now that I am thinking about it. But this week I yelled at her about a bill that was not paid on time. The thing was, I was the one who should have mailed the payment. It was actually my mistake, but I knew it was going to cause a bunch of problems so I just convinced myself that she was the one who had screwed up.

T:      I think you are making a very important point right now. Is there anyone else in the group who has done this?

In this example, one person's ability to confess and have insight into his behavior is quickly reinforced, and then used to move other group members to do the same kind of work. Further reinforcement is added if, at the end of the group session, the members are asked to describe one thing that they respect about the comments of some other group member. Group members usually compliment others for having the courage to make themselves vulnerable. This type of positive peer influence can be very powerful.

Sometimes the uncomfortableness of change causes clients to complain about behaviors that need to be reinforced and reframed as an important new skill.

C:     Things are really different. It used to be that I would just say things. Now I am almost nervous, like I'm not sure how I should say things.

T:     That is a really good sign. Can you understand how this new skill is helping you?

C:     Yeah. Now I am thinking about things before I talk. I try to think about how she is going to take it . . . how she will feel after I say it.

T:     Is this a better way of doing things, or would you prefer to go back to your old ways?

C:     No! (*Pause.*) I mean "Yes," it is a better way and "No," I do not want to go back to my old way of doing things.

T:     Could you tell the group what is so great about being more respectful of others?

In this example, the client reinforces his own behavior as he describes the benefits he is enjoying. His self-disclosure also serves to inspire other group members.

The therapist should be careful not to reinforce negative behaviors inadvertently. If a client becomes angry, and the therapist backs down on a particular issue, then the client's acting-out is reinforced. Instead, the therapist can respond by acknowledging the difficulty of participating in this type of counseling. The client can be congratulated on his or her willingness to attend. The willingness to confess to having a problem is framed as an act of courage. If the client has remained quiet long enough for these things to be said, then the therapist can also congratulate the client on his or her willingness to listen to things he or she might not want to hear. These types of statements make it easier for clients to give in, so they can continue to win.

## AIM FOR MINIMAL INTERVENTION

As in medicine, the mental health practitioner always strives for minimal intervention, in the least intrusive manner possible. While using confrontation, this guideline is especially important. Confrontation does not add anything to the client's behavioral repertoire. Rather, it is a means of limiting or constricting the range of behavior. Confrontation is used to show the client the behaviors that are problematic and the associated consequences. Direct confrontation is especially stressful for the client because it makes it impossible to agree with the therapist without accepting the idea that he or she was incorrect. This could be a problem for a client who is already defensive and suspicious of the therapist. When confrontation is used at an inopportune moment, the inevitable result is a power struggle between client and therapist. A client does not need too much confrontation, and certainly the therapist ought to have other means of intervention available, such as education and positive reinforcement.

Sometimes it is possible to have a tremendous impact on the client's thinking while using more subtle forms of confrontation. For instance, the confrontation might be delivered indirectly through the use of metaphor, or by simply expressing a vague sense of concern. For example, the question, "What did you just say?" is quickly followed by, "Are you sure you really think that?" While disconcerting, this type of question provides room for the client to decide what he or she should be thinking. A typical response is, "No, what I am trying to say is . . ." In this way, the client is able to change his or her line of reasoning but still save face. The most subtle of all is the confrontation that is entirely nonverbal. If a client is saying something that seems off-base, the therapist can silently shake his or her head, as if saying No. A client who is in close rapport will begin to correct himself or herself, or qualify his or her statements while remaining unaware that a confrontation has taken place. A similar method is simply to remain silent as the individual seeks agreement on a particular issue. The therapist's silence is much more powerful than any verbal argument, because there is no room for debate. As a rule, the most effective form of confrontation comes from the client's own lips and is based on his or her own understandings and subjective realities (Elms, 1966; Watts, 1967). This is perhaps the most sophisticated form of confrontation because the therapist formulates and delivers the confrontation in an entirely indirect fashion.

C:    An entire year has gone by since the last time I hit her.

T:    So what do you think went through her mind when you got angry and yelled at her last week?

C:     (*Pause.*) That I would hit her again?

T:     Does she have any way of knowing for sure that you won't?

C:     (*Hangs his head.*) Man ... what an asshole I've been ... every time
       I get mad, she's got to wonder whether or not I'm going to haul
       off and hit her.

T:     Do you want it to be this way?

C:     No! Of course not.

T:     Why not?

C:     Because it's wrong. That's no kind of life, always having to be
       afraid.

T:     You want her to be able to feel happy?

C:     Yeah ... I really do.

In this case, it was possible to initiate the confrontation simply by having
the client consider the consequences of his actions. This client is more
likely to accept this confrontation because it is based entirely upon information he has provided.

It is also helpful to remember that the therapist does not always have
to be doing something to the client. Watch for moments when it would
be beneficial to sit quietly and listen. The best times to demonstrate listening skills are moments when the client has just made himself or herself
psychologically vulnerable, or in some other way has taken a positive
risk. At some point, the client must leave therapy, and it is that end that
the therapist always keeps in mind.

T:     Long after you leave counseling, you will continue to face diffi-
       cult problems. That is simply how life is. So when you run into
       a bad situation, what are your two options?

C:     (*Pause.*) I'm not sure. What do you mean?

T:     You can either make a bad situation worse, or you can make a
       bad situation better. Those are your two options.

**In Summary**

- Begin with a commitment to change.
- Require a confession.
- Adhere to predetermined rules and procedures.
- Maintain therapeutic authority.
- Be specific and thorough.
- Create an atmosphere of safety.
- Do not accept responsibility for the client's choices.
- Demonstrate calmness and stability.
- Make it easy for the client to give in and win.
- Aim for minimal intervention.

## References

Aronson, E., & Mills, J. (1959). The effect of severity of initiation on liking for a group. *Journal of Abnormal and Social Psychology, 59*, 177–181.

Bem, D. J. (1967). Self-perception: An alternative explanation of cognitive dissonance phenomena. *Psychological Review, 74*, 183–200.

Boyd, H. S. (1993). Surviving treatment with borderline personality disorders. Lecture to Dallas Group Psychotherapy Society, November 12.

Carver, C. S., & Scheier, M. F. (1981). *Attention and self-regulation: A control theory approach to human behavior.* New York: Springer Verlag.

Deutsch, M., & Gerard, H. B. (1959). A study of normative and informational social influences upon individual judgment. *Journal of Abnormal and Social Psychology, 51*, 629–636.

Elms, A. C. (1966). Influence of fantasy ability on attitude change through role-playing. *Journal of Personality and Social Psychology, 4*, 36–43.

Erickson, M. H. (1963/1980). Hypnotically oriented psychotherapy in organic brain damage. In E. Rossi (Ed.), *The collected papers of Milton H. Erickson on hypnosis, Vol. IV: Innovative hypnotherapy* (pp. 283–311). New York: Irvington.

Haley, J. (1985). *Conversations with Milton H. Erickson, M.D., vol. III.* New York: Norton.

Hofling, C. K., Brotzman, E., Dalrymple, S., Graves, N., & Pierce, C. M. (1966). An experimental study of nurse–physician relationships. *Journal of Nervous and Mental Disease, 143*, 171–180.

Jourard, S. M. (1971). *The transparent self* (2nd ed.). New York: Van Nostrand Reinhold.

Petty, R. E., & Cacioppo, J. T. (1986). *Communication and persuasion: Central and peripheral routes to attitude change.* New York: Springer Verlag.

Rossi, E., & Ryan, M. (Eds.). (1992). *Mind–body communication in hypnosis. Vol. III. The seminars, workshops, and lectures of Milton H. Erickson.* New York: Irvington.

Watts, W. A. (1967). Relative persistence of opinion change induced by active compared to passive participation. *Journal of Personality and Social Psychology, 5,* 4–15.

Zanna, M. P., & Cooper, J. (1974). Dissonance and the pill: An attribution approach to studying the arousal properties of dissonance. *Journal of Personality and Social Psychology, 29,* 703–709.

Zeig, J. K. (1985). *Experiencing Erickson.* New York: Brunner/Mazel.

## 23

# Ericksonian Strategies
# for Successful Weight Loss

*Carol J. Kershaw*

In Vincent Ferrini's play "Shadows Talking" (1991), a character says:

> If you could forget
> Who you think you are
> You might catch up with
> What you really are
> And can't see—

Anxiety and compulsive eating frequently stimulate amnesia for the ability to maintain conscious choice and control over what is eaten. A serious issue for many, the problem of obesity in the United States has become steadily worse. The National Institutes of Health maintains that 33% of American adults are obese. Health-care costs attributable to obesity add up to $68 million annually. Obesity is a major contributory factor to hypertension, stroke, coronary heart disease, gall bladder disease, type 2 diabetes, some cancers, and respiratory problems (Bray, 1992).

## MANAGING EATING BEHAVIOR

Obesity can lead to feelings of being helpless and out of control, and may lock the overweight individual into a cycle of dieting and then regaining the pounds lost. Most dieters try every new food regimen for a short time, only to see the lost weight reappear. As one of my patients told me, "Everyone who has a weight problem is looking for the one program that will finally be the cure-all."

There are complex variables that play a role in weight gain: biochemical factors, the context and the system by which the individual is influenced, the "internal weight manager," susceptibility to external food cues when in a state of anxiety, learned trance phenomena, and brain dysregulation. These factors work together in an interactional system in which eating is adjusted in the interests of biological regulation and adaptation to the environment.

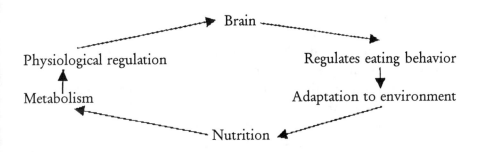

The brain regulates eating behavior, and foods stimulate the production of certain neurotransmitters. Researchers experimented with two groups of mice to determine the differences in response to walking over a hot plate with and without ingesting sugar. The mice in the group that ate a sugar solution prior to the experiment took twice as long to lift their feet from the hot surface (Blass & Ciaramitara, 1994). In a second experiment, researchers measured isolation distress in baby mice. The researchers noted that when the mice were taken away from the mother, they cried over 300 times in a six-minute period. However, eight baby mice given sugar water cried only 75 times in the same period. But when the second group was given the drug naloxone before drinking the sugar water, the chemical blocked the effect of the sugar (Cleary et al., 1996), and these baby mice cried as frequently as did those in the first group.

The researchers concluded that the sugar blocked emotional as well as physical pain. It slowed the response time to the painful stimulus of the hot plate. Additionally, sugar seemed to slow a painful reaction to being isolated from the mother (Blass, Fitzgerald, & Kehoe, 1986). Other researchers suggest that human beings may have a similar response to sugar. To increase one's serotonin levels and change states, one may crave carbohydrates, alcohol, or sweets. When an individual gives in to the craving multiple times, an addictive cycle is set up (Drewnowski & Rock, 1992). Once the problem cycle is in place, any environmental stressor medicated with food becomes self-reinforcing, slows metabolism, and places the brain in a state of dysregulation.

The brain's ability to work properly determines one's level of satisfaction with everyday living. How anxious, depressed, easily distracted, or sensitive to eating cues we are is the result of a variety of factors. How well the physiology of a person's brain operates affects the person's behavior. The part of the brain that is involved in eating disorders is the cingulate gyrus. Located longitudinally through the middle part of the frontal lobes, it allows people to shift attention and change thoughts and behaviors. When an individual is caught in loops of thought or compulsive behaviors, this part of the brain has become overactive.

Moreover, quantitative studies on people with weight problems have shown a decreased ability to create alpha frequency, the brain state associated with relaxation (Stroebel, 1997). Under stress, the automatic and trancelike behavior of eating may become activated. Frequently, patients report no memory for the act of eating, nor do they feel hungry. Amnesia, as well as analgesia, may be used unconsciously to keep anxiety low and awareness of overeating from the conscious mind. More often than not, the physical sensations of hunger and anxiety are confused. Because the act and ingestion of food may change a stressful state into a relaxed one, food becomes associated with relaxation. Carbohydrates specifically stimulate serotonin and send an opiatelike sensation to the body, and physical relaxation follows.

Another key element in the management of eating behavior is the system in which an individual lives. Frequently, patients report having had anxiety around mealtime when growing up. Either there was an overfocus on food, or food was synonymous with love, and the family rule dictated a clean plate at every meal no matter what signals one's body delivered. Usually, weight patients are aware of many conflicts surrounding food and have good insights. However, they may be less aware of the present system that reinforces negative behaviors and attitudes. A thorough history of the problem is always useful.

## Taking a Present History

1.  Collect a history of the problem and when it began.
2.  Have the patient describe any particular cravings or tendencies toward binges and the circumstances in which these occur.
3.  Record any family-of-origin messages regarding food.
4.  If the patient is married, ask about the contract made regarding food and how slim each partner would remain over the years. Sometimes weight gain becomes an arena for a power struggle.
5.  Listen for the "food" language patients unconsciously use. "I could really taste that success." "That idea is something you can really get your teeth into." "This is food for thought." This is the language the therapist may use in conversational hypnosis to focus attention on the impending change to becoming a slimmer individual.
6.  Discover the motivating anxiety within the problem. There has to be enough positive motivation to create change.
7.  Most people have an internal weight manager that tells how much weight gain is too much. This manager may be found by asking the patient how he or she maintains his or her present weight. Find out whether the patient knows how to feel full.
8.  Find out how the patient related to food when he or she weighed less.
9.  Ask about expectations regarding treatment.
10. Identify the trance phenomena the patient may be using to keep the problem going.

Milton Erickson was a master at utilizing a patient's reality and eliciting resourceful states. In treating a young obese woman, Erickson utilized her intense pain about her weight by asking her to stand in front of a full-length mirror and really notice how much she disliked all the fat. He continued, "And if you think hard enough and look through that layer of blubber that you've got wrapped around you, you will see a very pretty feminine figure, but it is buried rather deeply. And what do you think you ought to do to get that figure excavated?" Erickson reported that the woman "excavated" five pounds a week (Erickson, 1983). With his intervention, Erickson elicited positive motivating anxiety by using the patient's own pain and redirecting it toward action. He helped this woman find the real body she had long been unable to see.

What Erickson perhaps observed with this binge eater was that in an attempt to escape internal distress, she would narrow her attention to the immediate noxious stimulus in the environment and avoid a broader view that would allow for more options. The narrowing of one's cognitive focus onto specific food cues disengages the normal inhibitions against eating. This process could be thought of as hypnotic dissociation followed by time distortion for how long one engaged in eating and amnesia for the act itself.

## CASE STUDY: WEIGHTING FOR THE LIGHT

A health care professional referred for help with obesity was 100 pounds overweight and had struggled with eating problems all his life. Night bingeing had been a chronic problem for 30 years. In a family where anxiety was calmed by food, his mother, father, and brother were all obese. His father had died from a heart attack, and his brother had been hospitalized with heart problems. The patient reported that his overweight mother used to act like the "food police" and tell him what he should and should not eat. As many young people do, he responded with rebellion, anger, and resentment.

This professional had seen many previous therapists and nutritionists, and had tried many weight-loss programs. He had spent years in analysis and had insightful understandings about his problem, but just could not stop. He suffered terribly and told me he was waiting for the "light," just the right insight to propel him toward success. He had binged for years by stopping at four or five restaurants on the way home from work. Whenever he was surprised by being put on call at his job with little notice, the familiar anger and resentment toward authority triggered bingeing episodes. He felt victimized by his work, even though being on call came with the position.

In addition to his feelings about work, he resented his wife, who had begun to behave as his mother had. She became a spy, investigating when, what, and where he was eating. Secret kitchen eating followed by his wife's discovering crumbs on the counter and confronting him became a ritual. This pattern had to be interrupted.

I suggested a couple session to help support his wife's good intentions and to move her out of the problem. She was given an assignment to purchase a Sherlock Holmes type of hat. He was instructed to pretend to slink into the kitchen and binge on bagels, while she donned her hat and jumped through the door to announce boldly, "I caught you!" They began to joke about the Sherlock Holmes investigation. With this pattern interrupted, internal resources needed to be retrieved.

In the first hypnosis session, I suggested, "You can go back in time and discover two or three experiences where you were completely determined to succeed." Immediately, he described his "full" focus in medical school (food language) and his ability to complete the course work. Another resourceful memory was his determination not to give in when he divorced and his ex-wife attempted to keep their children from him. I suggested, "You can fully remember these feelings—first one event and then the other. Really savor the flavor of determination to succeed. Then remember what you looked like, felt like, how people responded to you, when you were 100 pounds lighter."

These resourceful memories "jump-started" the loss of weight. He began to follow a food program that had been successful in many cases, but the binges continued. After each frustrating day, he would stop at three or four restaurants and feel shame. Curiously, his report of these events lacked much emotion. When I asked him where the missing feelings were, he became aware of his lack of anxiety to resolve the problem. The pattern clearly had to be interrupted for him to succeed.

This health professional needed to find a way to manage his mental attitude regarding work, and a change in body state to interrupt the bingeing episodes. He reported that he always felt exhausted before he binged. He agreed to utilize a relaxation technique in order to calm his body and put himself in a more positive state.

The patient was cooperative and used the relaxation technique every evening before leaving work. In the process of entering a more positive state of relaxation and comfort, he rediscovered some ability consciously to choose to drive straight home. He was successful at passing up the food stops until he had a particularly upsetting and stressful day at work. He binged again. Obviously, more drastic measures were needed.

At the next session, I asked the patient to name the person or persons whom he hated the most. After much thought, he said that it had to be the American neo-Nazi party. I asked him what he could do if he had the motivation to take charge and manage his weight differently. He replied that he probably could easily lose one pound a week without any struggle or feeling of deprivation and could keep himself from bingeing. I then asked him to take out his checkbook and write a check for $1,000 to the American neo-Nazi party and give it to me. All of the color drained from his face. I told him that if he could not maintain his contract, the check would be sent. He could imagine being placed on the group's mailing list and receiving literature. What would the letter carrier think? Would word of this spread to his rabbi? Of course, he could blame it on his therapist. But would they really believe him? What would his Jewish neighbors think, much less his friends and family? "Perhaps you could imagine the swastika rotating behind you and a beam of light coming from its center each time you see an unhealthy food or a fa(s)t-food restaurant. Can you see the light?"

Because we did not know the address of the neo-Nazi group, I asked the patient to look it up on the Internet. He had the address at the next session and reported that he had searched the Internet late at night so that no one in the family would know. He lost three pounds the first week. Positive motivating anxiety was now activated, and at follow-up a year and a half later, the patient reported that he had not binged again.

### Food Management and Exercise

The patient began eating five times per day and included a protein and a complex carbohydrate each time he ate. Eating fibrous vegetables with protein in the evening and the last carbohydrates by 5:00 P.M. was encouraged. Exercising with light weights three times a week and at least 20–30 minutes of aerobics were suggested.

Each time the patient exercised, he was instructed to visualize himself as thin and enjoying others admiring his physique, and to develop an image of himself as healthy and old. Whenever he had lost weight before, he realized, he had visualized himself as heavy again.

To assist the hypnotic work, the patient used electroencephalographic (EEG) biofeedback or neurofeedback to practice developing the alpha frequency at will. This is a learning strategy that enables a person to normalize dysregulated brain waves and create desired changes in behavior and mental functioning. The EEG biofeedback training is a painless, noninvasive procedure. One or more sensors are placed on the scalp and one at each ear. Brain waves are monitored by means of an amplifier and a computer-based instrument that processes the signal and provides the proper feedback. This feedback is displayed to the patient by means of a video game operated by focusing attention to maintain certain frequencies. In the case of addictive problems, such as overeating, the alpha (8–11 hertz) and theta (4–7 hertz) are operantly conditioned by providing brain-relaxing sounds each time the correct frequencies are maintained (Peninston & Kulkosky, 1989).

During this treatment, hypnosis was used to practice various scenarios in which the patient made healthy food choices. Suggestions for the proper balance of protein, complex carbohydrates, and vegetables were paired with feelings of comfort, delight, fullness, and enjoyment of a lighter sensation (Blum, Tractenberg, & Cook, 1990). The patient responded by feeling less stress daily, being in a more positive mood, and losing weight (Fahrion, 1990). As a result of the hypnosis, he continues to maintain the weight loss two years later.

### Ericksonian Hypnosis

The case presented here illustrates a number of Ericksonian hypnotic principles.

1. Recognize that symptoms are frequently contextual.

    The system in which an individual operates may serve to keep a problem active. In this case, the patient's wife unintentionally played a role in the reinforcement of symptom behavior. He could be angry with her and have more reason to binge.

2. Assess the particular trance phenomenon negatively used to keep the problem going.

    As with many people with weight problems, this patient was skilled in using dissociation from body sensations. He could not distinguish anxiety from hunger or recognize feeling full. He employed amnesia for bingeing episodes and only later recalled the several restaurant stops. In trance, he was asked to attend to body sensations and become more conscious of how many restaurant stops he made and exactly what he ate. Using association to bring himself out of a dissociated state gave him more conscious choice.

3. Utilize and reframe the problem to expand the number of solutions.

A desire to be in control dominated the patient's thinking. While he experienced himself as out of control, I suggested he was demonstrating an amazing ability to binge only in a way to maintain his weight. Even though he was 100 pounds overweight, he had remained at this weight for the past five years.

This patient used food to calm anxiety and vent anger. Both of these motivating emotions were channeled positively through the fear that his check to the American neo-Nazi group might be mailed. His desire to receive the magic insight, the "light," to experience inner control was connected symbolically to the image of a spinning swastika with a light coming after him.

4. Retrieve resources to assist in a resolution of the problem.

This patient needed to experience a sense of renewed determination to succeed. By remembering several incidents where he strongly had this emotion, he transferred strong affect to resolve the problem. We built an association to these feelings by suggesting that his adult children continue to observe his success at every stage of life. The determination to stay in their lives and have a relationship was associated with the powerful feeling of wanting to demonstrate success in the area of food management. He was asked to bring a picture of himself at the target weight and remember how he felt. This image was later used in future orientation in time.

5. Use future orientation in time where the problem has been resolved.

In hypnosis, various scenarios of being thinner and enjoying looking as he did in the picture were employed. He practiced visualizing himself thin when exercising and eating.

Perceptual distortion and lost access to inner resources attributable to stressful life events may develop survival behavior to keep anxiety at bay. Later, this behavior results in negative consequences. Ericksonian hypnosis may stimulate a renewed ability for self-regulation so that "you might catch up with what you really are ..." (Ferrini, 1991).

## References

Amen, D. G. (1994). New directions in the theory, diagnosis, and treatment of mental disorders: The use of SPECT imaging in everyday clinical practice. In L. F. Koziol & C. E. Stout (Eds.), *The neuropsychology of mental disorders* (pp. 286–311). Springfield, IL: Charles C. Thomas.

Blass, E., & Ciaramitara, V. (1994, July). A new look at some old mechanisms in human newborn tastes and tactile determinants of state, affect, and action. *Monographs of the Society for FESE*. Chicago: University of Chicago Press.

Blass, E. M., Fitzgerald, E., & Kehoe, P. (1986). Interactions between sucrose, pain and isolation distress. *Pharmacology, Biochemistry & Behavior, 26*, 483–489.

Blum, K., Tractenberg, M., & Cook, D. (1990). Neuronutrient effects on weight loss in carbohydrate binges: An open clinical trial. *Current Therapeutic Research, 48*(2), 217–233.

Bray, G. A. (1992). Pathophysiology of obesity. *American Journal of Clinical Nutrition, 55*(suppl. 2), 488S–494S.

Cleary, J., et al. (1996). Naloxone effects on sucrose-motivated behavior. *Psychopharmacology, 176*, 110–114.

Drewnowski, A., & Rock, C. (1992). Taste responses and preferences for sweet high-fat foods: Evidence for opioid involvement. *Physiology & Behavior, 51*(2), 371–379.

Erickson, M. (1983). In E. Rossi, M. Ryan, & F. Sharp (Eds.), *Healing in hypnosis: The seminars, workshops, and lectures of Milton H. Erickson* (vol. 1, pp. 267–268). New York: Irvington.

Fahrion, S. (1990). Self-regulation of anxiety. *Bulletin of the Menninger Clinic, 54*(2), 217.

Ferrini, V. (1984). This other ocean. Books VI and VII of *Known fish*. Storrs, CT: University of Connecticut Library.

Peninston, E., & Kulkosky, P. (1989). Alpha-theta brainwave training and beta-endorphin levels in alcoholics. *Alcoholism: Clinical Experimental Research, 13*, 271–279.

Stroebel, C. (1997, August). Seminar on Weight Management Using EEG Biofeedback, New York.

# 24

# Addictions

## Cheryl Bell-Gadsby

The current movement in the direction of adopting a *harm reduction* approach to the treatment of addictions is both exciting and logical. The area of addictions is in a process of change that closely resembles the evolution of brief and solution-focused therapy. The traditional "disease model" of treating substance use/misuse is limiting, rigid, and one-dimensional. This conventional model lumps all clients into one class and directs them to one principle of treatment—abstinence. The "just say no" approach in drug and alcohol treatment is clearly ineffective and implies that anyone struggling with substance-abuse issues is weak-willed and/or in "denial."

Ericksonian principles of practice, such as utilization and the recognition of naturalistic processes, create a therapeutic environment of acceptance rather than judgment and of intrinsic health rather than pathology. Erickson's approach to treating addictions was no different from his approach to therapy in general: the client's unique personality, skills, and behaviors are utilized to facilitate change. Clients are encouraged to empower themselves by accessing inner resources and abilities that may have been dormant or frozen for a variety of reasons. The therapist, therefore, is an ally or coach who assists the client to co-create unique and tailor-made solutions to previously unresolved problems and stuck patterns of behavior.

There are many examples in Erickson's writings that deal with the treatment of addictions. All center around accepting the client at face value and utilizing what is presented at the outset of therapy. One such case example involved a man who had problems with alcohol and worked and lived within a mile of several bars. He couldn't walk or ride the bus down the street to his workplace and resist going into one of the bars. During a conversation with this man, Erickson pointed out that he (the client) felt perfectly free and had good intentions when he left his house, and that he could take an alternate, longer route where there were no bars. Erickson suggested that he could get within one block of a bar without going in. Soon, he was able to walk on the other side of the street without going in, and eventually, he could go back and forth across the street until he was able to walk "freely" down the street past the bars.

"Finally he said, 'I can walk down this street.' But why shouldn't he? He was a free citizen when he stepped outside the house" (Haley, 1985, pp. 113–114). Erickson was clearly validating the man's good intentions not to drink, as well as his freedom to stop drinking. There were many indirect suggestions during Erickson's conversation with the client, as well as positive support and validation for his wish to change his behavior.

It would be nice if we all had such elegant examples of successful brief interventions in our practices. While we may not have such quick resolution of addiction (or any) problems, we, too, can utilize these principles of acceptance and utilization to similar ends. One of the key ingredients of success in solution-focused interventions as illustrated in the previous example is pattern interruption. Erickson demonstrated this in a variety of ways and on many levels throughout his practice. By being curious and finding out how each individual behaves and altering that behavior in some way, we (client and therapist) can begin to shift the problematic pattern and co-create alternative ways of being.

By paying attention to what each individual brings into the therapist's office and observing how the person interacts with his or her internal and external environment, the therapist can seed the way to the desired change. "When patients come into my office, I greet them with a blank mind and I look them over to see who and what and why they are without taking anything for granted" (Haley, 1985, p. 114). It is rather like being a detective, helping the client to sort through all the pieces of the puzzle until the mystery is solved.

In *Working with the Problem Drinker: A Solution-Focused Approach,*

Insoo Kim Berg and Scott D. Miller (1992) write about recent developments in the treatment of alcohol problems and the utilization approach.
They emphasize that "this view stands in stark contrast to that of traditional alcohol treatment approaches, which have been based largely on the
client's accepting and then working within the frame of reference of the
*therapist* and/or treatment model" (p. 7).

Traditional models have viewed alcoholics as being all alike. "Each
person experiencing an alcohol problem is *different* ... In contrast with
the one-size-fits-all approach of traditional alcohol treatment, solution-
focused therapy, with its laser-like focus on what works, helps clients
identify and then implement their own individualized plans for recovery"
(Miller & Berg, 1995, p. 16).

While there is a growing movement toward solution-focused treatment
of addictions, because this is a new area, there is still not an abundance of
research available by which to measure positive outcome. Berg and Miller
(1992) cite numerous studies that support the success of brief versus traditional programs for alcohol abuse. "Moreover, some recent research in
the area of brief therapy indicates that alcohol abusing clients can experience positive change rapidly with only minimal or brief intervention
when treatment is targeted, individualized and focused [Berg & Gallagher,
1991; Hester & Miller, 1989; Institute of Medicine, 1990]" (p. xix).

The gradual but consistent movement toward a more positive, respectful, solution-oriented approach to addictions allows us to view addiction
in a more holistic context. This, in turn, opens the door to a more integrated and multidisciplinary view of substance use. The openness of the
Ericksonian approach lends itself to the integration of a variety of alternative methods of healing. Therefore, we are no longer limited to the
fragmentation of the mind from the body. The recent wave of mindbody
research has also helped loosen the rigid parameters of the traditional
medical model view of addictions as illnesses. Ericksonian hypnotherapy
has always emphasized the importance of balance and the interconnection
of all the sensory systems.

Rossi (1986/1993, 1996) also cites numerous cases of treating addiction
in which he introduces the mindbody connection as an added diminution
to this approach. By tracking the ultradian rhythms[1] of these clients, and

---

[1] Ultradian rhythms, a term coined by chronobiologist Franz Halberg, are generally regarded
as those that are 20 hours long or less; they describe rhythms that are faster or more frequent than

their association with the cravings for substances, Rossi uses hypnotic induction to ascertain whether or not feelings and cravings can be changed.

Rossi states the hypothesis that ultradian rhythms are a window through which we may view the chaotological patterns[2] of information and communication on all levels, from mind to gene. This is the scientific basis for the common observation that "mind" can influence "body," and vice versa. Hypnotherapeutic work facilitates mindbody healing by optimizing the flow of information transduction or communication between the cognitive-behavioral level of mind to the hormonal messenger molecules and genes of the body (Rossi, 1996, p. 328).

Rossi's hypothesis is supported by current research that views psychosomatic illness and stress as originating in the "chronic abuse of our natural mindbody rhythms of activity and rest" (Rossi, 1996, p. iii). He also discusses the importance of learning to recognize the natural signals that cue us to take brief breaks throughout the day to avoid chronic stress and other physiological symptoms and problems, including addictions. In my experience in working with substance-using clients, this ability to check in with oneself is a vital step in tracking and breaking patterns of addiction.

Neuroscientist Candice Pert has also done groundbreaking research on how the chemicals in our bodies construct an information network that links mind and body. The brain and the immune system continuously signal each other, often along the same pathways. This may explain how one's state of mind influences one's health, and why hypnotherapy can be instrumental in stimulating change. All of this new information supports and illustrates just how innovative Erickson's utilization approach was and is, and how the foundation he laid can assist us in understanding and integrating the current discoveries of how this new information enables us to bridge mind and matter.

If we believe that each person has within him or her the solutions to problems with which the person may be struggling, and that the unconscious mind tends to be naturally health-seeking, we are no longer limited to a cookie-cutter approach to therapy. We can weave a variety of techniques and modalities into the previously one-dimensional view of addic-

---

circadian (about a day) rhythm. Heart rate, breathing, and brain waves are all examples of ultradian rhythms (Rossi, 1996, p. 328).

[2] Chaotological processes are those in which nonlinear dynamics of deterministic chaos make it difficult to predict behavior over long periods of time (Rossi, 1996, p. 322).

tions. Rather than being helpless in the face of an addiction and giving in to the fact that individuals dealing with these problems are powerless, we can instead believe that each individual has the ability to intervene in and take an active role in his or her own healing.

For many years, I shied away from identifying myself as a therapist who dealt with addictions. But I had to look at my caseload more realistically as it became evident that even though clients may not present with addiction issues, a large part of my work was focusing on substance use/ misuse. For the last eight to ten years, my practice has centered on the area of childhood trauma and abuse. These clients have learned to survive by dissociating and numbing out via the use of a variety of substances and habits. Because of my Ericksonian training, I have always been uncomfortable in labeling their coping skills "dysfunctional." I have learned to have a great deal of respect for these coping skills as necessary ways of adapting to unnatural or unhealthy environments and circumstances. The challenge has always been to validate and acknowledge these problematic behaviors and to reframe them into more adaptive and healthier skill sets.

The following key assumptions upon which this work is based are relevant to utilizing these principles in therapy (Zeig, 1990, p. 372):

- The benevolent intent of the practitioner. This assumes that all healing takes place within the self and can be assisted by the therapist, but that the therapist follows the lead of the client and assesses and utilizes whatever the client presents.
- The unconscious contains solutions to problems that can be retrieved to help facilitate optimum health and functioning.
- By metaphor and other forms of indirect suggestion, the therapist may facilitate a series of internal responses that can lead to the desired change. The change may or may not be overt or immediately measurable or observable.
- The therapist assists in the facilitation of a reorganization of the client's inner world so that life can be experienced as less problematic and, therefore, the symptom may no longer be necessary.
- The unconscious mind tends to be benign and generally health-seeking.

How can all of this be applied to the treatment of addiction? The study of hypnosis has taught me that when emotions are flowing freely and all systems in the mindbody are in balance, one is able to function in a healthy manner. Most clients who have problems with addiction soothe themselves by using various substances, including prescribed medication and alcohol, in order to numb out from overwhelming and disturbing experiences and feelings. According to the research of Candice Pert (1997), "When emotions are repressed, denied, not allowed to be whatever they may be, our network pathways get blocked, stopping the flow of the vital feel-good, unifying chemicals that run both our biology and our behavior" (p. 273). Therefore, drugs and other substances interfere with the many natural feedback loops that help keep the psychosomatic network functioning in a balanced way. Hypnotherapy can help unblock these natural processes and assist the client to heal on many levels.

As Erickson taught us, the first step in the process of healing is to assess the nature of the problem by gleaning relevant information from the client, as well as by closely observing what the client presents in session. As each client is unique in the manifestation of problematic behaviors and responses, it is important to introduce the concept of being curious about how clients "do" the problem. By accepting what the client presents as valid in the context of his or her experience, the therapist can set the stage for reframing problematic coping skills, such as substance use, and provide an environment of hope for change.

Once the issue is named, the clinician can help to identify patterns and subsequently link those patterns with physiological experiences and responses, including emotional material that may have been out of conscious awareness for some time. It has been my observation that most clients are extremely fearful when it comes to facing many of the core issues that led them to abuse substances. The origins are often past traumas stemming from abuse or other life experiences. The key, therefore, is to assist them to self-soothe in more healthful ways, such as deep relaxation and trance. It is not necessary to process traumatic material or experiences consciously. Indeed, this can lead to retraumatizing clients and other abreaction. The therapist can access, reframe, and clear out the problematic material via indirect suggestion and metaphor.

Before I introduce hypnosis, I begin by presenting my beliefs, understanding, and experience of the healing process and the ways in which I utilize hypnosis to facilitate change. By inviting the client to discuss and explore new possibilities, and validating clients as experts on their own lives, the therapist can help create an atmosphere of hopefulness that sets the stage for co-creating change. This also builds rapport and trust with the client and indirectly presupposes that change can happen.

The following is a framework I developed to help delineate the treatment process.

### SOLUTION-FOCUSED TREATMENT PLANNING PROCESS

## Key Ingredients and Questions

1. What area(s) of the client's life are in need of change? Where does the client want to make changes? "Where do you want to be six months from now?"

   Establish goals:
   | | |
   |---|---|
   | *Hard* | • Stop drinking, smoking, bingeing. |
   | | • Identify skill(s) to be acknowledged, acquired, or re-activated. |
   | *Soft* | • How will the client feel and act differently? |
   | | • How will you know things have changed for the better? |

2. How will the client get where he or she wants to go?

   Identify strategies and tools:
   | | |
   |---|---|
   | *Existing tools* | • What is the client already doing that is healthy? |
   | | • Identify and explore existing strengths and abilities. |
   | *New tools* | • What new and more adaptive skills can be added to deal with the problem? |
   | | • Pattern interruption, inner resources. |
   | | • Hypnosis, guided imagery. |
   | | • Relaxation. |
   | | • Cognitive restructuring. |

3. What resources will be required and how can you assist the client to access inner resources to achieve the treatment goals?

- Hypnosis.
- Tailoring metaphor.
- Body centering and relaxation.

4. Where and how will the client experience change? What will be different?

- What areas of the client's life will be different?
- How might the client think, act, respond, and relate to his or her life differently?

5. What are the costs and benefits of this change (present and future)?

- How will the status quo (relationships, routines, work) change?
- How will the client's internal experience shift?
- How can the changes be maintained?
- How can the newly learned skills be further employed and generalized in the future?

The following case is an example of the integration of an Ericksonian utilization and the naturalistic approach.

## CASE REPORT

### Presenting Problem

Leslie, a 45-year-old nurse with a history of depression and substance use, was referred by her family doctor after attending several inpatient treatment programs without any sustained success. At the time she entered therapy, she had been on long-term disability from the hospital where she had worked for several years. Leslie was viewed by her family of origin as being depressed, erratic, and alcoholic. Her mother, who had also suffered from depression and alcohol use, had died a few years earlier. Leslie was being pressured by her sister and father to stop drinking or risk being cut off from any further financial or emotional support from her family. Leslie was also taking antidepressants and tranquilizers as prescribed by her psychiatrist.

## Treatment

During the first session, Leslie and I discussed her history of depression and substance use. She had already identified the goals of therapy—to stop drinking and, if possible, to manage her depression without the use of prescribed medication. A secondary gain would be an improved and empowered relationship with her father and sister. We explored her physiological symptoms and patterns, as well as her emotional needs and reactions. After a discussion of hypnosis, a brief hypnotic induction was employed at the request of the client. This included some suggestions for relaxation and imagery and Leslie was guided through a series of suggestions, such as: *"It might be interesting to imagine yourself in a different, more relaxed way. Where would you be? What might you be doing? In what part of your body would you experience that the most? How would you be acting differently? Sounding differently? How would you know something had changed?"*

The next three sessions centered on:

- Identification of strengths, successes, areas of enjoyment and interest.
- Validation of Leslie's motivation for wellness.
- The identification of patterns and behavioral associations of Leslie's substance use and depression—when, how, where, and with whom?
- Identification of triggers—isolation, arguments with family/peers, critical self-talk, no energy.
- The introduction of some new tools: self-hypnosis and relaxation techniques.

Hypnosis and the use of metaphor were carried out. The metaphor was created keeping in mind the treatment goals and utilizing the information gleaned from previous sessions. The theme was one of empowerment and freedom from emotional and physiological control (of addiction, as well as of family). Metaphors of nature, cycles, and seasonal changes were utilized, as Leslie enjoyed walking and this was one of her healthy habits. She had also enjoyed success in her career as a nurse for many years, a source of pride and accomplishment for her. So this, too, was used by inviting her to *"remember that sense of accomplishment and pride she experienced when she had graduated from the university."* Her motivation for change was utilized by reminding her during the trance/treatment of her desire for change, as well as by linking this desire to previous successes and healthy practices in her life. Specific suggestions were made to: *"Feel free to let go of anything you would like to sort through and let go of, and to hold on to those sensations of comfort and feelings of self-appreciation. Releasing anything you would like to let go of on every exhale, and holding on to the rest."* And to: *"Allow the relaxation to deepen and continue whenever necessary to relieve the tension, stress, and cravings."*

Throughout this process, the therapist was paying attention to any visible cues (breathing, change in color, facial expression, eye movement, etc.) and utilizing them to enhance the trance/treatment.

Subsequent sessions utilized anchoring[3] to pair the desired "tranquil" state and the ability to access strengths on an ongoing basis with those times when she felt triggered to use alcohol. Leslie wore a ring, a prized possession of her mother's; this was utilized in the anchoring process to recall warm and comforting thoughts and feelings associated with her mother (also a reframe of the negative and critical messages from her family connected to her mother and the alcohol use).

Additional sessions were spent reinforcing the process, as well as normalizing and dealing with the ongoing reactions of her family and periodic setbacks in her new behavior and emotions. After approximately 14 sessions, Leslie had established a new pattern of health that included being able to resist drinking in the presence of old triggers. Many of the symptoms of depression she previously experienced were diminished. Several sessions of hypnosis were audiotaped, so that Leslie could listen to them at home and reinforce the work between sessions. This was very helpful in sustaining pattern interruption between sessions, as well as in ratifying her ability to self-soothe in healthier ways. Leslie has sustained the new behavior and is now off the tranquilizers. She continues to work on improving her self-esteem and ending her need for antidepressants.

---

[3] Anchoring is a term used by Richard Bandler and John Grinder (1975) to describe the common occurrence of paired associations of certain internal states with specific external stimuli. It is stimulus response conditioning. A touch or signal of some sort can be used to associate with a desired experience or response.

The above case is a condensed version of the process, but illustrates possibilities for its use with other habits and addictions and psychotherapeutic issues. It should also be noted that not all clients are comfortable with trying hypnosis. However, many become curious enough to try it eventually, and all benefit from its relaxing effect once they feel comfortable enough to experience it.

In summary, it is evident that the area of addictions can greatly benefit from all of the mentioned dimensions of an Ericksonian solution-focused approach, and that more research and outcome measurement will enhance and confirm the growing trend to utilizing an integrated mindbody approach to help clients enhance awareness of their problematic patterns and implement lasting change that can enhance their quality of life and empower them to resolve their problems.

---

### Five Practical Ideas

- Validate, motivate, and utilize the client's experience.
- Access and enhance awareness of naturalistic processes.
- Utilize and enhance the integration of the mindbody connection.
- Ratify and heighten new responses and patterns.
- Practice and sustain new learning and behaviors.

---

### References

Alcoholics Anonymous. (1952). *Twelve steps & twelve traditions.* Alcoholics Anonymous World Services.

Bandler, R., & Grinder, J. (1975). *Structure of magic.* Palo Alto, CA: Science & Behavior.

Bell-Gadsby, C., & Siegenberg, A. (1996). *Reclaiming herstory: Ericksonian solution-focused treatment for sexual abuse.* New York: Brunner/Mazel.

Berg, I. K., & Miller, S. D. (1992). *Working with the problem drinker: A solution-focused approach.* New York: Norton.

Haley, J. (1985). *Conversations with Milton H. Erickson, M.D. Vol. I: Changing individuals.* New York: Triangle.

Institute of Medicine. (1990). *Broadening the base of treatment for alcohol problems.* Washington, DC: U.S. Government Printing Office.

Miller, S. D., & Berg, I. K. (1995). *The miracle method: A radically new approach to problem drinking.* New York: Norton.

Pert, C. B. (1997). *Molecules of emotion: Why you feel the way you feel*. New York: Scribner.

Rossi, E. (1986/1993). *The psychobiology of mindbody healing* (rev. ed.). New York: Norton.

Rossi, E. (1996). *The symptom path to enlightenment*. Pacific Palisades, CA: Palisades Gateway.

Zeig, J. K. (1990). Ericksonian psychotherapy. In J. K. Zeig & W. M. Munion (Eds.), *What is psychotherapy? Contemporary perspectives* (pp. 371–377). San Francisco: Jossey-Bass.

## Suggested Readings

Erickson, M. H., & Rossi, E. L. (1979). *Hypnotherapy: An exploratory casebook*. New York: Irvington.

Miller, S. D., & Berg, I. K. (1995). *The miracle method: A radically new approach to problem drinking*. New York: Norton.

Pert, C. B. (1997). *Molecules of emotion: Why you feel the way you feel*. New York: Scribner.

Rossi, E. (1986/1993). *The psychobiology of mindbody healing* (rev. ed.). New York: Norton.

Rossi, E. (1996). *The symptom path to enlightenment*. Pacific Palisades, CA: Palisades Gateway.

Weil, A. (1997). *Eight weeks to optimum health*. New York: Knopf.

# 25

# Enhancing Performance in Sports, Intellectual Activities, and Everyday Life

*Ronald A. Havens & Catherine Walters*

O ur purpose in this chapter is to describe a hypnotic technique we use to help our clients enhance their performance in almost any enterprise. Our approach remains fairly constant no matter what area of life a person wishes to improve. Whether a client wants to lower his or her golf score, become a better salesperson, develop new interpersonal skills, or simply feel better emotionally, we conduct our sessions in essentially the same manner.

## ENHANCING FUTURE PERFORMANCE

After an initial diagnostic interview to determine why the person is there and what he or she wants to accomplish, we use hypnosis to clarify the thoughts, sensations, emotions, and behaviors that individual associates with the desired outcome. During this trance session, the client is instructed to imagine how it will feel to accomplish the desired goal and to examine all of the elements of this imagined situation, including the events that led up to it. This utilization of the individual's own prior experiential learnings and understandings to establish the treatment outcome ensures that the particular objectives, personality, and background of that person are taken into account and that the prescribed changes truly suit the activity under consideration.

On the other hand, the client's reservoir of experiential learnings and understandings is not the only possible source of guidance at this point. Relevant information from the professional literature also may be incorporated into the hypnotic suggestion process if necessary. For example, an ever-growing body of research consistently shows that success in virtually every endeavor, including everyday life, depends on an optimistic attitude and a positive sense of self-efficacy (e.g., Taylor, 1989; Maddi & Kosaba, 1984). Accordingly, we routinely include suggestions regarding these attitudes as the person develops the imagined experience of a successful outcome.

We also routinely include suggestions designed to promote a condition of highly focused attention. Obviously, one must focus one's attention on an activity to perform it with any degree of success. What is less obvious, and less widely known, is that a particular state of highly focused attention is commonly associated with exceptional performances in virtually any area. For example, Gallwey (1974) taught tennis and golf players to enter into a state of "relaxed concentration" to improve their game. Lozanov (1978) found that students could learn a foreign language more efficiently in a similar state that he called "concert pseudopassiveness," and Gilligan (1987) attributed the "controlled spontaneity" frequently observed in the performances of professional musicians, athletes, and psychotherapists to this condition of absorbed attention. Zeig (1985) described the way in which Milton Erickson reportedly predicted the winners of a track meet. He would choose those who were "concentrating and focusing." Race car drivers refer to this state as "streaming" and athletes in general talk about being "on" or "in the zone." Given the similarity of this experience to the absorbed attention typical of a hypnotic state, it is natural and useful to incorporate a description of it as a desirable outcome of therapy for most clients.

Furthermore, individual activities, such as target shooting, require a narrow internal focus of attention for peak performance (Maxeiner, 1987), whereas team sports demand a more diffuse and external focus (Nettleton, 1986). When such information is available for the pursuit being considered, it is added to the client's own understandings via the suggestions we offer regarding the goal state.

The specific steps involved in this intervention are as follows:

1. Conduct a trance induction or any other procedure designed to stabilize and redirect the client's attention inward. Ideally, the person will be in a receptive, passively observant frame of mind before the therapist proceeds to the next step.

2. Explain to the person that in the same way that it is possible to remember and relive a past experience, it also is possible to use imagination to "remember" an event that has not yet happened. Quickly add that the person can, for example, "remember" what it will feel like when the person realizes that he or she accomplished whatever it was that brought the person to you in the first place. Indicate that the client already knows how it will feel to do so and suggest that they he or she pay attention to those feelings and sensations now. While he or she is locating and becoming familiar with how it feels to succeed, suggestions for different aspects of the experience can be provided, such as a sense of satisfaction, well-being, or excitement.

3. After the client begins to identify and experience the emotions and sensations associated with accomplishing the desired goal, the experience is expanded and clarified, one sensory pathway at a time. Details about that future situation are gradually filled in by asking the person to pay attention to physical sensations, sounds, and sights. Eventually the person is asked to take cognizance of where he or she is, who else is there, what the date is, and so on.

4. As the person vividly imagines being in that future situation, happy and satisfied with a successful outcome, he or she is asked to "remember" the actual experience of succeeding. This step can be omitted if the goal is a change in emotional or psychological state, because it is often difficult to identify exactly when such changes occur, but if the objective is enhanced performance of some specific mental or physical activity, then it is a useful part of the process. The client has an opportunity to "experience" (and thus rehearse) how it feels to perform in a successful manner, and the therapist has an opportunity to include suggestions for particular actions or states of mind that are known to enhance performance in that endeavor. For example, this is an appropriate time to suggest that the client "remember" how it felt to be effortlessly focused and undistracted, to be sure of himself or herself and yet amazed by his or her own abilities. This also

is an appropriate time to suggest that the client examine things about the situation that seemed to make it easier to perform so well, that is, to become aware of any changes in attitude or approach that apparently helped to create a positive outcome.

5. The next step is to ask the client to remember, from that future vantage point, some of the significant events that took place along the path leading from now, sitting in your office, to the desired result. These events are mentally "reviewed" to "remind" the person about what led to the hoped-for end product and to set the stage for their eventual occurrence, but there is no need for the events to be reviewed in sequential order, nor is it necessary for the client to understand how those happenings contributed to that conclusion. In fact, it is best if the client views them as a selection of unrelated events that simply pop into the mind. Throughout the entire process, the client is encouraged to wait for different aspects of the experience simply to emerge or appear and not to create them on purpose. Even if what springs to mind does not make sense or seem relevant, as is often the case, the person is asked to observe passively and allow things to unfold in whatever manner they do without interfering or attempting to alter them.

6. Finally, as the trance and the session are brought to a close, the client is told to forget about the things that have occurred and to allow the unconscious mind to assume responsibility for turning these imagined events into reality. Although some clients are able consciously and intentionally to follow their own "unconscious" advice, others tend to alter matters in a way that merely perpetuates previous patterns of action and reaction. Thus, whenever possible, it is desirable to elicit amnesia for these experiences and to offer a posthypnotic suggestion for their eventual accomplishment in a seemingly spontaneous manner. When this suggestion is successful, clients engage in the activities that lead to the desired outcome without realizing that there is a method to it. Looking back on it, they typically report, "One thing just led to another."

Although we would love to take credit for inventing this approach, the basic rationale and structure of the technique presented here were derived directly from the work of Milton Erickson.

## ERICKSON'S APPROACH

In our book on *Hypnotherapy for Health, Harmony, and Peak Performance* (Walters & Havens, 1993), we point out that Erickson was less concerned with what people were doing wrong in the present than with getting them to do things right in the future. He encouraged the development of attitudes and behaviors that would eventually result in successful adjustment and emotional well-being. He elicited the positive attitudes, states of mind, and behaviors that he knew would allow his clients to accomplish their goals, whether those goals involved enhanced athletic performance, academic performance, or performance in everyday life. Erickson concentrated on what people could do, and he devised an impressive array of techniques to help them build better futures for themselves. He used direct and indirect hypnotic suggestions, implications, metaphorical anecdotes, and straightforward behavioral assignments to get people to begin thinking and behaving in healthier, more productive ways. The approach outlined here is based on one of these many techniques, a technique Erickson called "pseudo-orientation in time" (Erickson, 1954).

Because Erickson usually devised a unique therapeutic intervention to suit the needs and personality of each unique person, it may seem somewhat presumptuous to reduce his approach to one specific strategy to be used with a broad range of problems. Nonetheless, we believe that it is appropriate to do so. Few practitioners can emulate Erickson's creativity or wisdom and, luckily, most of the time it is not necessary to do so. We propose that it is possible, instead, to use his pseudo-orientation-in-time technique with virtually every client because it is the one intervention that captures the underlying essence of Erickson's seemingly endless list of strategies. By concentrating on one particularly powerful Ericksonian hypnotherapeutic approach, it is possible to condense his insights and genius into a manageable procedure.

Pseudo-orientation in time is one of the few techniques Erickson used with more than one patient, and it is the only one of his techniques that seems to be useful for almost any presenting problem. In his original publication on the topic, Erickson (1954) described his use of this technique with five very different patients, all of whom enjoyed successful outcomes. Each patient eventually engaged in the activity he or she had foreseen in the age-progression visualizations, and each did so with no recognition that he or she was following his or her own self-generated prescription for success.

In another publication (Erickson & Rossi, 1977), Erickson even described using this approach on himself to prepare for the unpleasant situations he realized he would eventually encounter as a physician. He projected himself into an imagined future, figured out how to cope with the unfairness and unpleasantness of the events he was likely to face in his practice, and emerged from his reverie ready to continue with his career. Given the nature of that career, it is safe to conclude that his intervention worked.

Like most of Erickson's interventions, the pseudo-orientation-in-time approach focuses the client and the therapist fully and solely on the future. In addition, because it is centered around the client's self-generated imagined experience of accomplishing the desired objective, this technique relies heavily on the client's own "unconscious" learnings and observations to define both the goal state and the steps required to arrive at that goal. Once the desired future and the steps to that future are identified, then the client is instructed to forget about it and to allow this outcome to unfold automatically or "unconsciously." No other strategy seems to capture the essence of Erickson's approach more directly or completely, and no other approach seems to be more consistently successful.

## CASE EXAMPLE

Jason, a 17-year-old member of a local high-school track team, consulted our office to improve his performance in the 1,600-meter race. His coach suggested that he seek professional help because he repeatedly lost races that, theoretically, he should have won. During practices, his lap times were consistently fast. During actual competition, however, he was unable to maintain a fast pace throughout a race. He started and finished fast, but always faded during the middle laps and lost too much ground to catch up and win. As Jason described it, he was always fired up during the first third of the race, discouraged and ready to quit during the middle third, and then would become angry and try to do his best again for the final third of the way.

The intervention in this case was quite simple and brief. Following an induction process, Jason was asked to imagine himself talking to his coach after winning an upcoming race. He was able to do this with little trouble, and he was also able to offer a verbatim account of his conversation with the coach about that race. He was then asked to remember what was different about the way he had thought about the various parts of the race and to tell his unconscious to make sure that these new thoughts arose during the next track meet. Finally, he was told to wake up without remembering much, if any, of the session. He left with a promise to return the following week and report what happened.

Jason later said that he had won his next race, although he did not know why. As he described it, he was really fired up during the *first half* of the race, and by the *second half* was getting angry and determined, just as he always did. It was immediately obvious that he had stopped splitting the race into thirds. He had solved the problem of becoming discouraged and tired during the middle third of the race by simply eliminating it from his thoughts. Interestingly, this was exactly what he had said to his coach during his imagined winning experience.

## SUMMARY AND CONCLUSIONS

Peak performance in any field is a function of multiple variables, including attitudes, emotions, innate talents, and practice. People who succeed have a clear idea of an attainable goal. They also know what they must do to accomplish that goal, and they have the willingness or desire to do it. Finally, they have optimistic expectations that they can and will reach their objective; they trust themselves and know how to get out of their own way. The techniques presented here are designed to provide these ingredients of peak performance to those who want and/or need them.

Hypnotic trance allows people to establish attainable goals. During trance conscious concerns, inhibitions, misunderstandings, fantasies, or wishful thinking do not interfere with the construction of a viable outcome. People are able to review the potential disadvantages or advantages of various goals and actions in a detached and careful fashion. The end product springs into awareness before it can be censored or modified by ordinary conscious considerations. Consequently, the imagined future is almost invariably compatible with the person's needs and capacities.

This also is the case when trance is used to envision a series of actions or events that will lead to that imagined outcome. When conscious biases are bypassed, the end product is a set of activities, insights, or decisions that are quite appropriate for that individual and that lead almost inexorably to the desired outcome. Hypnotherapists merely help people discover what they already knew about their own abilities and potentials but were unable or unwilling to acknowledge.

People seek help from professionals because they want something different, something better, to occur. They want to change their thoughts, their feelings, their actions, and their lives, but those changes will take place only after they can envision them as happening in the future. Our vision of the future is a road map, a program, a guiding principle that modifies our present actions in ways that lead us toward that envisioned outcome. To explain his technique of pseudo-orientation in time, Erickson (1954) said, "Deeds are the offspring of hope and expectancy" (p. 261). When we expect more of the same, that is what our deeds create. But when we can imagine a better future so clearly that it actually seems possible, then we begin to think and behave in ways that lead us there.

Many different techniques can be used to attain enhanced performance, but few are as straightforward or as likely to meet the unique needs and capacities of each individual as the approach presented here. If you want to help others respond in ways that promote a better future, why not follow Erickson's lead? Imagine the changes your clients will experience, first in their imaginations, then in their lives. Once you have envisioned such outcomes, you will find this approach hard to resist.

---

### Points to Remember

- Focus on what will make things go right in the future, not on what made things go wrong in the past.
- Remember that people need to know where they are going in order to get there. Help them develop a clear picture of a successful outcome.
- Always assume that the client knows at some level what goals and strategies are most appropriate and useful, but also remember to mention relevant information from the research.
- Encourage the client to enter imagined future situations by thinking about how it will feel to succeed rather than about what to do.
- After the client has a clear picture of a successful outcome and reviews the events that led to to it, suggest that the unconscious mind can now accomplish these things and that the conscious mind can forget all about them.

## References

Erickson, M. H. (1954). Pseudo-orientation in time as a hypnotherapeutic procedure. *Journal of Clinical and Experimental Hypnosis, 2,* 261–283.

Erickson, M. H., & Rossi, E. (1977). Autohypnotic experiences of Milton H. Erickson. *American Journal of Clinical Hypnosis, 20,* 36–54.

Gallwey, W. T. (1974). *The inner game of tennis.* New York: Random House.

Gilligan, S. (1987). *Therapeutic trances: The cooperation principle in Ericksonian hypnotherapy.* New York: Brunner/Mazel.

Lozanov, G. (1978). *Suggestology and outlines of suggestopedy.* New York: Gordon & Breach.

Maddi, S., & Kosaba, S. (1984). *The hardy executive: Health under stress.* Homewood, IL: Dow Jones-Erwin.

Maxeiner, J. (1987). Concentration and distribution of attention in sport. *International Journal of Sports Psychology, 18,* 247–255.

Nettleton, B. (1986). Flexibility of attention and elite athletes' performance in "fastball games." *Perceptual and Motor Skills, 63,* 991–994.

Taylor, S. E. (1989). *Positive illusions.* New York: Basic Books.

Walters, C., & Havens, R. A. (1993). *Hypnotherapy for health, harmony, and peak performance: Expanding the goals of psychotherapy.* New York: Brunner/Mazel.

Zeig, J. (1985). *Experiencing Erickson: An introduction to the man and his work.* New York: Brunner/Mazel.

# 26

# My Daughter, My Self:
# On the Neglected Importance of the
# Clinician's Own Experience

*Joseph Barber*

In the Ericksonian world, our striving to be better clinicians is most often characterized by our focus on the refinement of our clinical technique—especially our use of language. In that context, we have a wealth of opportunities to learn how to use language more effectively and benignly to manipulate a patient's perception of his or her problem.

I wish to propose a different perspective on clinical improvement, however. Participation in meetings of the Erickson Foundation for nearly 20 years, combined with my own training and experience over that period and longer, has led me to believe that the clinician's awareness of his or her perceptual and emotional responses to patients—as a guide to effective treatment—have been greatly underappreciated. The following case illustrates the neglected importance of the clinician's—not only the patient's—experience of the psychotherapeutic process.

Although as psychotherapists, we are familiar with the complications of our emotional responses toward patients when they involve angry or romantic or sexual feelings, in my treatment of Andrea, I experienced other feelings that were surprisingly unfamiliar to me, both in kind and intensity, requiring me to enlarge my understanding of myself and my patient, as well as of the process of psychotherapy as it unfolded.


## THE CASE OF ANDREA

Andrea was 28 years old, a tall woman with wide-set eyes that were alive with intelligence and curiosity. She seemed confident and poised, with a clear mind and focused attention. When I came to know her, however, I discovered that she was also profoundly influenced by others' demands and needs, which often resulted in emotional upset and intellectual confusion. Thus, I felt the need to cautiously balance the necessity that effective treatment be influential against the equal necessity that the influence derive from her own growth in awareness and self-understanding. I think that Andrea's case illustrates that this requirement was well served by the integration of, rather than the avoidance of, hypnotic technique.

### Her History

Andrea, an aspiring actress, had had a series of short-lived roles on the stage. She had recently moved to the West Coast, hoping for greater success in television and films than she had experienced on Broadway. She sought treatment for a troubling romantic relationship, her disappointment and confusion about her unfulfilling career, and long-standing, pervasive feelings of loneliness and unhappiness. I also came to learn that her parents and her siblings (she was the youngest child) were continuously enmeshed in one another's lives. While Andrea enjoyed her parents' love and support, she also suffered the suffocating, interfering quality of that love when her parents persistently gave her advice about how she could live up to their expectations.

At the beginning of treatment, Andrea was sharing an apartment with her boyfriend, Rick, 42, who had given up an unsuccessful acting career to pursue a similarly unsuccessful writing career. Rick drove his motorcycle without wearing a helmet, regularly drank alcohol to excess—and argued with Andrea daily. He physically threatened her on more than one occasion. Andrea saw their difficulties as primarily her fault for not being more understanding and supportive of Rick, a view he seemed to endorse.

Her first romantic and sexual relationship had begun at the age of 14. She characterized it as an emotionally intense, painful four years. According to Andrea, Dennis was an ingenious and troubled 16-year-old who had

had a Svengali-like influence over her, which included severe physical and emotional brutality. However, she also felt deeply understood and loved by him, and she experienced a kind of romantic exaltation, which, even now, 14 years later, she remembered with both fondness and longing.

## Initial Impressions

I found Andrea appealing and likable, with an unusual imaginative capacity. I was concerned, however, about her use of alcohol as an emotional anesthetic, and that she trusted others indiscriminately and did not respect her own perceptions and judgment.

As she recounted her history and her current situation, Andrea revealed a complex, benevolent attitude toward others and a wholly magical optimism about the world. This beautiful, childlike faith created a fragility in her: Andrea was easily surprised and hurt by the reality of life's sharp edges for which her childlike optimism had not prepared her.

## Andrea's Clinical Problems

### Her Relationships

Andrea's romantic relationship with Rick was an unsatisfying one, and was her third abusive relationship. Common to all of these relationships was her deep feeling of responsibility for the other's happiness and the consequent submersion of her own needs.

### Her Suggestibility

Andrea's mind easily made real whatever she might imagine. Unlike most people who can, for instance, imagine an elephant when asked to do so, for Andrea, imagining the elephant would involve a vivid sensory experience, almost as real as actually being in the presence of an elephant. When she engaged her imagination, there was little distinction between fantasy and reality.

The advantages of such a capacious imagination for an actress are obvious. The disadvantage for Andrea was that this facility also made vividly real her doubts and fears. For example, if she merely imagined an emotionally troublesome encounter with someone, her perceptions and emotions would develop as if she had actually had that encounter. Similarly, if Andrea felt that someone was expressing a need or a demand, her experience was that it was actually so, with little capacity for reflection or consideration of alternative possibilities. Whereas most people have some imaginative ability, Andrea's imagination was far more vivid, operated more instantaneously and seamlessly, and left her with far less observing ego than most of us have.

## Her Career

Andrea felt deeply satisfied when acting, particularly during her college years. But the arduous struggle to find remunerative work in the field made it a frustrating and painful career choice. However, she persevered because of the satisfaction she felt when she did have the opportunity to act. Perhaps even more influential, however, was her need to satisfy her mother's own lost ambitions. Her mother had abandoned a successful acting career in order to raise her family, and Andrea felt the burden of reclaiming that loss. A further source of trouble was Andrea's uncommon capacity to enter into a role. For example, if the role involved expressing unhappiness, confusion, or other unpleasant emotions, Andrea might be troubled by these feelings for days thereafter.

## Her Family

Andrea was deeply and lovingly connected to her parents and her siblings, but she was also deeply troubled by their demands on her. This became evident when Andrea had a panic attack soon after boarding an airplane to return home after a holiday visit to her family. In our exploration of this traumatic experience, Andrea became aware that leaving her family was fraught with the painful recognition that they needed her in ways she did not fully understand, and that troubled her because she felt unable to satisfy them. Moreover, she began to realize that the family depended on her to entertain them in order to distract them from family problems. She began to express to me her ambivalent feelings about this situation.

It was to be more than a year into treatment before Andrea would reveal her father's chronic alcohol use. With her greater mental clarity and emotional strength, she subsequently inspired the rest of the family to confront the father, which ultimately led to his acceptance of treatment. This confrontation was extremely confusing and painful for Andrea, because it risked her idealization of her father.

## Her New Relationship

Twenty months into treatment, Andrea met Daniel. She described her reluctance to become romantically involved with him, partly because she had begun to enjoy the emotional independence she had been developing over recent months, but mostly because she feared engaging in still another unhappy relationship. Yet she felt excited by the promise for a happy future this relationship might hold.

## TREATMENT GOALS

In addition to the goal of establishing a trusting and safe alliance with Andrea, my initial intentions were to establish a safer living environment for her by (1) facilitating her clear understanding of the harmful consequences of her relationship with Rick (for whom she acknowledged feeling sympathy and emotional dependence, but not love); and (2) helping her gain control of her excessive use of alcohol.

Once these goals were met, I intended to help Andrea develop a healthier, more fully developed sense of her self and to better tolerate unhappy feelings. Subsequently, as the troublesomeness of her imagination became clear to me, I planned to assist her to manage it better.

### Highlights of Treatment

At the beginning of our third meeting, Andrea and I discussed her MMPI profile, which confirmed my impression of her vulnerability to alcohol abuse and to needs or demands expressed by others. The profile also emphasized her chaotic life, as well as her substantial ego strength and capacity to deal effectively with problems if she were in a sufficiently stable environment. Her problems with her family and her capacity for insight suggested the likely benefits of an interpersonally based, psychodynamically oriented psychotherapy.

Andrea was embarrassed by my discussion of her drinking and energetically tried to relieve my concerns, even while reporting that she became intoxicated almost nightly. Nonetheless, she agreed to abstain from alcohol for one month and to begin keeping a daily journal. I asked her specifically to include in her journal her thoughts and feelings about drinking—especially if she noticed occasions or circumstances when she particularly missed alcohol.

When I expressed my concern about her physical jeopardy in her violent confrontations with Rick, Andrea looked surprised and sad. When I asked what she was feeling, she began to cry softly. She said, "You don't even know me. It's so hard to believe you really care about what happens to me."

At the sixth meeting, Andrea told me that she had quarreled with Rick a few days earlier, when she realized for the first time that she was afraid that he might injure her physically. I was very relieved when she acknowledged that she no longer wanted to be a part of the relationship. (I was also concerned that her reaction might reflect her need to be confluent with my point of view, rather than an independent judgment of her own.) She told Rick he would have to move out and he did, although he left many of his possessions behind. Andrea felt great sympathy for his pain and confusion, she said, and her sympathy weakened her insistence that he complete his move.

Andrea's sympathetic response to Rick was my first glimpse into her unusual capacity for empathy. Unfortunately, her empathic experience was untempered by thoughts about its meaning. This leap from thinking to affect could occur almost instantaneously for her and seriously impaired her judgment. I felt a growing concern as I came to realize how distorted that judgment could be. I also thought it likely that my relief at the breakup of their relationship included elements of a paternal judgment—not necessarily a clinical one—that Rick was not good enough for her.

A month after Andrea stopped drinking, she said that she no longer missed alcohol, although she realized that it had been a comfort to her. Because she was now free of the daily stress of the conflict with Rick, however, she said she found little need for alcohol's balm. I was pleased when Andrea also reported how much clearer her mind was. She appreciated mornings free of hangovers, and her mood was brighter. She had also begun to exercise regularly, which probably was contributing to her improved sense of well-being.

But although Andrea's mood in general had improved, she was struggling with increasing disappointment after several months of being unable to find acting jobs. She began to discuss the possibility of giving up her career, an idea she had considered intermittently, but never seriously, over the years.

Andrea loved being able to make people feel what she felt, and she identified this dynamic as the primary source of her pleasure in acting. Also, she believed that her acting was the only way to satisfy her mother's expectations, which contributed substantially to her ambivalence. She felt confused about what to do about her career choice. However, as we explored the history and psychological foundation of her role as the family's "entertainer," Andrea became less enthusiastic about a theatrical career.

I was surprised to discover that, in addition to my empathy with Andrea's ambivalence about acting, I also felt disappointed that she probably would never be a successful actress. Surely, I believe, I was feeling a father's desire to see his daughter's happy attainment of her career goal. At the same time I recognized how liberating it would be for Andrea to find a career that did not involve so much rejection and pain.

Andrea struggled with this dilemma for three months without coming to any conclusion. After much discussion with me, she finally agreed to set a deadline for making a decision about her acting career: She proposed a date one year in the future. Taken aback by the impracticality of her suggestion, I asked her if this delay might not represent further denial of the need for a decision. She laughed and said that she would make her decision about acting three months from that day.

Andrea then became depressed. Unlike her direct, contactful behavior during our previous meetings, she now seemed shy and tended to avoid eye contact with me. When I did occasionally catch her eye, she appeared discomfited, even embarrassed. Although I was not certain what this meant, I thought it might be a result of her characteristic focus on others' needs and reactions to her. It seemed likely that she resented my pressure on her to make a career decision.

A week later, Andrea asked if she could lie on the couch, saying that she might find it easier to talk to me if she were not looking at me, "... if I could forget who you are."

This suggestion seemed to me both her way of being less aware of me and an expression of her resentment of me, but at the same time, it might be an opportunity for us to deepen the therapeutic work by accessing less conscious processes.

Lying on the couch with her eyes closed, her imagination readily blossomed. She lay quietly for a minute, and then, thinking I would not need to provide suggestions to create an alteration in her consciousness, I merely asked her what she saw in her mind's eye.

Her face became animated and her voice sounded childlike. "Oh, wow! It's so amazing that you ask me that! I don't think I can describe it. It's like having a kaleidoscope in my head. No, it's more like being *inside* a kaleidoscope! Weird. Do you know what I mean?"

"I think so. Can you tell me what you see in your mind's eye if you look to your left?"

"Oh! It's so beautiful!" She began to cry, softly at first, then gradually more fully, until, finally, she was sobbing loudly.

After a while, Andrea described happy childhood scenes that came to her, unbidden. She became quiet, and I thought she might have fallen asleep.

Very softly, I asked, "What is happening now?"

Without pausing, and without stirring, Andrea spoke, in a gentle and peaceful voice, "I'm drifting."

I let a few moments pass. Then I asked, "Andrea, is it pleasant or unpleasant to drift in this way?"

"Oh, yes," she said, "Pleasant. I'm a cloud, and I'm just drifting with other clouds, all around the earth. The earth is so beautiful!"

I was puzzled. On the one hand, I was perfectly satisfied with Andrea's enjoyment of the moment. On the other, I was not at all sure that this was effective treatment; I did not understand what her experience was about. I continued to listen carefully, working to understand what was happening, when she suddenly interrupted the silence.

"I remember now. I had a dream last night."

Now we were entering territory familiar to me. I felt clearer and more confident. "Yes? What did you dream?"

She began to describe the dream, but then she stopped, saying she could not remember anything further. Then, "I'm feeling bored. I'm sorry, I know that sounds awful, but I'm just feeling bored right now." She laughed, and I imagined her laughter might be in response to her thinking that she was being rude.

"You're feeling bored now," I said, careful to not weight my response with any particular expectation. I believed that her boredom was a defense against the feelings evoked by the dream.

"Well, not right now. Now, I'm feeling embarrassed."

"Now you're feeling embarrassed?"

"Yeah, I suddenly think, 'Oh, this is dumb!' You're trying to help me, I can't remember my dream, and now I tell you I'm bored, like some spoiled kid." Her self-recrimination sounded harsh to me.

"I'd like you to be free to feel whatever you feel and to express your experience in whatever way you feel inclined to express it." I wondered, then, if I might have overstated the case. Trying to clarify, I went on, "I mean, I'd prefer that you don't break the furniture, but I'd like you to feel as free as possible to just be yourself right here and now."

"Oh, what a concept!" Andrea laughed. "You sound just like a shrink."

I felt a sting. What had provoked her anger? I realized that, in my attempt to be reassuring, I had awkwardly misspoken. Should I comment on her anger, or let it pass? Would commenting on it distract us from this discussion of her freedom of mind, or was this comment an essential part of the process? As these thoughts filled my mind, I became increasingly convinced that my need to reassure Andrea had resulted in my distracting her. And insulting her.

Andrea quietly apologized for "being snotty," saying that I had hurt her feelings by suggesting that she might break the furniture. "Why did you say that?"

Why, indeed? My misstep had left me feeling awkward and doubtful about how best to see this through. I wanted to be honest and clear with her, yet I did not want to hurt or confuse her further. I heard myself rushing onward to explain myself, anxious to recover my balance. To be honest, I was more worried about me and my ability as a psychotherapist at that moment than I was about Andrea. I was overreacting to her misunderstanding of my intent and to her hurt feelings. I felt an inappropriate level of responsibility for her feelings, which was one way in which Andrea and I were similar—a similarity likely to heighten both positive transference and positive countertransference. As if in response to my silent concern, her response sounded more like a reassurance to me than an understanding of what I meant. As she left my office a few minutes later, I wished that I were a less clumsy psychotherapist. In subsequent meetings, however, I did not observe further consequences of this troubling conversation.

At the 16th meeting, Andrea was still reporting fatigue from restless nights and anxious days. Thinking both that it might be prudent to help alleviate these symptoms and that now might be a good time for Andrea to begin learning to manage her imagination better, I decided it would be an appropriate juncture at which to integrate hypnotic methods more actively. I suggested to her that we could use her imagination to help her with these problems.

Andrea was enthusiastic. In the ensuing conversation, I noticed that her unusual comfort with the imaginative world was for me a source of pleasure and pride. I found her highly imaginative mind quite charming. In this instance, her imaginative capacities were clearly a strength for her.

I suggested to her that, just as her imagination could create unpleasant anxieties, so, too, this capacity could be used to foster other, more pleasant thoughts and feelings. She responded quite readily to this intervention, which focused primarily on suggestions for comfort and relaxation. Afterward, she said that she greatly enjoyed the experience. Over the next several weeks, Andrea happily reported using self-hypnotic methods I had taught her to improve her sleep, and she was proud of this newly found self-control.

I had expected that, although Andrea continued to do well in a number of areas, when the deadline for making her career decision arrived, she would characteristically attempt to procrastinate. However, I was wrong. The week before the deadline, Andrea reported that she had applied for an administrative job. Further, she said, "If I get the job, I want to begin seeing you twice a week. There's a lot to talk about."

I was surprised at her enthusiasm for accelerating treatment; I hoped it reflected a greater comfort with the psychotherapeutic process. Andrea did not get the job, but she accepted my proposal that we meet twice a week anyway.

Although she had wide-ranging job interests, Andrea concentrated on finding work in a library. To this end, she first volunteered her time at the city library, and then effectively pressed whatever advantages she could in her capacity as a volunteer. She was soon hired as an administrative assistant. Although she thought of this job as a strategic step toward more challenging positions, she began to enjoy her work.

Over the next several months, Andrea's mood improved substantially. She no longer seemed anxious or depressed, she reported growing satisfaction with her new work, and she became more and more engaged in the process of exploring herself and in developing greater emotional independence.

It was soon after this that Andrea visited her family, carrying with her some newly acquired insights that had replaced her familiar, idealized sense of the family. It was during this visit that Andrea observed the seriousness of her father's drinking problem. Conversations with her siblings led to their unanimous insistence that their father undergo treatment for his alcoholism, and with their mother's reluctant support, he did so. This confrontation also led to Andrea's seeing her father as a somewhat pitiable man, overshadowed by his wife both intellectually and emotionally.

Andrea felt less helplessly bound to her family after this visit, and for the first time in her many visits with them, when it was time to leave, she was ready to do so. She did not feel the familiar painful longing to stay. "I guess I'll really make the West Coast my home now," she told me.

When Andrea arrived in my office several weeks later, the smile on her face reflected good news. Daniel was a struggling young architect, and the first man of her own age to whom she had ever been attracted. She did not really know how Daniel felt about her, but she was delighted that he had accepted her invitation to dinner later in the week.

Andrea was to feel both thrilled and frightened by Daniel as they became better acquainted. She loved his gentle, mature masculinity; was excited by the intensity of his emotional response to her; and yet felt frightened by the strength of her own response to him: She feared yet another painful romantic entanglement.

Sharing some of Andrea's own reactions, I was both delighted and wary. Rather than express my feelings, however, I tried to facilitate her growing awareness of the meaning of the emotional reactions this relationship evoked for her. I felt confident of her developing self-awareness, but I wanted to protect her from becoming involved in another unhealthy relationship. However, I did not act on my impulse to suggest that she bring Daniel to the office so that I could meet him (as a good father might, I thought).

In my view, with Andrea's growing ability to deal more effectively with her family and, in particular, with her father (who remained sober following inpatient treatment and ongoing participation in Alcoholics Anonymous meetings), she developed a greater ability to deal more effectively with the rest of her life. Andrea was growing up. She spoke less about the interpersonal difficulties that had been such an expected, routine part of her life, and more about her internal process. When I asked about particular work or social relationships, Andrea reported having substantially more satisfying interactions.

About four months after meeting Daniel, Andrea told me that they were discussing the possibility of buying a house together. She was excited about the potential for creating a happy home with Daniel, and less anxious about his growing importance in her life. My own delight increased correspondingly.

I asked her if this meant that they had discussed the future of their relationship. Andrea blushed and said, "I was just about to tell you! But

I'm a little worried as to what you'll think."

This eventuality was not really a surprise to me; the quality and intensity of their relationship had seemed increasingly healthy and happy, and I was privately hoping that it would continue to develop. I invited her to tell me about her worry.

"I feel worried, I guess, that you might think we don't know each other well enough yet. I feel worried that you might not want me to get married."

Now, this was a startling idea. Did I not want this, or was this Andrea's projection? "Have I said or done something that tells you I don't want you to get married?"

"No, not exactly. But whenever I talk with you about Daniel, I feel like you're searching for evidence that he's a creep, or something."

Perhaps this was not merely her projection. I was aware of concern for her, but I was not aware of anything more. How could I best convey my concern without also implying that I did not want her to marry? I felt quite paternal as I considered this.

"Well, you're certainly right, I always listen for anything that might be a source of trouble for you. This is true not only about Daniel, but about any other area of your life, I'm sure. Andrea, I do care about you, but I'm not worried about your relationship with Daniel."

"I guess I'm glad that you're concerned. I just wondered if there was something you knew about Daniel that I don't know."

"If you had told me something that made me worry about Daniel as a partner for you, I'd certainly let you know, but you haven't. On the contrary, you've told me how gentle, loving, and respectful he is toward you. You've told me how easily and quickly the two of you connected. What is it, four or five months now? You've told me about arguments you've had, and how the two of you were able to handle your hurt and angry feelings. So far, from what you tell me, this sounds like a pretty terrific relationship."

Andrea smiled, opened her eyes, and turned her head to look at me as she continued to lie on the sofa. "You're so sweet. You knew just what I needed to hear."

Did I? Was I being manipulated here, like a father by a daughter? I hoped not, but I was not sure. "What are you feeling right now about what I've said?"

She spoke through tears. "I feel so lucky that you've helped me to be ready for meeting Daniel."

I was touched, again, by Andrea's openness and generosity of spirit. I did not know what to say, so I remained quiet, basking in the glow of her happiness.

A few months later, after she told me that she and Daniel were engaged, Andrea was trying to tell me something else, but was having difficulty finding the words. Finally, she said, "I really want to send you a wedding invitation, but I would feel truly uncomfortable if you came. Oh, I feel so ungrateful! I mean, I'd like you to be there in spirit."

I felt very much the same way. "Andrea, I would be delighted to receive an invitation, but I can understand that my actually being at your wedding might feel very strange."

She sighed deeply. "I'm so glad you understand. I mean, I'd really like you to be there, but when I imagine it, it seems so weird—I mean, to have *my shrink* at my wedding! Like I'm mentally ill, or something. Or worse—a Hollywood actress!"

We both laughed.

She went on, "At the same time, you've been such an important part of my life, and I feel like you're part of my family. Oh, I don't know how to say what I want to say."

I felt grateful and relieved. And I felt liberated by her acknowledging her feeling that I was part of her family. After all, I was not Andrea's father, I was her psychologist. Her own father would be there—and sober—to be a part of her wedding.

## MY PERSONAL EXPERIENCE AND REACTIONS

What was it about my time with Andrea that stirred primitive feelings of paternal tenderness in me?

Upon my first meeting Andrea, I had felt a normal human interest in her, and I had a professional interest in helping her with her problems. As I began to know her better, I also observed the colorful intricacies of her unusual mind and I felt both a fascination with her imaginal capacities and an admiration for her lack of defensiveness. I had misgivings, as well, as I learned of the difficulties she sometimes faced as a result of being undefended against the harshness of the world.

Over time, I began to feel as if Andrea were a child who needed someone (me) to take care of her—as if she were my daughter. When she made progress, I felt fatherly pride in her. Sometimes, I realize now, I felt too protective. I wanted to keep her safe from harm—as well as from sadness, loss, and pain. At the same time, though, I recognized that this was impossible and I knew she had to learn for herself how to handle life's challenges. This process meant that I had to come to grips with, recognize, and accept my own paternal feelings, and yet despite their satisfying quality, to move beyond them to what was helpful to Andrea. Several times, over the months, I reminded myself that I was her psychologist, not her father.

Prior to my treating Andrea, I had not had such strong feelings of tenderness and affection for any patient. Over time, I found I could tolerate, and eventually even enjoy, these feelings. I think it was, in part, Andrea's openness and vulnerability that drew me further into this nurturing mode than I was used to, that created a new acceptance in me. More and more, I could delight in the experience, too. It also helped me to see how much growth and change this nurturance produced in Andrea. Although I tried to keep my overprotective impulses out of the treatment, I was not wholly successful in doing so. Andrea's concern about my feelings relating to her involvement with Daniel was just one of the indications that reminded me to remain vigilant as to my motivations.

In addition, a kind of wish identification with Andrea stimulated an even stronger set of paternal feelings. It was as if, in growing to know Andrea, I was meeting, in some respects, an ideal, younger, female version of myself, and I felt, as we sometimes feel about our children: "Here is someone who carries the hopes I have had for who I might have become." Just as this wish poses hazards for our children, so, too, my response to Andrea, while fostering potential therapeutic qualities in myself, was also fraught with potential difficulties.

Four of Andrea's characteristics evoked this wish identification: (1) She came from a privileged background. In particular, she had received an unusually fine undergraduate education. This was an opportunity I wished I myself had been given. (2) She had a rare and vivid imagination. Although I also have good imaginative capacities, I wished that mine were as unlimited as Andrea's. (3) Andrea's empathic ability was remarkable. Whereas I believe my own to be ample, I wished mine were as substantial as hers. (4) Andrea's lack of defensiveness when confronting troublesome qualities of her self and her life was a characteristic I admired and wished for in myself.

As I would come to learn, my experience of treating Andrea was also an opportunity for growth in my capacity for self-awareness and for greater comfort and familiarity with these particular, tender emotions and wishes as they emerged in treatment, and as they continue to develop.

### EPILOGUE

In the years since they met, Andrea and Daniel have developed a happy and satisfying partnership. Although I am pleased for them, I also feel a pride in the courage Andrea demonstrated in her psychotherapy, with her family, in her initial struggles with Daniel, and in her enduring commitment to their partnership. I notice that this pride is not entirely unpaternal.

Even now, many years later, I sometimes find myself thinking about Andrea, wondering how she and Daniel and their children are faring. When I was her psychologist, I felt appropriately constrained from expressing my own paternal needs with her. Although I refrain from intruding in her life, I enjoy responding (carefully) when she writes to me. So it is with special pleasure that I receive a card from Andrea each year around holiday time.

Before meeting Andrea, I had never harbored paternal feelings for my patients. However, that has changed. Perhaps my treatment of Andrea freed me to enjoy those qualities of tenderness and uncritical affection that both are intrinsically rewarding and foster easy interactions with patients, especially with those who will benefit from my nurturance. My experience with this special patient did more than broaden my capacity to nurture; it also taught me, like a father, when and how to let her go when she was ready to move more fully and independently into a healthy adult life.

## 27

# The Problem Is the Solution:
# The Principle of Sponsorship
# in Psychotherapy

*Stephen Gilligan*

"Wake up to find out
that you are the eyes of the world."
— Robert Hunter

In the movie "Pleasantville," two adolescent siblings from the 1990s find themselves transported into a 1950s black-and-white TV sitcom landscape based on the old show "Father Knows Best." While on the surface everything seems perfect, there is no depth, mystery, color, or soul in this world. Everyone lives in an enclosed "pleasant trance" devoid of real liveliness, a sort of mindless "brave new world." The two "visitors" instigate a series of happenings that precipitate awakenings in each person, including themselves. Each awakening occurs when a person connects with a hidden or undeveloped part of his or her being. For a teenage athlete, it happens via love and romance; for the kids' "mother," it comes from discovering the sensuality of her body; for the father, it comes from recognizing his longings; for the girl, it comes from reading classics; for the boy, it comes from finding his fierceness. In each case, the experience and expression of undeveloped parts of the self transform the person into living "color." They and others around them have to deal with the myriad responses that arise in response to this awakening.

Pleasantville is all around us. It keeps us asleep through false smiles, violent threats, unspoken fears, disembodied thinking, numbness, consumerism, and other practices of the modern and postmodern world. A corporate woman in a poetry workshop (cited by Whyte, 1994, p. 31) wrote:

"Ten years ago . . .
I turned my face for a moment
And it became my life."

We have all suffered those 10-year "gaps" in our lives, where we thought we were present but then, in hindsight, realized we weren't.

The damming of life cannot continue forever. Sooner or later, the river leaks through, bringing with it a myriad of memories, dreams, and reflections. This can be a frightening time, for the fear in exile is that we will be overwhelmed, perhaps even die, if we allow these currents to wash over and through us. New defenses arise—more dissociation, more compulsive behaviors, more "playing dead," more intellectualization, more violence against self and others—all desperate attempts to regain control and expel the "negative otherness" that presses upon us. At some point, it becomes clear that we're losing the battle—we're dealing with a presence stronger than our ego, and our vaunted defenses no longer can keep separate from it. In desperation, we may turn to a therapist in the hope of fortifying our ego and its defenses.

When clients visit us, how we regard the disturbances in their lives—the experiences and events that are throwing them into "organized chaos"—makes a great deal of difference. The traditional view is generally that we should help the client overcome these "pathological" forces that threaten well-being. This view regards the "problem" as an "enemy" that should be defeated, through any means possible. Milton Erickson (1980a, 1980b) pioneered an entirely different approach, one based on accepting and working with a person's "problems" as unique presences that could, under the proper conditions, be the basis for new learning and growth. For example, a young secretary was utterly convinced that a large gap in her teeth made her ugly and undesirable. Erickson had her learn to squirt water through the gap in her teeth until she was able to hit a distant target. He then got her to wait at the office water cooler to "ambush" a young man (to whom she was attracted) with a squirt of water. One thing led to another, and the couple lived happily ever after.

The legacy of Milton Erickson has been elaborated on and deepened in many ways in the last 20 years. My own work has moved from a more mainstream Ericksonian emphasis (see Gilligan, 1987) to the development of a neo-Ericksonian approach I call self-relations psychotherapy (see Gilligan, 1997). Like Erickson's work, self-relations emphasizes the positive aspects of problems and symptoms. It sees such disturbances of the "normal order" as evidence that "something is waking up" in the life of a person or community. Such disturbances are double-edged crises. On the one side, they are (often hidden) opportunities for major growth. Most of us, for example, can recall negative events—a death, divorce, illness, or addiction—that led to a significant positive change in our lives. On the other side, such disturbances can be very destructive; we *can* get lost in depression, acting out, or other problematic behaviors. Self-relations suggests that the difference lies in whether or not a disturbance can be "sponsored" by a skillful human presence.

The principle and processes of sponsorship are the cornerstone of self-relations. The word "sponsorship" comes from the Latin *spondere*, meaning "to pledge solemnly." So sponsorship is a vow to help a person (including one's self) to use each and every event and experience to awaken to the goodness and gifts of the self, the world, and the connections between the two. Self-relations suggests that experiences that come into a person's life are not yet fully human; they have no human value until the person is able to "sponsor them." Via sponsorship, experiences and behaviors that are problematic may be realized as resources and gifts. In this way, what had been framed and seen as a problem is recognized as a "solution."

The motto for therapeutic sponsorship may be found on the Statue of Liberty in New York Harbor:

> "Give me your tired, your poor,
> Your huddled masses yearning to breathe free,
> The wretched refuse of your teeming shore,
> Send these, the homeless, tempest-tost to me.
> I life my lamp beside the golden door."
> — Emma Lazarus, 1849–1887

In self-relations, this motto not only refers to people, but to experiences and behaviors as well. For example, Fred was an academic who was seeing me for what he described as "low-grade, long-time depression." He arrived at one session complaining of being "a sexual pervert." Taking a sabbatical year off to write and to stay home with his baby son, Fred found himself downloading pornography from the Internet for up to three hours a day. He explained that it took him this long partly because his fear of being "caught" would not allow him to give his credit card number; instead, he would search for sites featuring free "teaser pictures," download them, and then meticulously organize them into a library that had to be constantly updated. I had been working with him for about three months on his presenting problems of feeling depressed and anxious in some work-related matters. He had let me know in general terms about the pornography interests when I previously inquired about his sexual and social life, but had strongly rebuffed my attempts to engage him around those topics.

In bringing it up now, he said it was draining his energy and he desperately wanted to do something about it. As I listened to him, I noticed that my early Catholic guilt had come back to visit me, suggesting I send Fred to Father McCarthy for confession, followed by a lifetime of very cold showers. I also noticed that this "suggestion" led to my feeling off-center and rigid, so I allowed it to pass. (A major benefit of both hypnosis and meditation is that they teach you a "just let it happen" attitude toward your mind, so you can compassionately observe each thought or feeling without identification, and then decide how you'd like to proceed.) I worked to develop a receptive state in which I felt connected, open, and curious as to the positive gift that was awakening in Fred. After several minutes, l became aware of what a beautiful man Fred was, something I had somehow overlooked previously. I found myself talking with him about how sexual energy is perhaps the most powerful, undefeatable energy in the world. I suggested that finding one's deep sexual identity is a lifelong challenge that takes everything one has. I complimented Fred on the amazing depth and intensity of his sexual presence, but said that I had little confidence in his repressing it.

The relational "field" seemed filled with a deep connection, probably the most connected I'd felt with Fred. He seemed touched and receptive to my compliments, and developed a light hypnotic state in response to them. I talked some more about how, for whatever reasons, his sexuality seemed to be calling him to a deeper awareness. He agreed, but said he was scared. I acknowledged that he was scared, noting with special emphasis, "Yes, Fred, as a sexual being, you are scared." Pausing to let this stand on its own, I then asked: "As a sexual being, who else are you?" He laughed a bit nervously before saying, "I'm also very horny!" I paused to sense this part of his sexual self before feeding back, "Yes, Fred, as a sexual being, you are also horny!" I then suggested that he continue with further answers to, "Who am I as a sexual being?" It took a little coaching for Fred to settle down so he could speak, feel, hold, and make visible one sexual identity at a time. For example, he might say, "As a sexual being, I am really ashamed," then be encouraged to let go, feel that identity in his bodymind as I fed it back and acknowledged the importance of that truth. The next one might be, "As a sexual being, I really get turned on by looking at beautiful naked female bodies." As he spoke it, I would see it, nonverbally connect with it, gently name it, encourage him to know it, and nonverbally witness it. After 10 seconds or so of silence, I would ask, "Who else are you as a sexual being?" This continued for about eight identities, including "I am . . . afraid, really turned on, interested in touch, numb, obsessed, paranoid, and intense." Each identity was individually sensed, felt, made visible, properly named, blessed, and allowed its special place.

Somewhere during the process, Fred looked so beautiful, the way people look in therapy when they're no longer dissociating. It was as though he somehow had found a way to begin to make room and to reveal the deepest parts of his sexual identity. We talked about how sexual identity had so many different emotional truths and other identities enfolded in it. I suggested that what really distinguished a "pervert" from a vital, healthy sexual being was the ability to sense the relational connections between these diverse identities, as well as to feel the "unitary field" of self that held all of them. (For example, many identities might be contradictory, but all can have a place in the field of self.) We talked about a few technical ways (extensions of the exercise) in which he could practice this sponsorship of sexual identity.

Two weeks later, at the next session, Fred shared his surprise that, for whatever reason, his preoccupation with Internet pornography had been virtually absent. At the same time, he began to focus on concerns regarding his wife and their relationship. Further sessions focused on couples work, especially in terms of the relation between intimacy and sexuality.

## IDEAS ABOUT SPONSORSHIP

This small example provides a few hints about a number of ideas of therapeutic sponsorship. We might note three basic ideas here.

1.    There are two modes of experience: the *fressen* of nature and the *essen* of culture. In German, there are two words for eating: *fressen* and *essen*. *Fressen* means to eat like an animal, a pig; *essen* is to eat like a human being. As anybody who has raised a child can attest, the road from *fressen* to *essen* is a long one. It takes tremendous acts of sponsorship to help a child learn to eat like a person!

If we take this distinction and generalize it to other human activities, we can see that each aspect of being a person comes to us as "not ready for prime time" *fressen* energies. It is the "re-spons-ability" of the community to help a person develop social-cognitive relational skills to transform these energies into *essen* forms that have value to the person and the community. Thus, the fierceness that reveals itself as temper tantrums in a toddler can, if properly sponsored, developmentally progress into the admirable fierceness of the mature individual. If negatively sponsored, the same tantrums may later reveal themselves as rage, passive aggressiveness, violence, or other social forms that seem to have little or no value.

I discussed at length in *The Courage to Love* (Gilligan, 1997) what some of these sponsorship practices involve, including the following.

- Centering/opening attention
- Deep listening/proper naming
- Being touched by/touching
- Challenging/accepting
- Connecting with resources and traditions
- Developing multiple frames/practicing behavioral skills
- Cultivating fierceness, tenderness, and playfulness

These practices, some of which are elaborated below, are the ways and the social/cognitive/experiential means by which a *fressen* energy is awakened into consciousness and cultivated into the human value of an *essen* form.

2. A generative self develops each time *essen* and *fressen* integrate. In this view, the experience of a self arises at each moment that the *essen* mind—the *cognitive self* that performs acts of meaning and value—integrates with the *fressen* mind—the *somatic self* organized within the archetypal, experiential language of the body. The generative self is not a given, nor is it always present: it is a dynamic realization that awakens each time the cognitive and somatic selves are cooperating. A good example of this creative/created self can be found in artists. Most artists—writers, painters, poets, dancers—emphasize that their creative energies come from some place other than their cognitive (conscious) self. The task of the artist is to find ways in which to receive those energies and cultivate a relationship with them. This relationship is neither one of domination nor one of submission; the artist neither totally "controls" the creative energy nor has the

luxury of just "passing out" and being overwhelmed. Rather, he or she must find a way to "sponsor" these energies, to midwife them into creative form.

In the same way, each person is a performance artist, and is visited regularly by creative but chaotic life energies that are calling the person to do something interesting. If he or she can develop sponsorship skills, these energies can take helpful forms in the social world. If not, they may become persistent, troubling feelings or behaviors—anxiety, depression, agitation, and the like.

3.   Symptoms and other acts of violence arise each time *essen* ignores, curses, or exploits *fressen* energies. We can begin to see that while life flows through you, giving you everything you'll need to become a person, your presence also is deeply needed. If you do not "sponsor" the *fressen* gifts given in the moment, they will persist and repeat themselves with an even greater intensity. If you curse them, they will take on negative forms. If you exploit them, they will take on distorted forms. At some point, they seem to be a presence greater than the social/cognitive self, a repetitive experience or behavior beyond your control. The more you try to get rid of it, the deeper it becomes entrenched. This is what we call a "clinical symptom": a disturbing *fressen* energy that has not yet been therapeutically sponsored into a helpful *essen* form.

As therapists, we look for the unsponsored *fressen* energies. We become intensely curious about the disturbing experiences and behaviors by which a person feels overwhelmed, and welcome them as the basis for creative new developments. We realize that efforts to resist or overcome these "problems" not only are futile but typically have the effect of sustaining them. As Watzlawick, Weakland, and Fisch (1974) emphasized, the attempted solution is the problem. For example, a person who tried to overcome nagging doubts by obsessive "positive thinking" became even more agitated, self-absorbed, and ineffective. Self-relations posits that the opposite is equally true: the problem is the solution. That is, what seems at first glance to be a terrible experience to be avoided at all costs is that which provides, under proper conditions and effective sponsorship, exactly what the person needs in order to grow and develop further. For example, the client with "nagging doubts" was invited to welcome them while in a deeply relaxed state. While doing so, the client noticed a tender presence within the heart that had been ignored. Integration of this tender presence led to a calmer, more centered presence, one that was neither negative nor positive.

The presence of "proper conditions and effective sponsorship" is the key here. Without them, more ineffective suffering (Merton, 1964) and disturbing events will be the case. So our major challenge in psychotherapy is to define and effectively create the ways and means of transformational sponsorship.

### ASPECTS OF THERAPEUTIC SPONSORSHIP

### Active Non-doing

When clients enter therapy, they are often caught up in an obsessive mode of "What do I do? What do I do? What do I do?" Often therapists react to these anxious demands with the response, "What do *I* do? What do *I* do? What do *I* do?" The compulsive problem solving that results is a major reason why therapy remains stuck. So one of the important things for a therapist (and client) to do is "nothing." The Chinese call this state *wu-wei*, or "active non-doing."

*Wu-wei* does not mean falling asleep, collapsing, resigning oneself, or withdrawing. On the contrary, it is an alert, yet relaxed, mode in which one feels centered and open to the entire field of activity. Erickson had this in mind when he said: "Too many psychotherapists try to plan what thinking they will do instead of waiting to see what the stimulus they receive is, and then letting their unconscious mind respond to that stimulus" (in Gordon & Meyers-Anderson, 1981, p. 17).

So *wu-wei* is a sort of a relational meditation process. It is what an artist does to invoke the creative spirit or an athlete does before a big event.

The therapist practicing active non-doing feels connected to the self and client, deeply curious about whatever is "waking up" in the client's consciousness. The interest is in letting the client's spirit touch you, find you, and guide you. There are many ways to enter this process; most involve conscious breathing, somatic relaxing, attentional opening, and cognitive curiosity (see Gilligan, 1997). Sometimes I even say a little prayer to let whatever needs to be sponsored find me and teach me how to love it and support it.

A major skill being cultivated via *wu-wei* is attentional stability. In problem spaces, one of the first casualties is the destabilization of attention. When disturbing experiences arise, the result is often overrigidity, fragmenting, spaciness, constricting, and so on. A person loses his or her center, forgets about his or her embeddedness within larger fields, and becomes unhelpfully reactive (rather than responsive). *Wu-wei* is a relational meditation that allows one to reconnect with whatever is happening while regaining one's center. From there, helpful responses can arise.

Active non-doing is especially helpful for both client and therapist at the beginning of each session. It can be introduced through a meditation, light trance, or other simple mindfulness practices. It can be consciously returned to throughout the session, especially when it seems that the experience is stuck.

## Therapeutic Focusing

Eugene Gendlin (1996) found that one of the best predictors of the helpfulness of a therapy session is whether or not the client can develop, within the first part of the session, a "felt sense" of the problem. Gendlin (1996) points out that felt sense is distinct from simply emotions, physical sensations, or perceptions:

> A felt sense is the wholistic, implicit bodily sense of a complex situation. It includes many factors, some of which have never been separated before ... A felt sense contains a maze of meanings, a whole texture of facets, a Persian rug of patterning—more than could be said or thought ... One single thing, one statement, or next step can arise from the whole of it, if we allowed it to form. (p. 58)

In Gendlin's "focusing" approach, a client is asked to develop a "felt sense" by letting go of trying to figure things out and then sensing how the body is representing the problem. Further listening and dialoguing with the felt sense are the basis for therapeutic progress.

In the self-relations method of *therapeutic focusing*, both client *and* therapist are asked to connect with and track their respective felt senses. In the first step of this process, the therapist gives primary attention to the felt sense in his or her own body as the client talks about his or her problem. For example, the therapist may notice a sense of tightness, or emptiness, in the belly as he or she listens receptively to the client's presentation. The therapist allows his or her attention to drop into that place, making it a listening center. Mindfulness of this center continues throughout the method.

In the second step, the therapist also attends to the *client's* center of disturbance. The therapist might find the client's voice tonality leading to the center. Or he or she might look at the midline of the client's torso, noticing where the energy seems to be either intense (anxiety) or withdrawn (depression). Tuning into that place (while maintaining his or her own felt sense), the therapist gently asks the client to take a few moments of silence to sense where in his or her body he or she most feels the center of disturbances. The client is invited to gently place a hand on that center to bring more attention to it.

The simultaneous sensing and tracking of the two centers are then continued for the duration of the session. One value is that this centers and stabilizes the attention of both therapist and client. One of the major problems with problems is that they tend to destabilize attention; it can become fragmented, disconnected, too narrow, too intellectual, and so on. Therapeutic focusing can keep bringing both the therapist and client back to their felt senses.

Therapeutic focusing also helps the therapist to listen to the story without being involved with it. It is important to appreciate that the problem narrative typically leads one away from connection, not deeper into it. It is easy to get caught up in "talking about" the problem, or even forgetting it; therapeutic focusing teaches you a way to "be with it" without being affected by the explanations or "story line." In this sense, self-relations sees problems in terms of a disconnection between the stories of the cognitive self and the felt sense of the somatic self.

Therapeutic focusing also establishes a center-to-center relational connection between the therapist and client that can be used to track what's happening. For example, I was talking with a client about some difficult aspects of his marriage. We had established some form of therapeutic focusing, and the man seemed very connected. But after several minutes, I suddenly felt a disconnection to my own center. I noted this aloud to him, and wondered what he was feeling in his center. He started talking faster, but I gently asked him again. He said that he felt the same, that he had gone off somewhere. This awareness allowed us to reconnect with the felt center, so that what was being talked about was connected to felt sense.

## Providing Sanctuary, Proper Naming, and Blessings

As you connect with felt sense, you can begin to midwife new life into a person's being. Felt sense is a first stage of a new identity-related process that can be more fully developed through such sponsorship practice as providing sanctuary, proper naming, and blessings.

Providing sanctuary means offering a safe place, both in the bodymind and in the community, for a person or experience. This requires touching it with human presence, allowing it to be, listening deeply, and extending connection to it. It is what an artist does in welcoming creative impulses, or what a parent does when a child approaches with a skinned knee. If these felt senses are ignored, rejected, or cursed, they can turn nasty and unbearable. Their human value will go unrealized, and real suffering will result. So the stakes are enormously high.

Thinking in terms of sanctuaries suggests that we think of a person's center as having two levels: emotional context and emotional content. Virginia Satir pointed to this difference when she would ask a person two questions: (1) How do you feel about that? (2) How do you feel about feeling that way? The first regards emotional content; the second relates to the feeling context in which the content is held. The latter is especially important: The person who develops a bodymind sanctuary within which any experience can visit a feeling context has made it safe both for the experience and for the person(s) involved to "just let it happen."

A major value of creating a sanctuary is that it differentiates the experience from the person experiencing it. This is a central goal of many bodymind practices, including hypnosis, meditation, EMDR, and self-relations. For example, as the experience of rage arises, providing it with a place (say, in the belly) allows the person to bear witness to the rage without identifying with it. At the same time, providing sanctuary within a mindbody center (heart, solar plexus, or belly) gives it a specific container so that it doesn't spill out, project, or overwhelm the person or others.

As the person can bear witness to it, proper naming may develop. This does not mean an objective classification, but rather a touching of a felt sense with language. It is not an act of separation or dissection, but one of communion of subject with object. Naming adds an entirely human level to an archetypal experience, transforming it and extending it into the realm of human consciousness. (Without language, an experience is living but not human.) With most symptoms, a significant experience has not been properly named, held, and blessed; it is, therefore, dominant but seems to have no human value, for the simple reason that the sponsors involved have not properly welcomed and named it as "value-able."

For example, a man who had spent much of his adult life as a top-notch, hard-working lawyer began to slow down as he hit the age of 70. He was exhausted at night, his body wracked with anxiety, fear, and worries. His attempts to muscle the tiredness into submission just made matters worse.

When he finally slowed down and listened to the felt sense in his heart, the presence of "death" was sensed and named. He broke out sobbing, continuing for some time. As the sobs subsided, he talked about how he had been running from death and that it was overtaking him. Further conversations with "death" clarified his interests in living and enjoying quality time as long as possible, which led to a significant change in his lifestyle, and the relationship of his "head" with his "heart."

There are many ways in which to name experiences properly that are felt but not sponsored. For example, a simple exercise that I often use with couples, and sometimes with individual clients, involves having the clients get comfortable, centered, open to the field, and tuned to each other. Partner A makes the following statements:

- Today my woundedness is about _____.
- Today my longing is for _____.
- Today my strength is about _____.

For each blank, the person lets a word or phrase come to mind, and then speaks it. It is important that it not be planned; the response should just come from listening to one's center and letting it happen. For example, the person might say: "Today my woundedness is about *missing my daughter* ... Today my longing is *to be held* ... Today my strength is about *reaching out to others.*" In speaking each experience, the person seeks to let the energy lift from his or her center and extend into the relational field holding both partners. This is then released, a silent pause ensues, and the next sentence is undertaken. After Partner A finishes three statements, Partner B responds with his or her own three. This cycle can be repeated a number of times, five or six being typical.

Such an exercise, which can also be practiced alone or silently during a conversation, is a simple way to bring sponsorship to whatever is arising in one's center. Bringing mindfulness to an activated experience gives it place, and the connection between the cognitive self and the somatic center can allow each experience to be a valuable resource rather than a distracting or symptom-causing nuisance. This is the difference that sponsorship makes.

## Cultivating Archetypal Energies: Fierceness, Tenderness, and Mischievousness

Effective sponsorship, whether of one's self or of another person, requires the use of a number of complementary energies. For example, a helpful spon-sor must be able to embody and extend fierceness in many ways: staying committed, seeing through "bullshit," remaining focused, taking a person ser-iously, respecting and defending boundaries, and so forth. A good sponsor must equally cultivate tenderness in the self and others via a soothing pres-ence, an ability to touch and be touched emotionally, a gentle and kind presence, compassion, and so on. Effective sponsorship also requires a sense of playfulness or mischievousness: a twinkle in the eye, a sense of humor, a capacity to hold multiple perspectives and shift gracefully among them, and the like.

A sponsor lacking any of these energies might run into difficulty. Fierce-ness alone deteriorates into rigidity and crankiness. Tenderness by itself can sink into a sort of Barry Manilow–like sentimentality. Mischievousness in iso-lation makes everything a cynical game. Tender fierceness interspersed with timely humor has a much more powerful effect. Thus, an effective sponsor-ship works to cultivate and blend these complementary energies within one centered approach.

At the beginning of a session, I typically check in with myself to ensure the presence of a felt sense of each of these energies. If there is not, I take a few moments to access each of them within me. I then look to sense the pres-ence of each energy within the client. This may be challenging initially, as a client may seemingly present only one. For example, a new client recently presented primarily in a helpless, regressed, vulnerable mode. While accepting that mode as valid and genuine, I sought to sense her hidden fierceness and her "inner rascal" before proceeding any further. Once I could sense them, I felt a much deeper connection, respect, and calmness with her.

There are many ways in which to cultivate these archetypal energies. For example, one training exercise done in dyads is as follows:

1.  Partners get comfortable, centered, open to field, tuned to each other.
2.  Partner A says:          See my tenderness . . .
                             See my fierceness . . .
                             See my mischievousness . . .
                             See me.
3.  Partner B says:          See my tenderness . . .
                             See my fierceness . . .
                             See my mischievousness . . .
                             See me.

| | | |
|---|---|---|
| 4. | Partner A says: | I see your tenderness ... |
| | | I see your fierceness ... |
| | | I see your mischievousness ... |
| | | I see you. |
| 5. | Partner B says: | I see your tenderness ... |
| | | I see your fierceness ... |
| | | I see your mischievousness ... |
| | | I see you. |
| 6. | Partner A says: | May tenderness remain with us ... |
| | | May fierceness remain with us ... |
| | | May mischievousness remain with us ... |
| | | May each of us remain with us. |
| 7. | Partner B says: | May tenderness remain with us ... |
| | | May fierceness remain with us ... |
| | | May mishievousness remain with us ... |
| | | May each of us remain with us. |

As with the "today my woundedness" exercise, the major interest is in relaxing, dropping into center, connecting with the partner, using the mindfulness of speech to touch and awaken an emotional center, and then extending the energy into the interpersonal field. This is the purpose not only of hypnosis, but also of other performance arts: to develop and express an embodied experience within an energetic relational field. In this embodied relationality, old patterns may be reorganized into new meanings.

Each archetypal energy has many forms: integrated or unintegrated, undeveloped or mature, and so on. By recognizing this, the therapist can sense a "problem" as an undeveloped or unintegrated form of an essential human resource. Thus, an angry person can be deeply appreciated for his or her fierceness, and encouraged to "do it more, do it better," in ways that connect it with the other energies and allow new, more helpful forms to develop. Again, a basic principle of self-relations is that the problem is the solution: What seems to have no value may, under proper sponsorship conditions, be transformed into a deeply valuable expression.

### Replacing Negative Sponsorship with Positive Sponsorship

Each of us carries many sponsors within our head, some positive and some negative. A positive sponsor is one who (1) helps awaken awareness of the goodness and gifts of self, (2) helps awaken awareness of the goodness and gifts of the world, and (3) helps develop practices and understandings that connect the two domains. A negative sponsor is one who (1) turns awareness away from the goodness and gifts of the self, (2) turns awareness away from the goodness and gifts of the world, and (3) promotes practices and traditions of neglect or abuse against self, others, and the world. Using these definitions, it is easy for most people to identify examples of both positive and negative sponsors in their lives.

In exploring sensitive areas in therapy, it is common for negative sponsors to become activated. Self-relations suggests that a difficult experience becomes a clinical symptom when three things happen: (1) the somatic/archetypal self feels a disturbance (what we call the activation of a "neglected self"), (2) the normal cognitive self disconnects or dissociates, and (3) negative sponsors overtake the "neglected self." The therapist should be sensitive to when this happens, and work to replace negative sponsorship messages with positive ones.

One straightforward way to do this is by (1) identifying a repetitive problem sequence in a person's life, (2) tuning into where in the sequence the person accesses a felt sense of somatic disturbance (i.e., a neglected self), (3) identifying the negative sponsorship messages that are influencing the neglected self, and (4) replacing them with positive sponsors. For example, Jill was a 51-year-old woman building a successful business consulting practice. She complained about becoming anxious when talking to new clients. We explored an example of this, and she noticed herself beginning to feel "tension and fear" centered in her solar plexus about 30 minutes before an appointment. Self-relations emphasizes that such disturbing experiences are not the problem; the problem (or solution) arises in terms of how they are sponsored. To identify the negative sponsorship messages, Jill was requested:

1.  As you experience those difficult experiences, just take a moment and sense the presence of your mother in the room. And as you do, just notice what she would say or do in response to witnessing the struggle you are voicing here right now.

Jill imagined her mother to be very silent and depressed, with an implicit message of, "You're asking too much of yourself, you're going to get hurt." When asked, she noted that her solar plexus responded to that message with a sinking feeling of fear. I commented, "That's good to know ... that when you hear that message, your inner self feels that way."

She was next requested:

2.  As you return to sensing yourself struggling with that experience of anxiety, just take a moment and sense the presence of your father in the room. And as you do, just notice what he would say or do in response to witnessing your experience here.

Jill sensed her father getting tense, telling her just to focus on what needed to be done and to forget about her feelings. She felt her solar plexus respond to this message with a feeling of greater fear and confusion. I encouraged her simply to study and note each inner response to each sponsorship message.

I then suggested that this feeling of fear would probably revisit her many more times during her life. She was learning how her mother sponsored it and how her father sponsored it, and how her inner self responded to such sponsorship messages. While that was good to know, even better was that it was her turn now: She now had "first options" in terms of how to sponsor that feeling when it returned. We examined how positive sponsorship might involve creating a place for the feeling, touching it with kindness, deeply listening, properly naming it, and having a collaborative conversation with it. I pointed out that when the feeling came, her cognitive self could remain, with a resulting bodymind integration that would allow creative new responses.

As she developed this embodied relationality, a deep calm spread through her. She looked radiant and at peace. I suggested that she imagine herself going through the problem sequence while maintaining this positive sponsorship of herself. She successfully navigated the process, not only in the session, but also when facing actual challenges over the following several weeks.

This example suggests just one of many ways in which positive sponsorship can replace negative sponsorship (see Gilligan, 1997, for other examples). In encouraging this process, it is important to recognize that resistance sometimes occurs. A person might say, for example, that he or she doesn't deserve kindness or respect. In such instances, it can be helpful first to access that person's patterns of positive sponsorship toward significant others—for example, a child, pet, or best friend. (Most people know how to nurture others much better than they know how to nurture themselves.) For instance, Ray was a client who was feeling extremely insecure about losing his job. He flatly refused to provide positive sponsorship for his feelings of confusion and fear, claiming that they were undeserving of attention. I asked him if he had children, and he softened as he told me of his three young boys. Were one of his sons to experience confusion and fear, I asked, how would he respond? Would he scold him? Hit him? Electroshock him? Tell him to go to his room and not come out until he lost those feelings?

To each of my questions Ray responded "No," he would never do that. Each time, I acknowledged with a tender fierceness, "Yes, I see that you would not do that to your son." I then asked him how he would respond if it were a different son, or a friend, or anybody else? Would he hurt, punish, or ignore the person? To each question he again answered "No," which I continued to acknowledge. When asked what he would do in such situations, he replied earnestly that he would want to support and comfort the person in need. I said I believed deeply that he would provide tender support to anybody in that situation, so the real question remained: Wasn't he somebody too? Wasn't he a human being deserving of respect, love, and kindness? As tears fell from his eyes, I suggested he go inside himself, touch the place where he most felt the confusion, and provide positive sponsorship. Thus began a process of reconnecting with the center of his being, a process that continued in many positive ways over the next months.

## DISCUSSION

Each person is given a life to be lived and enjoyed. As this great gift opens across time, a multitude of primary experiences are brought through a person's center and into the field of awareness. Sponsorship is the relationship process that gives form, meaning, and value to each of these core experiences. Sponsorship can be positive—that is, it can awaken awareness of the goodness and gifts of the self and the world—or it can be negative, in the form of curses or inattentiveness that numbs or darkens awareness of the soul and the world. Sponsorship initially is held entirely by outsiders, but as psychological growth develops, the possibility of self-sponsorship is added. Positive sponsorship allows an experiential pattern to change and grow over time, while negative sponsorship freezes a pattern in form and meaning, forcing it to repeat itself over and over in a process that Thomas Merton called "ineffective suffering."

When the suffering from negative sponsorship becomes unbearable, disturbing behaviors may arise as unsuccessful attempts to resolve it. What seem like irrational or incomprehensible behaviors from the outside can be compassionately sensed as important efforts at healing. By demonstrating and encouraging positive sponsorship of these disturbing experiences, a wonderful transformation can occur. A life lived in fear and oppression can shift to one lived in courage, self-acceptance, and delight. Such is the difference that positive sponsorship can make.

## References

Erickson, M. H. (1980a). *The nature of hypnosis and suggestion: The collected papers of Milton Erickson on hypnosis, Vol. 1* (E. L. Rossi, Ed.). New York: Irvington.

Erickson, M. H. (1980b). *Innovative hypnotherapy: The collected papers of Milton Erickson on hypnosis, Vol. IV* (E. L. Rossi, Ed.). New York: Irvington.

Gendlin, E. T. (1996). *Focusing-oriented psychotherapy: A manual of the experiential method.* New York: Guilford.

Gilligan, S. G. (1987). *Therapeutic trances: The cooperation principle in Ericksonian hypnotherapy.* New York: Brunner/Mazel.

Gilligan, S. G. (1997). *The courage to love: Principles and practices of self-relations psychotherapy.* New York: Norton.

Gordon, D., & Meyers-Anderson, M. (1981). *Phoenix: Therapeutic patterns of Milton H. Erickson.* Cupertino, CA: Meta Publications.

Merton, T. (1964). *Gandhi on non-violence: A selection from the writings of Mahatma Gandhi.* New York: New Directions.

Watzlawick, P., Weakland, J., & Fisch. R. (1974). *Change: Principles of problem formation and problem resolution.* New York: Norton.

Whyte, D. (1994). *The heart aroused: Poetry and the preservation of the soul in corporate America.* New York: Currency Doubleday.

# 28

# Marriage Contracts That Work

## Carol Lankton

When stories of Milton Erickson's therapy are told, they typically include the outcome that the clients got married, had lots of children, and lived happily ever after, thus proving the technique's success. And why not? This is a tangible indicator that the clients moved appropriately through the family life cycle and normal developmental stages. In *Uncommon Therapy*, Jay Haley (1973) superimposed this life-cycle structure over countless case examples in which Erickson had successfully treated patients manifesting a broad range of symptoms. Erickson had not placed his therapy in a framework of family therapy, although strong family orientation was implicit in his work. Haley viewed human problems as inevitable when a family normally develops over time (or fails to do so). Erickson's characteristic commonsense approach was to intervene so that clients could get past whatever obstacles prevented them from moving freely, whether this involved courtship, entering marriage, creating harmonious and satisfying marriage contracts, having children, rearing children, or launching children.

### ERICKSON'S POSITION ON MARRIAGE THERAPY

This chapter focuses on the stage of creating, maintaining, and revising healthy marriage contracts that work to the mutual satisfaction of both partners. In Haley's (1985a) *Conversations with Milton H. Erickson: Changing Couples*, Erickson described a good marriage as one in which both partners experience mature love, which is the capacity to find enjoyment in the other person's enjoyment. Happiness in marriage is enhanced when both partners honor the other person's privilege of enjoying whatever special, peculiar pleasures he or she desires and simply appreciating the fact that the other person is happy. The partners don't have to share, or even understand, each other's pleasures. Erickson emphasized to couples that they could not (and need not aspire to) share equally in all things because biologically they are totally different creatures and have many different interests. They just need enough mutual interests and pleasures to create a healthy balance between autonomy and relationship. In that balance, both individuals are accomplishing certain things for the self, for each other, and for their lives together.

Like much of Erickson's wisdom, this notion of balance sounds simple in theory. And yet it can be too complex for many people to put into practice. Erickson explained that many people "grow up in the conviction of the goodness of their ideas ... They never learn to respect the goodness of separate ideas ... and they get into difficulty when they try to influence each other" (Haley, 1985a, p. 5). In this framework, problems in marriage result from too much effort on the part of each spouse to convert the other spouse. Furthermore, each holds the faulty belief that it is his or her right to reform the other. In a wedding ceremony Erickson conducted for us in 1979, he said: "The first thing I want to do is admonish both of you because you're both blind. But don't worry, it will clear up and you will begin to see one another's faults. And when you do, don't either of you give up any of your faults because you're going to need them to understand and accept the faults of your partner!" This paradoxical instruction to accept each other, faults and all, is incompatible with impulses to correct the other. And the faults can even be utilized for their value in promoting tolerance and understanding.

Erickson's approach to marriage therapy basically reflects the same principles of utilization, positive framing, symptom prescription, redirection, distraction, getting clients active, and reassociation of experiential life evident in all of his work. Various techniques, such as hypnosis, confusion, metaphor, assignments, and reframing, are equally likely, as well as possibly absent from either mode of therapy. The assumption that people have psychological problems because they do not know how to put desired experiences into contexts in which they are needed can easily be applied to any stage of the life cycle or of marriage. In dealing with a client, Erickson would assess the requirements of the particular context and what experiences were needed. Then, drawing upon any technique suitable for that client, he would facilitate a "reassociation of experiential life" that generally resolved the dilemma. He usually didn't bother to discuss why those experiences had not been conditioned to occur in the context. He just acted in the most efficient manner to get clients moving normally past previous obstacles.

## POSITIONS OF
## VARIOUS ERICKSONIAN PRACTITIONERS

Haley (1973, 1985a, 1985b) is usually recognized as the chief expositor of Erickson's work as it applies to marriage and families because of his extensive exposure to Erickson over two decades, and because of his own interest in family therapy as part of a health-oriented developmental framework. Haley first developed the term "strategic" to describe therapy in which the therapist is active and assumes the responsibility for initiating movement toward change. He described the way Erickson exemplified this element in his highly distinctive approach to families. In so doing, Haley influenced many others who have attempted to clarify and discuss Erickson's work in terms of specific systemic factors (Araoz, 1988; Czech, 1988; Dammann, 1982; Loriedo, 1985; Malarewicz, 1988; Ritterman, 1983; Schmidt & Trenkle, 1985). Bateson (1972, 1979), Watzlawick (1976), Bandler, Grinder, & Satir (1976), Fisch, Weakland, & Segal (1982), Madanes (1983), Kershaw (1991), Wiener-Davis (1986), and DeShazer (1988) have all described Erickson's creative and pioneering contributions to marriage and family therapy in terms of language patterns, solution focus, and epistemological stance. All of these practitioners have placed their unique fingerprints on aspects of influence congruent with individual style. Erickson's work has functioned as a projection screen for theorists and provided the data they framed in varying conceptual formulations. Yet each diverse application derives from fundamental beliefs about people, such as that every behavior is an attempt to solve some problem or to accomplish a legitimate goal. While different intervention strategies will be favored, the implicit ecosystems orientation and aspects of Ericksonian influence are far-reaching and profound (Fisch, 1990).

## CREATING MARRIAGE CONTRACTS THAT WORK

As an Ericksonian therapist, I tell a lot of stories to clients. When couples are in a crisis of transition, I assess whether or not they feel allowed to outgrow, and capable of outgrowing, an old pattern and to revise an obsolete contract without leaving the marriage. Many couples I see are caught in a marriage contract that they don't remember consciously creating. Yet it binds them, and because they are hardly aware of its control over their various actions and interpretations, they feel helpless and confused. They may present some problem for therapy without recognizing it as a symptom of their inherited, unexamined, usually limiting, or antiquated marriage contract that ill fits them now. Neither do they think much in terms of what they want to accomplish or how they would know if they succeeded. Often each believes the other to be the enemy or the one who is causing the problems and selectively perceives "evidence" to support that belief. Communication about what they both want is nonexistent or ineffective.

I frequently relate to such couples Erickson's story of a case in which a woman requested hypnosis to help her stop smoking. She then volunteered the irrelevant information that she had been married for 20 years and had two teenage children, that her husband was a 56-year-old university professor, and that she was a 52-year-old mental health professional who made just as much money as her husband did. Erickson said to her: "Women your age who want to use hypnosis to stop smoking usually aren't sincere. To demonstrate your sincerity to me, I'd like you to climb Squaw Peak every morning at sunrise for a week and come to see me next Saturday" (Erickson, 1979). When the woman arrived for the appointment, Erickson confiscated her cigarettes and matches, and told her that they would be placed on the compost heap if not reclaimed in two weeks. She suggested getting her cigarettes from home, which Erickson complimented as a good idea. These also were taken. She was then told that her time was up and asked if she wanted to pay in cash or by check. She made her choice, left the session, went home, and assertively demanded cooperation from her husband and persevered until he complied. This was unheard of in their 20-year marriage. She asked him to type something for her and he, accustomed to being the one who received services, refused. He did not realize that he was on the precipice of an entire contract reorganization and that his whole world was about to change.

How or why had the wife suddenly become unwilling to continue in the role she had played for so long without complaint? Perhaps her congruent insistence was stimulated by all that literal perseverance required in climbing the mountain. Or maybe it was the way Erickson demonstrated the kind of comfort you can have when you make a request, insisting that she climb the mountain to display sincerity, telling her to bring her cigarettes and leave them in his office, or even telling her that her time was up and asking how she preferred to pay. The influence of Erickson's directives, challenges, and encouragement cannot be measured directly, but for whatever combination of reasons, when her husband refused her request, she persevered, and even insisted. She reported that after much grumbling on his part, the husband begrudgingly produced a letter that "had more mistakes in it than is humanly possible to make in one letter." The wife pronounced it unacceptable and insisted that he do it correctly. He turned off the light and went to bed. She turned the light back on, pulled the covers down, grabbed him by the ankles, and put his feet on the floor, literally dragging him out of bed. She told him, "I want that letter typed tonight." Convinced that body snatchers had taken the woman he knew, he decided to comply with her simple request. As the wife shared this account with Erickson, she admitted that things were not right in the marriage. As evidence, she described years of tyrannical rule by the husband, his domination of her and the children, his not allowing the children to play their music or have friends visit. She reported that when they married, her husband had insisted that she learn gourmet cooking and had agreed to cook every other week. "But in 20 years of marriage, his week to cook has not yet arrived," she complained to Erickson.

At this point, Erickson told her to go home and inform her husband that his week to cook had finally arrived. She objected that he would simply boil potatoes and fry hamburgers. She was instructed to bring home takeout gourmet meals for herself and the children, and let the husband eat what he had prepared. The wife, now in too deep to do otherwise, followed the instructions and came back the next week to report the results. The husband had cooked as anticipated and glared at them while they ate their gourmet dinners. It would now be her turn to cook again, and since her husband had spent a careful week teaching her the kind of gourmet cooking he really preferred, Erickson explained to her that she was to continue the takeout gourmet meals for herself, son, and daughter, but prepare boiled potatoes and fried hamburgers for the husband. Miraculously, by the third week, when it was again his turn to cook, the husband had learned to prepare acceptable gourmet meals. And, of course, nothing was ever the same in that home again. The wife had come to recognize that her needs were legitimate and that she was no longer willing to play the complementary roles that keep a dictator in power. Almost simultaneously, the husband discovered an unknown flexibility in that he could play a cooperative role rather than that of an unchallenged tyrant. The children were allowed to play music with friends. Smoking was never mentioned again, and the cigarettes most likely were composted.

This story makes several compelling points about the possibility of one's making drastic changes in one's habits without even knowing why; it illustrates the humorous behaviors of asking for what you want and persevering confidently until you get it, and the amazing fact that people whom you never suspected of it can, in fact, be quite flexible if given the chance. I tell this story because I want to make the point that entering therapy is an opportunity for the partners to discover that they are essentially free to negotiate between the two of them any marriage contract they want! The only requirement is that they create a contract that works for both of them. So what do they both want? I ask this and wait expectantly for them to tell me but, unfortunately, few couples know exactly what it is that they want. Even if they do, there are often conditioned inhibitions against expressing it. They don't want to appear selfish or demanding. And often they simply lack practice in motivating action by setting goals.

Asking a couple to imagine themselves in a relationship that truly fits and satisfies them will occasionally result in their identifying desired elements and enthusiastically sharing them with the partner who passionately agrees. More often, however, the request will be met with blank stares, expectant looks at each other, shrugging of shoulders, and turning to the therapist for the "right" answer! They will not have this paralysis if they are asked to describe the things they dislike about each other. With couples thus blocked, I am quite willing to utilize their awareness of what they don't want as a means to discover what they do want. Using a problem as an information-gathering device to clarify wishes sometimes makes the problem worth having. I might ask them silently to review their complaints and privately identify the "go to" goal implied in each one and share that information with the partner. They exchange "I want you to ..." or "I like it when you ..." statements that begin to detail an ideal relationship.

As the partners begin to ask each other for what each needs in a direct manner, I often urge them to specify desired behaviors far more clearly than they normally would, even including a script of words they want to hear from each other. Language is potentially vague and abstract and people use words to mean different things. Partners may feel that they have made their needs known to the other, when, in fact, that person may have missed the message entirely. For example, "I need your support" can translate into a wide variety of specific actions. One spouse may say these words wanting the partner to give him or her a massage while the other interprets the words to mean that he or she should give advice. Or perhaps the spouse decides the other to "support" the other by refraining from criticism when the other just wants to be held. Partners need to help each other with such questions as "How exactly would you like your support right now?" With greater specificity on a routine basis, couples significantly improve their odds of getting their needs met.

## BELIEFS THAT MAKE CONTRACTS WORK

There are several beliefs that are conducive to upgrading marriage contracts. The belief by both people that their needs are acceptable, and that they can actually take action to get them met, leads the list. It is also extremely helpful for them to believe that they can depend on each other to cooperate, to care, to be sensitive to expressed needs and feelings, to be able to survive and even benefit from the expression of negative feelings, and to tell the truth as they come to know it about their own needs, feelings, likes, and dislikes. Although many couples present superficial accusations to the contrary, they usually agree that they wouldn't be staying in the relationship if they congruently believed that the other didn't care, couldn't be trusted to be honest, or intended them harm. Getting them to agree on terms of a marriage mission statement helps to solidify these wispy beliefs. A basic version might be: We are a team dedicated to getting more of our individual needs met than either of us could accomplish independently. Membership of this team implies that we accept each other as adding value and that we both accept the validity and importance of each other's needs. It is very affirming for each partner to believe that the other genuinely supports the other's getting what he or she wants, even if the partner does not share that need or understand its importance.

## UPDATING THE VOWS

Nothing commemorates a "new" marriage contract like updating the vows, adding important features that likely were overlooked in the original ceremony. If they elect to accept the mission, I ask spouses to solemnly vow to tell the truth to each other as they come to know it about how they feel and what they want, need, and dislike. If they had the courage to take the first vow, they take the next, usually harder, vow to believe each other when they share how they feel and what they need. After all, each is the undisputed expert on his or her feelings and perceptions and has just vowed to tell the truth to the trusted partner. What reason would they possibly have to lie? Fear of conflict or hurting the other is often mentioned in answer. So a third level to the vow is for the spouses to reassure each other that they can handle hearing even "unpopular" truths or "bad news" about dislikes, hurt feelings, anger, and so on. They may not like it, but they can deal with it. They don't need to be protected from the other's feelings, good or bad. If they want to protect each other from something, have them agree to protect each other from the demoralizing implication that they won't or can't handle the truth or be sensitive to feelings.

With these vows in place, couples win a turn in the "lightning round." That is, they get to discover how educational and instructive "workable conflict" can be. Expressing what they want and feel obviously increases the chances of needs being met and the partner is seen as motivated (even honored) to be trusted, included, and allowed to participate in helping the loved one meet those needs. It is comforting and feels safe to be partnered with someone who can be depended on to clarify his or her needs, thus minimizing the need for haphazard guessing about what is wanted. But, at the same time, the more that spouses take this risk, the more they create the chance of direct conflict when it is revealed that they have opposite preferences or incompatible needs. However, in a loving and equal relationship, this is simply the stimulus for finding the middle ground where they both get as much as possible of what they want. Or when it is an "all or nothing" kind of decision, they evaluate whose need is the most urgent and the other yields. Obviously, it will not work if one spouse does all the yielding every time.

## THE CASE OF THE OCEAN AND THE RIVER

One of the arenas for potential conflict concerns how much intimacy each spouse wants. Of course, there is no correct amount and people vary according to character, upbringing, culture, stage of life, and time of day with regard to perceived need for intimacy with another person. Carol and Walt were clients who personified this dilemma. Their arguments about incompatible intimacy needs were pervasive. Carol *highly* valued intimacy and craved an "ocean of it" she said, to encompass, surround, and embrace her all of the time. Walt, however, had come from an *extremely* private, emotionally reserved family and highly valued his personal space which he would happily withdraw for hours at a time. Because Carol's dissatisfaction with this arrangement was so strong, she was considering divorce and initiated therapy as a last resort. Because Walt did, in fact, love Carol very much (in his way) and did not want to divorce, he made great efforts to engage in intimate exchanges that were difficult and awkward for him. These efforts resulted in a steady trickle, or a "river," of intimacy that Carol welcomed, depended on, and even came to accept as a satisfactory amount of intimacy. She reevaluated her earlier need for constant togetherness as an indicator of insecurity and need for approval that no longer applied to her. She freed herself from an obsolete obsessive craving and simultaneously helped her husband to develop the life-enhancing option of connecting in a more emotionally revealing manner. They co-created a mutually satisfying contract.

They worked long and hard to achieve this success. They carefully and systematically communicated specific needs, grievances, frustrations, and fears in manageable bits, such that the other could hear, remember, and respond. They both framed what they wanted the partner to understand in a goal-oriented manner, describing feelings and needs without blaming or attacking. They accomplished this even when the feeling being shared was anger, hurt, or sadness. They became skilled with compound sentence structures, such as: "I feel angry at you when you criticize me *and* what I want is for you to tell me that you love me." They expressed negative feelings and used them as springboards that led to logically related but previously unstated needs. Detecting anger became an opportunity to focus inward, identify the need, and then tell the other partner.

Effective communication is a cyclical process. I have discussed the benefits of spouses' identifying and sharing needs with each other, which requires their participation as empathic, active listeners as well. In couples therapy, the goal is to have the spouses learn to listen to each other at least as empathically as the therapist does. This should be possible because the spouses presumably love each other whereas the therapist simply cares in an impersonal, detached way. Spouses can acquire this response style by modeling the therapist's interacting with each of them, and also by directives in the session to earn a turn to speak only after having successfully understood (not necessarily agreed with) what the other speaker was attempting to convey. They may have to paraphrase what was heard in order to correct misunderstandings, and sometimes inspire the speaker to greater clarity in the process. The listener can ask questions for understanding or to help the speaker stay focused on what he or she wants. The listener has already vowed to believe whatever the speaker is sharing, but this agreement does not necessarily mean understanding or liking this truth.

Carol and Walt faced a challenge in this regard when Walt planned to stay an extra day at a conference he was attending. Carol could not understand this decision as she would have taken the first flight out. She struggled not simply to decide that Walt must not value their relationship as much as she did and instead listened to his take on the situation. He was initially tempted to yield to her implied pressure to come home as she would have done to prove that he loved her. But this action would have caused resentment. Instead, he explained that he did value the relationship and had a perfectly valid desire to stay the extra day for reasons she did not understand but accepted. It was an example of the mature love Erickson spoke about making a breakthrough. She gained happiness from his enjoying himself.

## PRESUPPOSING SUCCESS AND POSITIVE EXPECTANCY

Positive framing comes from the fundamental belief that every behavior is an attempt to solve some problem or accomplish a legitimate objective. It is one of the common denominators among otherwise diverse Ericksonian therapists. This belief is the basis for utilizing whatever is presented as a means of reaching relevant goals. It is manifested almost continuously in every phase of therapy, and, indeed, creates the therapeutic atmosphere of hope and possibility. Behaviors described as problems are accepted as valid and the inevitability of the desired behavior is presupposed, precisely by means of being able to display what had been considered the problem. Almost any personality orientation, symptom, or concern can be framed as an ability that leads in some requisite way to its desired opposite. It is a matter of accepting clients and affirming the presence of strength even in what they had considered a weakness, fault, or problem. "Don't either of you give up any of your faults because you are going to need them to understand and accept the faults of your partner."

Developing an ongoing new marriage contract depends on understanding what the couple can agree they want to happen. If this understanding can develop only by means of addressing the apparent here-and-now function of a symptom, then this is a valid method. The partners can be asked to imagine themselves in a future in which the presenting problem has been solved in a most satisfactory and comprehensive manner. As they share what they see in this future, a tentative marriage contract emerges. Using a future perfect verb tense ("Look into the future when you *will have* accomplished . . .") presupposes success that they were able to create precisely as a result of the stalemate that led them to therapy. Then it is simply a matter of fine-tuning the details and making sure that they both support the options being discussed and that the picture encompasses all desired resources.

But they should not restrict themselves simply to reviewing how they resolved presenting problems. They might want to see themselves as deserving and trustworthy and imagine how they will have created new levels of intimacy, sharing, and mutual support through respectful and trusting interaction. They may see themselves setting limits and boundaries, taking responsibility for choices, creating opportunities for connecting and for being alone. They can see themselves revising the new marriage contract when it has become obsolete in the future. When couples agree that such pictures look good to them, an unconscious prophecy is beginning even if they consciously doubt that the picture is an attainable reality. However, it is no longer an unexamined unconscious prophecy like the one they had been influenced by earlier. It is a self-fulfilling prophecy that holds agreed-upon wishes slightly outside of ordinary consciousness by "haunting" them until the dream is a reality. Yet they can take full responsibility and credit for having engineered it from their wishes made conscious and shared in therapy.

The conviction that whatever the other is doing represents the best choice organized thus far for solving some problem or need puts partners in a position to question how they can engineer a better choice that will best fit them both. For some couples, this may include mutual agreement that their different, and perhaps incompatible, individual needs and goals would best be met by ending their marriage. Even termination can be accomplished without blame: no good guys, no bad guys, just you and me, and we just disagree. The clients in the ocean-and-river case might well have been in this group, except for their agreement that what they both wanted was more similar than different. They decided to tolerate the distinctive differences and preferences that were never going to go away, no matter how much change occurred. Some couples can even learn to truly delight in those differences, be inspired by them, and nurture and appreciate them as aspects of their partner that are essential to who the partner is and what makes the person loveable. Then they can have lots of children and live happily ever after, just like the folks in Erickson's cases.

---

### Practical Ideas

- Spouses need to accept, not reform, each other. They can take joy in their differences.
- Spouses can have any marriage contract they want (and can agree on)! They can leave the roles of an old marriage but keep the marriage. Updating wedding vows to include profound honesty about needs leads them to a modern mission statement.
- Therapists can utilize any presented problem as a means to accomplish desired outcomes. The more the spouses were able to have the problem, the more they are capable of creating a true and unique solution.
- All must presuppose the success they will have accomplished when current problems have been resolved.
- Therapists can encourage the motivation strategy in which wanting to is a good-enough reason. Get the partners to believe that it is acceptable to change their minds and outgrow what had worked before just because they want to!
- Therapists can build the expectancy that the partners will review, revise, and upgrade marriage contracts that work in an *ongoing* manner.

---

## References

Araoz, D. (1988). *The new hypnosis in family therapy.* New York: Brunner/Mazel.

Bandura, A. (1969). *Principles of behavior modification.* New York: Holt Rinehart & Winston.

Bateson, G. (1972). *Steps to an ecology of mind.* New York: Ballantine Books.

Bateson, G. (1979). *Mind and nature.* New York: Dutton.

Berne, E. (1972). *What do you say after you say hello?: The psychology of human destiny.* New York: Grove.

Czech, N. (1988). Family therapy with adolescent sex offenders. In J. Zeig & S. Lankton (Eds.), *Developing Ericksonian psychotherapy: State of the arts. Proceedings of the Third International Congress on Ericksonian Therapy.* New York: Brunner/ Mazel.

Dammann, C. (1982). Family therapy: Erickson's contribution. In J. Zeig (Ed.), *Ericksonian approaches to hypnosis and psychotherapy* (pp. 193–200). New York: Brunner/Mazel.

Dell, P. (1985). Understanding Bateson and Maturana. *Journal of Marital and Family Therapy, 11,* 1–20.

De Shazer, S. (1988). Utilization: The foundation of solutions. In J. Zeig & S. Lankton (Eds.), *Developing Ericksonian psychotherapy: State of the arts. Proceedings of the Third International Congress on Ericksonian Therapy.* New York: Brunner/Mazel.

Erickson, M. (1979). Personal communication.

Erickson, M. (1983). *Healing in hypnosis: The seminars, workshops, and lectures of Milton H. Erickson, Vol. 1* (E. L. Rossi, M. O. Ryan, & F. A. Sharp, Eds.). New York: Irvington.

Erickson, M. (1985). *Life reframing in hypnosis: The seminars, workshops, and lectures of Milton H. Erickson, Vol. 2* (E. L. Rossi, M. O. Ryan, & F. A. Sharp, Eds.). New York: Irvington.

Erickson, M., & Rossi, E. (1981). *Experiencing hypnosis: Therapeutic approaches to altered state.* New York: Irvington.

Erickson, M. H., Rossi, E. L., & Rossi, S. I. (1976). *Hypnotic realities: The induction of clinical hypnosis and forms of indirect suggestion.* New York: Irvington.

Fisch, R. (1990). The broader interpretation of Milton H. Erickson's work. In S. Lankton (Ed.), *The Ericksonian monographs, no. 7: The issue of broader implications of Ericksonian therapy* (pp. 1–5). New York: Brunner/Mazel.

Fisch, R., Weakland, J., & Segal, L. (1982). *The tactics of change: Doing therapy briefly.* San Francisco: Jossey-Bass.

Godin, J. (1988). Evocation and indirect suggestion in the communication patterns of Milton H. Erickson. In S. Lankton, & J. Zeig (Eds.), *The Ericksonian monographs, no. 4: Research, comparisons and medical applications of Ericksonian techniques* (pp. 5–11). New York: Brunner/Mazel.

Haley, J. (1963). *Strategies of psychotherapy*. New York: Grune & Stratton.

Haley, J. (Ed.). (1967). *Advanced techniques of hypnosis and therapy: Selected papers of Milton H. Erickson, M.D.* New York: Grune & Stratton.

Haley, J. (1973). *Uncommon therapy: The psychiatric techniques of Milton H. Erickson, M.D.* New York: Norton.

Haley, J. (1976). *Problem solving therapy*. San Francisco: Jossey-Bass.

Haley, J. (1984). *Ordeal therapy*. San Francisco: Jossey-Bass.

Haley, J. (1985a) *Conversations with Milton H. Erickson, M.D.: Vol. 2: Changing couples*. New York: Norton.

Haley, J. (1985b) *Conversations with Milton H. Erickson, M.D. Vol. 3: Changing children and families*. New York: Norton.

Havens, R. (1985). *The wisdom of Milton H. Erickson*. New York: Irvington.

Jackson, D. (Ed.). (1968a). *Communication, family, and marriage: 1*. Palo Alto, CA: Science & Behavior Books.

Jackson, D. (Ed.). (1968b). *Therapy, communication, and change: 2*. Palo Alto, CA: Science & Behavior Books.

Kershaw, C. (1992).*The couple's hypnotic dance*. New York: Brunner/Mazel.

Laing, R. D. (1967). *The politics of experience*. New York: Ballantine Books.

Laing, R. D. (1972). *The politics of the family*. New York: Ballantine Books.

Lankton, C. (1985). Elements of an Ericksonian approach. In S. Lankton (Ed.), *Ericksonian monographs, no. 1* (pp. 61–75). New York: Brunner/Mazel.

Lankton, C., & Lankton, S. (1989). *Tales of enchantment: Goal-oriented metaphors for adults and children in therapy*. New York: Brunner/Mazel.

Lankton, S. (1988). Ericksonian systemic approach. In S. Lankton & J. Zeig (Eds.), *Developing Ericksonian psychotherapy: State of the arts. Proceedings of the Third International Congress on Ericksonian Approaches to Psychotherapy* (pp. 417–437). New York: Brunner/Mazel.

Lankton, S., & Lankton, C. (1983). *The answer within: A clinical framework of Ericksonian hypnotherapy*. New York: Brunner/Mazel.

Lankton, S., & Lankton C. (1985). Ericksonian styles of paradoxical therapy. In G. Weeks (Ed.), *Promoting change through paradoxical therapy* (pp. 134–186). Homewood, IL: Dorsey Press.

Lankton, S., & Lankton, C. (1986). *Enchantment and intervention in family therapy: Training in Ericksonian approaches*. New York: Brunner/Mazel.

Loriedo, C. (1985). Tailoring suggestions in family therapy. In J. Zeig (Ed.), *Ericksonian approaches in psychotherapy, Vol. 2: Application* (pp. 155–162). New York: Brunner/Mazel.

Lustig, H. (1975). *The artistry of Milton H. Erickson, M.D., part I and part II* (videotape). Haverford, PA: Lustig.

Madanes, C. (1983). *Strategic family therapy*. San Francisco: Jossey-Bass.

Malarewicz, J. (1988). Ericksonian techniques in family therapy. In J. Zeig & S. Lankton (Eds.), *Developing Ericksonian psychotherapy: State of the arts. Proceedings of the Third International Congress on Ericksonian Psychotherapy* (pp. 446–451). New York: Brunner/Mazel.

Matthews, B., Bennett, H., Bean, W., & Gallagher, M. (1985). Indirect versus direct hypnotic suggestions—an initial investigation: A brief communication. *International Journal of Clinical and Experimental Hypnosis, 33*(3), 219–223.

Matthews, B., Kirsch, I., & Allen, G. (1984). Posthypnotic conflict and psychopathology—controlling for the effects of posthypnotic suggestion: A brief communication. *International Journal of Clinical and Experimental Hypnosis 32*(4), 362–365.

Matthews, W. (1985). A cybernetic model of Ericksonian hypnotherapy: One hand draws the other. In S. Lankton (Ed.), *The Ericksonian monographs, no. 1* (pp. 42–60). New York: Brunner/Mazel.

Maturana, H., & Varela, F. (1987). *The tree of knowledge*. Boston: New Science Library, Shambhala.

Murphy, M. (1988). A linguistic-structural model for the investigation of indirect suggestion. In S. Lankton, & J. Zeig, (Eds.), *The Ericksonian monographs, no. 4: Research, comparisons and medical applications of Ericksonian techniques* (pp. 12–27). New York: Brunner/Mazel.

O'Hanlon, W. (1987). *Taproots*. New York: Norton.

Otani, A. (1989). An empirical investigation of Milton H. Erickson's approach to trance induction: A Markov chain analysis of two published cases. In S. Lankton (Ed.), *The Ericksonian monographs, no. 5: Ericksonian hypnosis: Application, preparation and research* (pp. 35–54). New York: Brunner/Mazel.

Ritterman, M. (1983). *Using hypnosis in family therapy*. San Francisco: Jossey-Bass

Rosen, S. (1980). *My voice will go with you*. New York: Norton.

Rossi, E. L. (Ed.). (1980). *The collected papers of Milton H. Erickson on hypnosis: Vol. 1. The nature of hypnosis and suggestion; Vol. 2. Hypnotic alteration of sensory, perceptual and psychophysical processes; Vol. 3. Hypnotic investigation of psychodynamic processes; Vol. 4. Innovative hypnotherapy*. New York: Irvington.

Satir, V. (1964). *Conjoint family therapy*. Palo Alto, CA: Science & Behavior Books.

Schmidt, G., & Trenkle, B. (1985). An integration of Ericksonian techniques with concepts of family therapy. In J. Zeig (Ed.), *Ericksonian approaches to psychotherapy, Vol. 2: Application* (pp. 132–154). New York: Brunner/Mazel.

Szasz, T. (1961). *The myth of mental illness, foundations of a theory of personal conduct.* New York: Hoeber-Harper.

Watzlawick, P. (1976). *How real is real? Confusion, disinformation, communication.* New York: Vintage Books.

Watzlawick, P., Beavin, J. & Jackson, D. (1967). *Pragmatics of human communication.* New York: Norton.

Watzlawick, P., Weakland, J., & Fisch R. (1974). *Change.* New York: Norton.

Weakland, J., Fisch, R., Watzlawick, P., & Bodin, A. (1974). Brief therapy: Focused problem resolution. *Family Process, 13,* 141–168.

Weiner-Davis, M. (1986). What's new at BFTC? *The Underground Railroad, 6*(2), 7–8.

Yapko, M. (1990). *Therapeutic trances.* New York: Brunner/Mazel.

Zeig, J. (Ed.). (1980). *A teaching seminar with Milton H. Erickson.* New York: Brunner/Mazel.

Zeig, J. (Ed.). (1982). *Ericksonian approaches to hypnosis and psychotherapy.* New York: Brunner/Mazel.

Zeig, J. (Ed.). (1985a). *Ericksonian approaches to psychotherapy, Vol. 1: Structures.* New York: Brunner/Mazel.

Zeig, J. (Ed.). (1985b). *Ericksonian approaches to psychotherapy, Vol. 2: Application.* New York: Brunner/Mazel.

Zeig, J. (1985c). *Experiencing Erickson: An introduction to the man and his work.* New York: Brunner/Mazel.

Zeig, J. (1985d). Ethical issues in Ericksonian hypnosis: Informed consent and training standards. In J. Zeig (Ed.), *Ericksonian approaches to psychotherapy, Vol. 1: Structures* (pp. 451–474). New York: Brunner/Mazel.

Zeig, J., & Lankton, S. (Eds.). (1988). *Developing Ericksonian psychotherapy: State of the arts. Proceedings of the Third International Congress on Ericksonian Psychotherapy.* New York: Brunner/Mazel.

29

# The Hidden Symptom
# in Sex Therapy

*Daniel L. Araoz*

T he key difference between ordinary sex therapy and hypnotherapy lies in the so-called hidden symptom (Araoz, 1998). Walen (1980) was the first to point out the symptom in sexual dysfunctions. Because the hidden symptom is mostly unconscious and thus manifested in imagery, metaphors, and symbols, it is also a very Ericksonian concept. Both in theory and in its applications, it is one of those psychotherapeutic maneuvers, based on clinical observation and discovery, that Erickson himself could have used. Beahrs (1990) rightly claims that all psychotherapy is ultimately self-therapy. And the first condition for engaging in effective self-therapy is to stop giving ourselves negative messages about our problems, which is what we do to ourselves with the hidden symptom.

Before doing anything else, however, we must define the hidden symptom, limiting ourselves here to its relevance to sex therapy. The hidden symptom has three important elements: *self-talk*, *imagery*, and *non-consciousness*. A description of the process might clarify the definition. When people experience sexual difficulties of any kind, it typically happens that they start "to say" things about the symptom to themselves. In the majority of those who seek therapy, what they say to themselves is not positive, understanding, or constructive. On the contrary, it usually is the opposite. They blame themselves, they predict the worst, they foster fear and insecurity. But self-talk triggers mental imagery. And the images that the symptomatic person allows into his or her mind are catastrophic, self-fulfilling prophecies of doom and utter failure. By non-consciousness, I mean that the person is not doing this deliberately or intentionally. He or she is not fully aware of the negativism in which he or she is engaging.

Thus, a 54-year-old heterosexual man was having a period of low sexual desire, not reacting as before to the sight of a beautiful woman. He was less interested in sexual matters and in sexual activity than he had been in the past. Before he decided to seek professional help, he would say to himself such things as, "I'm getting old and sex is becoming a thing of the past." Or, even worse, "I'm like a 'castrato' and I guess my sexual drive is gone. Maybe I have a brain tumor or something. My wife has noticed this and she may find herself a lover." Many more such statements, including self-denigration and blame, are often typical: "It's all my fault. It's that drinking and smoking I've been doing for so long, like that article in the paper said." And these statements, inevitably, elicit memories and mental imagery of future grief.

The man may test himself by looking at erotic material or reading it without experiencing the expected positive sexual reaction. Or he may try to masturbate, and take longer than usual to obtain an erection. Finally, when he gives up the effort for lack of interest, he strengthens his conviction that there is no hope. Add to this the dark images that follow. He might see himself as standing flaccid in front of an inviting woman; as lying disinterested and motionless while his wife is trying to arouse him; as engaging in a homosexual encounter with a youngster but not feeling any sexual reaction. This may panic him even further, causing fear that he is changing his sexual orientation. In other words, the initial problem tends to escalate with the hidden symptom.

By the time the man shows up for the first sex-therapy appointment, his anxiety has grown and he has started to feel depressed as a result of the self-made tragedy inspired by his sexual difficulties. The differential diagnosis is inhibited sexual desire (or ISD), but he has catastrophized it, to use Albert Ellis' verb, into a major, perhaps insoluble, problem. He is afraid that there might be no solution to his plight.

From this description, the definition of the hidden symptom can be deduced. It consists of *a semiconscious or fully unconscious negative mental activity made up of self-defeating self-talk and mental images of greater problems and devastation.* The images usually appear before the self-talk, but the person is not aware of them until he or she recognizes the negative words being said to himself or herself. This mental process is the same preconscious cognitive behavior that I have called, more generally, negative self-hypnosis, or NSH (Araoz, 1995). Although NSH applies to many nonclinical areas, such as learning, concentration, self-confidence, creativity, marketing, promotion, and sales, when it is found clinically as a component of a particular problem, I prefer to indicate it more specifically as the hidden symptom.

When it comes to sexual dysfunctions, it takes the form of self-criticism, self-blame, and self-fulfilling prophecies. Patients see themselves failing again the next time they have a sexual experience, with their partners either laughing at them or rejecting them. And they actually say to themselves such negative things as, "This is never going to get better; it's getting worse."

For an explanation of this reaction, which is not limited to sexual dysfunction symptoms, but is found in many alterations of the normal functioning of our bodies, Mahoney's (1991) cognitive model of meaning and self-reference is helpful. Basically, it comes down to the epistemological fact that the human observer alters the objective reality observed by his or her own beliefs and expectations. "Knowing reflects the deep structures of the knowing organism," in the words of Quiñones and Zagmutt (1996). Consequently, one's "knowledge" of the objective reality may be distorted or erroneous. This is what happens in the case of the hidden symptom. The perception of the external symptom is distorted and interpreted negatively. Perception and knowledge being both active and proactive, the hidden symptom "makes" the external reality even more difficult to cope with and more damaging than it really is.

Another important element in the understanding of the hidden symptom is found in Goleman's (1998) emotional intelligence, which has three components: *emotional awareness, accurate self-assessment,* and *self-confidence.* The hidden symptom is an indication of not recognizing one's emotions and how they affect one's performance. It is also a sign of poor self-assessment, allowing the current sexual difficulty to become magnified and distorted. Finally, it is a manifestation of a weak self-worth under the pressure of a concrete difficulty in one's life. The intellectual understanding of the sexual problem is taken over by the emotional components, and thus interferes with one's personal (sexual) competence, aggravating the "real," differential diagnosis problem.

Finally, from a depth-psychology perspective, NSH in general seems to be related to poor object relations in early childhood, with the trauma that it implies. A study still in progress involves ten psychotherapists who are conducting research on 60 patients who showed high NSH in the first two therapy sessions. On the hypothesis that early object relations trauma may predispose people to NSH, they are asked about early traumas in their lives. The initial results of this investigation seem to show a strong correlation between early trauma and NSH in later life. It is as if the archaic and fragmented personality (see Kohut, 1971, 1978) has adopted a negative style and is unable to perceive clearly the positive aspects of life. In these cases, brief therapy would be contraindicated because these people need a reorganization of their personalities or a restoration of the self, in Kohut's (1977) words.

## CLINICAL APPLICATIONS

The sex therapist who ignores the hidden symptom does so to the detriment of the patient. To avoid missing this important element of the sexual dysfunction dynamics, the therapist always starts by asking the patient to concentrate on the problem that inspired him or her to consult a sex therapist. Experience has taught me to do this in an experiential manner, requesting that patients stop talking, close their eyes and mentally transport themselves to the last time they had the problem, to see themselves there. When a clinician then asks them to say aloud what comes to mind, inevitably they report the negative situation, the failure. Then, without any comments, questions, or interpretations, the therapist immediately adds, "And what do you say to yourself about this situation?" Here is where the negative statements begin to emerge.

Before starting any specific "sex therapy," the clinician makes sure that patients recognize the parts they play (certainly without full awareness of it) in keeping the symptoms active. The practical consequence is that a client can correct this aspect of the problem right away by a minor change in his or her mental attitude. To attain this goal, the therapist asks if there are other true things, but less negative ones, the client can honestly say about the sexual problem. Patience on the part of the therapist is especially needed here. Rather than feeding the answers, such as, "Your husband is sensitive and understanding," it is more direct and effective to demand, "Think of one thing about your problem that is not negative and bad."

When the client comes up with even the simplest item that is positive, the therapist can work on it. Let's assume that the patient states that the physical closeness with the partner felt good at the start of the encounter. In this case, the person is encouraged to focus his or her attention on the memory of that good feeling and to "put himself or herself there again," using hypnotic revivification. Then the client is asked to repeat this statement with enthusiasm. Often it is helpful to request that the client change bodily position (from just sitting there to sitting straight and erect, as most people do when they state something important and positive) and to say it with pride and vigor or with love and tenderness.

This is a significant step because an overwhelming number of clients spontaneously embellish the initial statement and add to it, making it even more positive and hopeful. It must be stressed that this maneuver is not meant to distract the person from the problem to be resolved or to give false reassurance. The purpose is to change the focus of attention from being problem-centered to a solution orientation and to emphasize that some progress can be made right away by not taking for granted the positive elements of the sexual situation. It is as if clients, centered on the problem, don't want to consider the true, positive, elements in the total picture. Reflecting again on Goleman's (1998) ideas, my suspicion is that those whose emotional intelligence is poor become our sex therapy patients, whereas the others handle their sexual problems effectively by themselves without escalating them by a counterproductive mental attitude.

## MOVING ON TO THE SPECIFIC PROBLEM

Once the client has recognized his or her role in the sexual problem, he or she is prepared to recognize two important components of that problem. The first is the negative "messages" (in words and mental images) he or she might be giving to himself or herself. The second is what the client can do (and how he or she can do it) to de-escalate the problem by changing the NSH into other, true and more constructive messages.

Two clinical vignettes might be helpful in affording a better understanding of how to work effectively with the hidden symptom for the benefit of the client.

## THE IDEALISTIC COUPLE

Married only two and a half months, a couple came to therapy very upset because sex was "no good." He was 44 and she was 32. In describing their problem, it became evident that they had unreasonable expectations about their sexual functioning. Strongly religious, they believed that they had to have children as soon as possible after the marriage. When they married, she was a virgin, but he had led a rather libertine life in his 20s and early 30s, before "converting" to strictly observing the tenets of his religion. The therapist asked them to spend a moment silently thinking about what "good sex" meant. After a brief period of silent concentration, they verbalized what they had "thought." She said she wanted every sex act to be "a glorious experience," but that she was worried about not respond-ing quickly enough to his efforts to turn her on. He stated that he wanted to be "fully concentrated on her, feeling passionate and completely turned on," but that he could not get into it because he was worried about her reaction and noted that she was not responding completely to his efforts.

When asked what each was saying to himself or herself during the sexual encounter, he indicated that he was blaming himself, saying that he was expecting her to react like women he had been with in the past, be-fore his religious conversion. She, on the other hand, felt that she was a failure, not satisfying him and afraid that he would tire of her and leave her, emotionally. It was beneficial for them to describe these reactions in each other's presence. He expressed compunction for his past "evil ways" and she was reassured, recognizing the foolishness of trying to be perfect, as he put it.

At this point, the therapist asked them again to concentrate silently for a moment and think of at least one good thing about their lovemaking. After a brief silence, she said, "I want him to be perfectly happy with me sexually." And he responded, "I also want her to have the best possible sexual experience since she had reserved herself for me for all these years." In discussing these statements, they realized that each had positive wishes concerning the other, but also that they were unrealistic expecta-tions. The therapist used the metaphor of the spoiled and stubborn child who is still part of the adult personality, and worked briefly on identify-ing wishes of the child as different from those of the adult.

This is an example of the need for sex education in many sex therapy cases. They were told that for every committed couple attaining good sex takes more time than just a few months. Consequently, they were encouraged to assess the progress they had made in the sexual area since they were married. They had to admit that things had slowly improved; that they actually were sexually satisfied when they did not evaluate, assess, or critique their "performance." They were also reminded that their religion's emphasis on procreation had to do with the importance of having a strong family and that it was very difficult to have such a family unless the parents truly knew each other, respected each other's differences, and were genuinely loving toward each other. This helped them to recognize that they still had a long way to go. The final destination was something to strive for patiently, not something that they should have expected to have accomplished already.

In this case, the importance of the hidden symptom is evident. If the therapist had focused only or mainly on improving the couple's sexual functioning, emphasizing behavioral techniques to help them do so, the expectations stemming from unreasonable beliefs would have continued to sabotage any real progress. Once they changed those expectations and accepted the need to allow the sexual relationship to develop, the couple felt a great sense of relief. They continued growing in their relationship, and, in a matter of months, were truly ready to become parents.

## "TRAPPED IN THE WRONG BODY"

A brief outline of this case of transsexualism is presented elsewhere (Araoz, Burte, & Carrese, 1998). Here I will concentrate on the hidden symptom and its treatment. Those interested in this condition are directed to Benjamin (1966), Money and Wiedeking (1980), Fausto-Sterling (1985), and Green and Fleming (1990).

Hal was 35 and still living with his parents when he finally started therapy in desperation. His life had been a series of sad and painful events related to sexual identity. Despite his male external organs, he had been convinced from the age of three or four that he was a girl, and now a woman. Although he solemnly promised in front of a rabbi never to dress in women's clothes again, he had not been able to abide by his parents' wishes. Now his father had a serious heart condition and Hal lived in dread of being found out and so causing his father's death.

The therapist evaluated the client by means of a battery of psychological tests before establishing the diagnosis of transsexualism in order to start meaningful treatment. The therapist expected the client to attain the following goals: (1) accepting his sexual identity and taking the first steps toward achieving that end, (2) involving his parents in the decision to change his sex, (3) starting the necessary steps to becoming a woman physically, as he already was one in his mind. When the therapist asked about the hidden symptom, the following emerged. He said he felt "like a freak" and kept calling himself that, as well as other appellations, such as monster, criminal, and lunatic. For many years, he had had nightmares of being severely beaten and left to die. When he felt despondent about his situation, he fantasized about harming himself in such ways as running in front of a speeding truck, cutting himself, castrating himself, or taking poison. He also had fantasies of setting his parents' house on fire and letting them die in it.

What needs to be emphasized is that by being aware of the existence of a hidden symptom, using the basic questions mentioned earlier, the therapist gets to these important matters much quicker and more directly than when this is not done. In the first part of treatment, the therapist directed Hal to the necessary information and to a group of serious transsexuals who were at the presurgery stage in the long process of sex change. This stage includes personality evaluations, living and dressing in the new role for one full year, and nine months of estrogen treatment, plus continued medical and psychological supervision. The therapist also used the metaphor, common among transsexuals, of a prison, which Hal had used in the very first session. During the years of therapy and based on what his life history had told him about his sexual identity, the client mentally rehearsed what it would feel like to be a woman in our society and to be freed from that confining anatomical prison. The negative self-hypnosis of the hidden symptom easily changed, a good sign that his images of violence and death were not the result of serious pathology, but came from desperation.

In four family therapy sessions, the parents made peace with the situation, accepting what both had suspected for a long time and giving him the loving acceptance and support he needed to proceed with the sex change. A few more family therapy sessions were used to discuss many details concerning his drastic decision. The individual therapy continued intermittently for the following five years, until Nancy (formerly Hal) was a well-adjusted woman working successfully in commercial real estate and enjoying a large circle of friends who respected and admired her courage.

It is only fair to assume that the concentration on the hidden symptom and the handling of it made the long process of sex change smoother and easier. To have left Nancy with her hidden symptom would not have been helpful to her, and would have made her ordeal even more difficult and painful.

## CONCLUSIONS

The purpose of this chapter was to bring to the attention of hypnotherapists the hidden symptom, an especially convenient hypnotic phenomenon that can be used beneficially in all forms of therapy, and particularly in sex therapy. The hidden symptom is called *hypnotic* (much as the self-fulfilling prophecy may be called hypnotic) because it bypasses reason and makes the mental images of failure, aggravation of the condition, self-blame, and the like appear as objective reality. It is also called *convenient* from the point of view of therapy, because it is frequently there, and with it the therapist has a positive starting point from which to proceed toward change and personal growth. Because humans engage in self-talk, asking the client what he or she is saying to himself or herself about the problem is never a threatening directive. Just by finding out that there is negativism, we convey understanding, caring, and sensitivity to the other person—important elements in quickly establishing a working alliance in therapy.

This is illustrated by a last example in a case not related to sexual behavior. A highly intelligent woman in her early 50s felt depressed and helpless, while blaming herself for not being able to handle the most important people in her life. She did not realize she was engaged in this self-defeating mental activity, and when she stopped it she became much more efficient in handling the difficult problems that faced her. Without the NSH, she was able to engage in self-therapy, mentioned earlier, and to use her mental resources to objectify what was really going on. The reality involved the following characters: a clinically depressed spouse 20 years her senior who refused treatment for his condition, a dying mother with Alzheimer's disease, a materialistic 25-year-old daughter who tried to take advantage of her at every turn, and a son, 28, who insisted on becoming the head of the family because of his father's passivity. She could handle these difficulties as long as she was not blaming herself for them. The problems were real, but her NSH, the hidden symptom, made them worse. The hidden symptom is more common than many mental health providers believe.

In every case of sex therapy, because the issue is so personal and sensitive, the client engages in NSH. Those who do not never become patients. The first intervention is to help them change their minds about their problems by changing their self-talk, with all the negative images it creates. This is what hypnotherapy can help clients do: change their NHS, reframe, use positive metaphors, trust therir unconscious, and use their inner resources. In doing away with the hidden symptom, we find a wide-open space in which to work constructively for the benefit of the client.

The ongoing research, mentioned earlier, seems to confirm what Seligman (1991) teaches us about optimism. It produces many good things, from better relationships to more life insurance sales. But optimism must be learned—or, rather the negativism must be unlearned. However, in order to unlearn negativism, we must discover it, acknowledge it, and find new ways of relating to the environment and what it brings to us. This is what we do when we work on the hidden symptom.

## References

Araoz, D. L. (1995). *The new hypnosis*. Northvale, NJ: Jason Aronson. (Formerly, [1985]. *The new hypnosis*. New York: Brunner/Mazel.)

Araoz, D. L. (1998) *The new hypnosis in sex therapy*. Northvale, NJ: Jason Aronson. (Formerly, [1982]. *Hypnosis and sex therapy*. New York: Brunner/Mazel.)

Araoz, D. L., Burte, J., & Carrese, M. A. (1998). The new hypnosis of Milton H. Erickson and sex therapy. Presentation at the Brief Therapy Conference, M. H. Erickson Foundation, New York, August 1998.

Beahrs, J. O. (1990). Strategic self-therapy. In J. K. Zeig & W. M. Munion (Eds.), *What is psychotherapy? Contemporary perspectives*. San Francisco: Jossey-Bass.

Benjamin, N. (1966). *The transsexual phenomenon*. New York: Julian Press.

Fausto-Sterling, A. (1985). *Myths of gender: Biological theories about women and men*. New York: Basic Books.

Goleman, D. (1998). *Working with emotional intelligence*. New York: Bantam Books.

Green, R., & Fleming, D. T. (1990). Transsexual surgery follow-up: Status in the 1990s. *Annual Review of Sex Research, 1*, 163–174.

Kohut, H. (1971). *The analysis of the self*. New York: International Universities Press.

Kohut, H. (1977). *The restoration of the self*. New York: International Universities Press.

Kohut, H. (1978). *The search for the self.* New York: International Universities Press.

Mahoney, M. J. (1991). *Human change processes: The scientific foundations of psychotherapy.* New York: Basic Books.

Money, J., & Wiedeking, C. (1980). Gender identity/role: Normal differentiation and its transpositions. In B. B. Wolman & J. Money (Eds.), *Handbook of human sexuality.* Englewood Cliffs, NJ: Prentice-Hall.

Quiñones Bergeret, A., & Zagmutt Cahbar, A. (1996). *Revista Americana Psicologica,* XIII, vol. 6, no. 25, 55–70.

Seligman, M. E. P. (1991). *Learned optimism.* New York: Knopf.

Walen, S. R. (1980). Cognitive factors in sexual behavior. *Journal of Sex and Marital Therapy, 6,* 87–101.

# 30

# Indirect Work with Couples[1]

## *Teresa Robles*

In applying Ericksonian principles and techniques to couples work, we must note that for Milton Erickson, the crises that emerge out of the natural development of the couple may become difficulties because of their intimate context, meaning that the conflicts of the couple are contextual. Even if he did not explicitly use a systemic approach, he always considered the reciprocity of the behaviors, the way in which a certain behavior affects another behavior, and vice versa. He suggested that a hypnotic trance may emerge from the interactions and that the visible conjugal conflict is often a metaphor for something deeper.

It is possible to study the work of Erickson with couples via Jay Haley's (1973) *Uncommon Therapy* and O'Hanlon and Hexum's (1990) *An Uncommon Casebook*. In both works, it is possible to observe the way in which Erickson used direct and indirect suggestions with couples, as well as all of his techniques. He was always very careful not to establish coalitions, to stop recursive communication between the couple in his office, and to confront them in a benign way in order to give them the chance to review and modify their ideas.

[1] I would like to thank Adriana Barroso, Dipl. Psych., for helping me with the translation into English, and Marina Castañeda, M.A., for her assistance with the use of idioms.

## WHAT SOME OF THE EXPERTS SAY

What these respected therapists have in common is their appreciation of, and interest in applying, Ericksonian approaches and principles, such as searching for resources, showing confidence in the unconscious mind, avoiding labeling the patient and his or her behaviors, and promoting new learning.

Jay Haley (1973), in his classic *Uncommon Therapy*, systematizes Erickson's work according to the family's life cycles.

William H. O'Hanlon (O'Hanlon & Hudson, 1995) developed a solution-oriented therapy that may be applied to individuals, as well as to families and couples. It emphasizes discovering and changing patterns.

Carol Kershaw (1992) proposes that couples' interactions create a hypnotic dance. Through it, they induce in each other a trance state. She says that the symptoms are ways of communication that show a lack of equilibrium in the relationship. Crises are opportunities for personal and conjugal growth. From the symptomatic trance, a healing trance may be induced. The therapeutic work consists of interrupting this dance to allow the unconscious mind to facilitate new ways in which to dance in an intimate and unique experience.

David L. Calof and Robin Simons (1996) work with the inner voices (internalizations of parental voices) to modify and transform them in inner resources or parts that collaborate in assuring the person's well-being.

Camillo Loriedo (1995) has developed a therapist-centered therapy that states that if the therapist changes, the couple changes. The therapy is blocked whenever the therapist is blocked, and it is necessary for him or her to change if the therapy is to go on. That is, in addition to using personal life experiences as resources, there is an intention to generate in the therapist the inner change that is necessary to the therapeutic process.

## A MODEL FOR INDIRECT WORK WITH COUPLES

I grew up in an upper-middle-class Mexican family, a family in which everyone smiled and was always courteous to each other, while participating in an unspoken pact to keep hidden any "shameful secrets." That is, in essence, we were a conflict-avoiding family. As a result, I have learned to manage indirect communication in a natural way. These lessons have enabled me to handle in therapy conflict-avoiding couples who use indirect modes of communication. And they also have helped me to train couples who live in a permanent situation of direct complaints and quarrels to develop indirect ways of communicating.

## Some Theoretical Reflections

Before becoming a clinical psychologist, I earned a master's degree in social anthropology. As an anthropologist, I could observe how social and cultural patterns and values unconsciously are transmitted from one generation to another, thus making it very difficult for us to recognize and change both the process of transmission and the transmitted contents (values and patterns) because they are out of awareness. For example, we are taught to perceive the world as if it were divided into halves: good and evil, mind and body, rational and emotional. And we are taught that the first half of each pair is first rate and the second is second rate, and so the latter must be under the control of the former. We all have learned that love is sacrifice and that we must control (that is, hide or not perceive) pain and bad emotions. And we become involved in social and cultural double binds. Because love is sacrifice, if I love, I suffer, because I am making a sacrifice and I am not O.K. But if I do not love, I am not O.K. either.

I believe that most of a couple's conflicts, and even most of the so-called pathology according to different theoretical approaches, can be attributed to those social and cultural lessons and double binds (Robles, 1995a). Through my clinical work and research, I have found that some topics appear to be universal, at least in Western society, because they arise from the internalization of those values and patterns.

The model I propose consists of a general outline for working with Ericksonian hypnosis, universal topics, and cultural lessons that are tailored to each couple (Robles, 1991).

Gregory Bateson (1979) reminds us that, if we observe something through various lenses, we may have a more complete view of it. For me, Ericksonian epistemology, cybernetic epistemology, psychoanalysis, systems theory, constructivism, and social anthropology are very useful lenses through which to observe couples from different angles and, therefore, to derive a multidimensional perspective.

Freud (1915/1956) proposed that all life experiences are registered in the unconscious as memory traces that are formed by: a representation, the memory itself, and the emotion or energy that this trace contains, and that can shift to other traces. As a result of this shifting, sometimes a representation accumulates the emotions of many other, similar traces. This is the mechanism of condensation.

Because the unconscious works on the basis of the pleasure principle, or the avoiding of pain, it represses painful memories and disguises them so that they emerge in the consciousness in a protected way; that is, they are symbolized.

If, instead of trying to make the unconscious conscious, or provoking a catharsis, we use the mechanisms of the unconscious mind and transform the symbols or solve them in trance without trying to interpret them, we obtain the following results.

- We flow with the pleasure principle, and this facilitates change.
- Resistance becomes unnecessary and disappears.
- When we solve or alter a symbol, we solve all the experiences that were condensed in it (Robles, 1997).

This is what Erickson did when he used metaphoric language, stories, and anecdotes as indirect suggestions. In this way, therapy becomes pleasant for both therapists and client, and that is important because behind all symptoms there lies a difficulty in enjoying life. And if we enjoy therapy, we are promoting health in an indirect way (Robles, 1995).

Twenty years ago, I began to use breathing as a metaphor for the mechanism of inner change. To the rational mind, it is a metaphor, but to the unconscious mind, through condensation, breathing *is* the mechanism of inner change. This mechanism works all the time, automatically and always healthfully. Freud suggested that the emotion, which I call "life energy," is only one, but it may take on different characteristics (LaPlanche & Pontalis, 1978). As a popular Mexican saying puts it, "From love to hatred is only one step." People who hate each other already are linked energetically. When they love each other, they continue being linked by this same energy, which has only changed its quality.

Breathing can be used, for example, to digest a negative emotion, keeping its raw material and transforming it into life energy, which remains available for building other emotions or pleasant sensations, or just to be used to live as one wants to live.

Although each member of the couple may have inner repressed conflicts, it is useless, tiring, and unnecessary to go directly through them. It is possible to solve them in a bearable, comfortable, and, therefore, efficient way by using symbolization and condensation. When conflicts are solved, repression and resistance are no longer necessary.

From my experience with systemic therapy, I learned to see—beyond the content—the reciprocity of the behaviors, as Erickson did. I learned that difficulties become problems when we repeatedly consider only one solution, and that both partners are involved in these problems. In this model, I break, like Erickson did, recursive interactions and dysfunctional patterns through unexpected proposals that lead to confusion, open new options, and enable each person to take on his or her own responsibilities.

## General Outline

*Before Each Session*

I try to build a hypothesis about what is going on with the couple, and I plan strategies that will be adjusted, changed, or tailored during the session.

*During the Session*

I observe what happens during the first five minutes of the session, asking myself: What is the underlying universal topic that is creating this situation? Then I begin to work, introducing the topic either by saying something like: "This couple, as any other couple ...," or by telling a personal anecdote or using a metaphor. For example, "We all have suffered injuries during our lives, and when we have open wounds, they hurt, and we even attack our loved ones." And I continue, looking for minimal cues to tailor the intervention to the couple.

I make proposals that break patterns, provoke confusion, present options. Some become the therapy rules; that is, "It is disrespectful to ask others to change," or "I'm not interested in getting involved in anyone's life. Here, we are not going to talk about problems or about personal things; we are going to do something different, we are going to build for the future."

At the end of the session, I always suggest that a change has already begun and that it will continue beyond the session. Sometimes I reinforce the process with homework—tasks that have to be done between sessions.

I have seen from my experience that, after several sessions, conflict-avoiding couples start to talk about things they didn't dare to discuss before; and couples who lived with constant, open conflict stop quarreling and start using different ways to communicate.

## Metaphors for Universal Topics
*One's Own and Inherited Wounds*[2]

When two people come to therapy arguing about everything and each overreacting to any comment by his or her partner, I tell them: "We all suffer wounds throughout our lives. And the wounds heal if we let them heal; but there are some that remain open, maybe because we are afraid of looking at them and we cover them, maybe because we are touching them, picking the scabs off, and they hurt even more.

"We all have natural mechanisms to heal wounds and every wound becomes a scar if we allow it to heal. And scars are painless memories that remind us that we have survived difficult situations and that we have grown up and developed new abilities."

I propose: "It seems to me that before going on, it is better to heal your wounds." I invite them to close their eyes and to imagine the kind of wounds they have and in which part of the body they would be. I suggest that they observe how, without doing anything, their breathing is cleaning, drying, and healing their wounds.

Whenever they tell me that their wounds are already healing, I continue, saying, "We all have wounds that we have suffered throughout our lives, but there are others that we have inherited from our parents, our grandparents, our other relatives, and those wounds also hurt. Observe those beloved people whose open wounds have also hurt you. Explain to them all the things that I have explained to you about the wounds. Suggest to them that they use their breathing to heal their wounds inside of you. If they don't want to do so, tell them: 'I have already told you how to heal your wounds. If you do not want to, it is your problem. I will be all right, living and enjoying my life as I want to, even if you continue feeling bad.'"

### Settling Accounts

I start a hypnotic conversation by saying, "It seems to me that all human relationships, but especially couple ones, should have a tune-up, just as we do for cars.

"When I do something that bothers the other, first of all, I ask myself what I did wrong in order to be able to change it. But I have also learned

---

[2] The idea of wounds was developed by the author (Abia & Robles, 1985). Later, Rafael Núñez added the idea that part of our wounds are inherited.

that the other's reactions have to do with his or her own problems, as happens to me. If I get angry or hurt because of something the other did, it is due to my own story. And by working with my feelings and solving my inner conflicts, I have discovered that I can stay still even if others keep acting in a way that in the past used to bother me. In my important relationships, I make a *leap of faith* and decide that whenever a beloved and reliable person does something that hurts me, he or she is not doing it against me, but because of what he or she is living and feeling in that moment, even if I don't understand it."

I ask the couple: "Do you think you can make a *leap of faith* and believe that no matter what the other does, it is not against you, even if you don't like it or don't understand it?"

If they agree, I continue: "In order to start a healthier relationship, maybe closer, maybe farther apart, at whatever distance you want to stay, you need to settle the accounts of your relationship up until now. Do it in silence, in your imagination, without any comments, because comments would only bring pain and problems, and what you need now is to be at peace with yourselves and with each other." I ask them to promise not to make any comment on the exercise.

I start a formal hypnotic trance by saying: "With your eyes closed, imagine yourself in a comfortable place settling accounts with your partner, talking about all those things that you have not talked about and that it is useless to talk about in real life. Now, in your imagination, air your grievances. As you are doing so, your breathing is digesting all the blocked feelings that you had about him or her. And also thank your partner for all the things for which you should be thankful, for the pleasant moments lived together, for the things he or she has given to you, for what he or she has taught you. Thank him or her too—even if it is your own doing—for how you have grown with that relationship. And while you are airing your grievances, digesting all the blocked feelings, thanking him or her, and keeping inside you all the good things that this relationship gave you, your breathing is doing a very important job for you. Your breathing is also giving him or her back all the energy that he or she expended on you, completing his or her energy, setting you free. And at the same time, your breathing is bringing back to you all the energy you had expended on him or her, and in this way, both of you are completing yourselves."

Through this exercise, the couple digests the blocked emotions that interfered with their relationship. It also helps the partners to see each other as all in one piece.[3] Once they know they have retrieved all their life energy, and keep inside things from the other that are now part of themselves, they feel more comfortable with whatever decision they make—whether to stay together or to separate.

It is very useful to help the couple to settle accounts with all the other people with whom they have problems, for example, with their parents and parents-in-law.

### The Other Is All in One Piece

Frequently, when couples come to therapy, each partner has a list of things that he or she thinks the other would have to change to make the relationship better. In these cases, I tell them categorically: "I think it is disrespectful to ask the other to change. What gives you the right to tell another how he or she has to be? Are you in love with the person himself or herself, or with the person you would like him or her to be? Because the latter does not exist! Furthermore, people don't change because someone wants them to change, they change because they feel bad as they are. You know how difficult it is to change yourself; now imagine how difficult it would be to make someone else change."

I invite them to open their eyes: "Observe how the other is. *He or she is like that.* He or she is all in one piece, with particular qualities, imperfections, and personal characteristics. You can take it or leave it; you can learn to live with him or her at a comfortable and protected distance, but *he or she is like that.* And now, knowing that he or she is like that, ask yourself: 'Do I love this person or not? Do I want to stay with him or her or not? Do I have physical and emotional security with him or her?' " If the answers are Yes, I continue: "Instead of asking your partner to change, why don't you ask yourself, 'What can I change in myself to feel more comfortable in this relationship? What can I do to be all right even if my partner does not want to change?' "

I explain: "All the imperfections have quality, if we know how to adjust their volume and if we use them in the right moment." And I ask them: "What would you like to learn from the other's 'supposed imperfections'?"

---

[3] For Melanie Klein, to see the person as a whole is to "integrate relations with total objects" and it is for her a synonym for mental health (see Roudinesco & Plon, 1997).

In a formal trance, I help them to rehearse that they are acting and feeling as they wish because each has already changed inside himself or herself what he or she wanted to change in order to live with the other in the way he or she wants to live.

## Difficulties in the Relationship as a Couple

Through hypnotic conversation, I introduce the following ideas.

"Problems are produced because we tend to establish relationships that start from our own needs and our hope that the other will satisfy them. We try to satisfy the other's needs at the expense of our own; we sacrifice so the other will do the same for us. This way, the relationship becomes an obligation instead of an opportunity to grow together, supporting and sharing with each other, and learning about one another.

"No one can compensate for another's deficiencies. Each behaves, reacts, and loves as he or she can, not as he or she would like to. Instead of receiving what the other can give to us, we are used to rejecting it when it does not correspond to what we want. We even get angry because we are not loved as we want to be loved. And, therefore, we do not accept all the good things the other is able to give to us.

"Each has a version of the problem, and both are equally valid. We are not going to discuss them. Each one sees the problem from his or her own point of view, from his or her own story."

Afterward, I present a hypnotic exercise for working with the difficulties that have turned the relationship into an obligation, for transforming it again as a chance to grow, whether together or separated.

## Building and/or Reinforcing Boundaries

I tell them that there are two important tasks that every couple should accomplish:

1. To permit each to keep on being himself or herself, as well as a member of a couple.
2. To decide how they will function differently from their families.

I use the metaphor of a fence that, like the skin, clearly delineates where each person and his or her interests and wishes end, and where the other's start.

I explain: "Just as we all have a skin that clearly shows that from this point [I mimic a movement from my skin to the inside part of my body] to the inside is ME, and from this point [I point to my skin again] to the outside is NOT-ME, we need to build a fence to define that from my fence to the inside is ME—with my desires, my interests, my emotions— and from my fence to the outside is NOT-ME. We need to build a distinctive, protecting fence, like the skin that, instead of isolating us, allows us to touch each other in a protected way and allows the entrance of what is part of us or what is good for us and leaves aside the things that would interfere with our well-being."

Then I tell them: "Close your eyes and imagine how that fence defines that from it to the inside is YOU and from it to the outside is NOT-YOU. Please look at it. What kind of fence is it? Of what is it made? What is its height? Does it surround you?

"Feel your breathing and see how, without doing anything, your breathing is rebuilding it, completing it, strengthening it, automatically. And it is allowing to enter, in a protected way, all those things that are YOU and that for some reason were outside; and, at the same time, your breathing is removing all those parts that are NOT-YOU, and that, for some reason, were inside of you. Your breathing is helping those parts to find their place, so that once they find it, they will continue having a healthy harmonious relationship with you. Your breathing is removing— in a protected way—all those things that would interfere with your complete well-being."

Once each has built a boundary around himself or herself, I invite them to build the couple's boundary. I suggest that they imagine their fences whenever they feel they need them.

### The Metaphor of the Couple

Metaphors can be used whenever the topic mentioned by the couple is not directly related to a universal topic, when one of the partners uses metaphorical expressions, or when the therapist spontaneously thinks of a metaphor that represents the situation of the couple at that moment.

I may tell them: "You have already talked about your problems many times, you have already analyzed them, reflected on them, so let's do something different." And I continue, saying: "Just as he or she says, this couple looks like ..." and I repeat the metaphorical expression mentioned by one of them. Or I may tell them: "I was thinking about you and imagined you as ..." or, "How can we represent through a metaphor the situation in which you are living now?"

I help them to build a metaphor, and from that moment on, we work with it, looking at the problem they are living as part of a natural process, and discovering the options, resources, and ways this process offers. (This is a very important Ericksonian technique. See, among others: Barker, 1985; Combs & Freedman, 1990; Mills & Crowley, 1986.)

If no ideas come to their minds, I invite them to close their eyes. I induce a formal trance and suggest to them that, without any effort, as they breathe, the metaphor for their difficulties will appear. Whatever they perceive, no matter what it is, it is the way in which the unconscious mind is representing the difficulties between them. Then I invite them to observe how their breathing is digesting the images, transforming the difficulties into new kinds of relationship.

I continue working with the metaphor in subsequent sessions.

## CASE STUDY

Joe and Mary have been married for two years. They live in a small cottage in the garden of Joe's parents' house. Living with Joe's parents are two unmarried daughters and a married daughter with her husband and children.

Mary complains about Joe because he works constantly, even at night and on weekends. And when he comes home, he still has work to do. He is never with her and she feels very lonely. The situation was the same before they were married, but Mary thought that marriage would give them more time together.

Mary says she does her best to be a good homemaker, cleaning the house and cooking nutritious meals. However, she frequently has problems with her sisters-in-law and feels that Joe doesn't defend her. She would like to have a child, but Joe says they will have to wait until his job is more secure and their economic situation is better. In his eyes, they have no difficulties in their relationship. He thinks that Mary is the one with problems and that she needs an activity to occupy her time.

I started the session by saying that it seemed to me that it is disrespectful to ask the other to change. I asked them to observe how the other is, as a whole, with his or her good qualities and imperfections, with the characteristics they like or dislike in the other. Next, I invited them to ask themselves: "Just as he or she is, without asking him or her to change anything: Do I love him or her or not? Am I interested or not in living with him or her?"

Both answered immediately that they loved each other and that they wanted to stay together. They had known each other since they were children and had always been very close.

Then I told them that the fact that Joe spends so much time working doesn't mean that he does not want to be with Mary. Rather, Joe may think that that's the way things should be; or he may act this way because of some personal reasons we do not understand and that may be unclear to him as well. If Mary spends all day at home waiting for Joe, it is not to complain about his absence, but because she thinks that's the way it should be or for some reason from her own story that may not clear to her in that moment. I asked them if they could understand that whatever one partner does is not against the other, but arises out of what the other is going through as the result of his or her inner needs or story. They both agreed that they could.

I explained that their misunderstandings have hurt them, that they are open wounds, and that even if all the wounds heal if we allow them to, whenever those misunderstandings arise, one after the other, the wounds remain open.

We all bear wounds that have been inflicted throughout our lives. And sometimes wounds made by the partner are superimposed on old, open ones, and so we suffer too much. We also inherit wounds from our parents and grandparents that bring us pain.

I invited Joe and Mary to close their eyes and to imagine their wounds and observe how they were in that moment. I invited them to observe how, without doing anything, their breathing was healing them. Then I suggested that they imagine their parents and grandparents standing in front of them, with their own wounds. I told them to teach them to heal their wounds through their breathing. Joe said that, in his mind, his father makes fun of him, and, of course, refuses to see his own wounds. I suggested that Joe tell his father internally: "I've explained to you how to heal your wounds so you can be all right; but if you don't want to do it, that's your business. But I want you to know that I will live my life as I want to live it, enjoying it, even if you don't enjoy yours."

When the exercise was over, they talked about the wounds of their childhood and about their parents' wounds. When Joe was born, he had breathing difficulties, which, the doctor said, might have affected his brain. His father became depressed upon hearing that he had a mentally defective child, and so he rejected Joe. Joe and his mother struggled to show the others that in spite of Joe's handicap, he was capable of succeeding. Actually, Joe was always a good student, graduating with an engineering degree and finishing his Ph.D. with honors. Nevertheless, it was not enough for his father. For him, Joe was still the mentally defective son. Joe admitted that in his job he always worked harder than his colleagues, to the point of taking on their tasks because he was afraid of being told that what he did was not enough, and that he would be fired. His father was an orphan who had to work even as a child to support his brothers and so was unable to attend college.

After Mary was born, her father abandoned the family. Her mother had to find employment, and as she had no training, she had to work as a maid. She left Mary alone all day in the attic room in which they lived. When Mary grew up, she still spent most of her time alone. She met Joe at school, and they would walk together to school and back home. She dreamed of having a family, a cozy house permeated by the friendly smells of home-cooked meals, a house full of people.

When they came to the second session, they looked better. They said that they hadn't argued much. On Sunday, Joe had stayed at home. Mary had invited her mother over twice and thanked her for all the things she had done for her. They talked about her mother's feelings when Mary was a little girl and they had a good time together. However, the problems with Joe's family had not yet been resolved.

We worked so that each could build a fence in his or her mind to defend and protect his or her own place and to distinguish it from the other's place. We also settled accounts between them and I gave them a tape of the exercise so that they could repeat it at home with their families, and with Joe's boss and co-workers.

They came back a month later. They said they were looking for an apartment and that Mary had started handicraft lessons and had made some friends at the school. Joe was spending more time at home. We commented on the importance of seeing one's partner just as he or she is and of receiving what he or she can give us. We talked about how the relationship may afford an opportunity for growing together. We finished the therapeutic process.

Joe and Mary returned again two years later. Mary was pregnant and they wanted to work with their fears of not being good parents. I still keep in touch with them; they have attended courses at our clinic, including self-hypnosis, improving creativity, and management of stress. They also have participated in groups for personal growth and workshops on such topics as sex education. They said they are well, and that whenever they have difficulties in their own relationship or with other people, they repeat the exercise for settling accounts.

---

### Practical Ideas

• To introduce breathing as a natural mechanism for inner change, for digesting emotions and for transforming the images in trance.
• To invite partners in a couple to settle accounts in their imagination.
• To help people heal their wounds.
• To emphasize that they must not ask each other to change.
• To propose that they look at the partner as a whole.
• To transform the couple relationship from an obligation into an opportunity.

---

### References

Abia, J., & Robles, T. (1995). *Autohipnosis, aprendiendo a caminar por la vida.* Mexico: Alom Editores.

Barker, P. (1983). *Using metaphors in psychotherapy.* New York: Brunner/Mazel.

Bateson, G. (1979). *Mind and nature. A necessary unity* (Chap. 3). New York: Dutton.

Calof, D. (1985). Hypnosis in marital therapy: Toward a transgenerational approach. In J. K. Zeig (Ed.), *Ericksonian psychotherapy: Clinical applications* (vol. II, pp. 74–89). New York: Brunner/Mazel.

Calof, D., & Simons, R. (1996). *The couple who became each other.* New York: Bantam Books.

Coombs, G., & Freedman, J. (1990). *Symbol, story and ceremony. Using metaphor in individual and family therapy.* New York: Norton.

Freud, S. (1915/1952). The unconscious. In *Metapsychologie* (pp. 91–161). Paris: Gallimard.

Haley, J. (1973). *Uncommon therapy: The psychiatric techniques of Milton H. Erickson.* New York: Norton.

Kershaw, C. J. (1992). *The couple's hypnotic dance. Creating Ericksonian strategies.* New York: Brunner/Mazel.

LaPlanche, J., & Pontalis, J. B. (1978). *Vocabulaire de la psychanalyse* (pp. 12–13). Paris: Presses Universitaires de France.

Loriedo, C. (1996). Psicoterapia centrade en el terapeuta. In E. Mendez (Ed.), *Compartiendo experiencias de terapía con hipnosis*. Mexico: Alom Editores.

Mills, J. C., & Crowley, R. J. (1986). *Therapeutic metaphors for children and the child within*. New York: Brunner/Mazel.

O'Hanlon, W. H., & Hudson, P. (1995). *Love is a verb. How to stop analyzing your relationship and start making it great*. New York: Norton.

O'Hanlon, W. H., & Hexum, A. (1990). Marital, family and relationship problems. In *An uncommon case book. The complete clinical work of Milton H. Erickson, M.D.* (pp. 243-260). New York: Norton.

Robles, T. (1991). *Terapía contada a la medida*. An Ericksonian Seminar with Jeffrey K. Zeig. Mexico: Alom Editores.

Robles, T. (1995a). *Concert for four brain hemispheres in psychotherapy*. New York: Vantage Press.

Robles, T. (1995b). *La magia de nuestros disfraces*. Mexico: Alom Editores.

Robles, T. (1996). *Revisando el pasado para construir el futuro*. Mexico: Alom Editores.

Robles, T. (1997). Reflections on how hypnosis works. Presented at the Congress of the International Society of Hypnosis, San Diego, CA.

Roudinesco, E., & Plon, M. (1997). In *Dictionnaire de la psychanalyse* (pp. 570-574). Paris: Fayard.

Zeig, J. K., & Lankton, S. R. (1986). *Developing Ericksonian therapy* (pp. 431-426). New York: Brunner/Mazel.

# 31

# The Hypnotic Language
# of Couples

*Jane A. Parsons-Fein*

## INTRODUCTION

Falling in love: a dance between two people whose conscious and unconscious rhythms move in harmony. But as time goes by, each begins to transfer or displace onto the other the intense, unresolved unconscious feelings that arose in the early years, when the partners were vulnerable to the myths, messages and unconscious inductions of their parents, and sometimes their siblings, in their families of origin. As they begin to experience inevitable obstacles and difficulties of life as a couple, some of the early imprinted patterns recur, and the beautiful flow of their falling in love automatically begins to congeal into hardened loops that move recursively back and forth between the erstwhile lovers. Each couple is unique in its infinite ability to create replays of each of the families of origin. The misunderstandings, misperceptions, and conflicts go back to the state-dependent memories, learnings, and behaviors of each spouse, often unrecognized and exterior to conscious awareness. Approaches pioneered by Milton H. Erickson can be effective in working with couples.

## ERICKSON'S POSITION

Milton Erickson demystified and redefined hypnosis. He believed that trance is a natural daily occurrence for everyone, and that when we are in trance, we learn on unconscious levels and take in suggestions uncritically, unaware of the power they can have over our unconscious thinking. Since, in childhood, we spend about 85% of our attention in the state of trance learning, much of what we take in and observe drops back into an area of the unconscious that is amnesic. Those memories that are formed in intense emotional states are called imprints. An imprint is a single-impact idea or suggestion that can become fixed in the unconscious and is carried out in exactly the same way as in a posthypnotic suggestion, although we do not consciously remember it.

In adulthood, when people shift into automatic behavior, they have been triggered into a forgotten childhood imprint. The family is a hypnotic unit and the parents are hypnotists who themselves were hypnotized as children. Alice Miller has described how family messages are transferred from the unconscious of one generation to the unconscious of the next generation. Each member of the couple brings these transgenerational imprints into the relationship.

Erickson considered every individual unique and so took care to see each person who walked into his office from a fresh perceptive. He often helped couples individuate themselves out of a marriage symbiosis, discovering in themselves and in each other new interests and new connections. In many of his task assignments, he created the context for each to discover facets hitherto unavailable.

He also believed that every person has within his or her own system the capacity to move toward health, and that it is possible to generate one small strategic change[1] that would have a ripple effect on the whole pattern. He often worked with the system without acknowledging to the patient the specific problem. Sometimes he prescribed or exaggerated the

---

[1] An example of this is a case I had many years ago, before I met Erickson. A young woman who was in treatment could not become pregnant, although the couple had been medically cleared after years of tests. One day she mentioned that her mother had been severely depressed when the client was two years old. Why? "Well," she replied flatly, "my mother's sister had just died in childbirth . . ." and she continued talking. I interrupted her and asked, "I wonder what a little two-year old, terrified at the sudden change in her mother's behavior, would think about death and childbirth? What are you thinking right now?" I remember her staring at me wide-eyed. Within two months, she became pregnant. I now realize that one moment of illumination helped her adult mind to reframe the unconscious child perception that had been trying to protect her from death.

symptom. He joined the metaphor of the patient or couple, was precise in his use of hypnotic language, direct and conversational, and paced[2] the unconscious processes flowing between the partners. Many of his task assignments reflected the paradoxical nature of the patterns the husband and wife had developed.

## OTHER PERSPECTIVES

I was trained in psychoanalytic psychotherapy and later explored Gestalt, transactional analysis, multimodal therapy, and neurolinguistic programming. It was a revelation to me to study with Milton Erickson, to learn from him how we communicate consciously and unconsciously with one another, and how powerful our connections are on linguistic and physical levels. Trance state for me became a path to self-understanding rather than something mysterious.

Jay Haley's study of Erickson, *Uncommon Therapy* (1973), also led me to believe that the family is a hypnotic unit. He writes: "Erickson's family orientation is implicit in his work, and talking with him and examining his cases helped me toward a new view of the family as a center of human dilemmas. When I began to think of human problems as inevitable in the way a family develops over time, I realized that Dr. Erickson's therapy was largely based upon that assumption."

I studied with Virginia Satir, who developed the family reconstruction model, and I recognized that she confirmed and amplified this theory on a practical level using genograms[3] and the dissociation techniques of role playing and sculpting[4] in her work. She tracked what she called "the family's myths and messages," often going back three generations.

Satir reframed these family transgenerational inductions. She enabled people to go into trance with her meditations[5] (which always preceded

---

[2] To pace is to align oneself with the verbal and nonverbal behavior of the client, feeding back words, moving with body language, joining the client's metaphor, and harmonizing with his or her rhythm. This mirroring is nonjudgmental. It is simply a multilevel dance between two people.

[3] A genogram is a family map that diagrams the history of generations of a family. It can reveal patterns and connections that highlight hitherto unrecognized repetitive themes.

[4] Sculpting is used by Satir in groups. I have adapted it to couples therapy. Each spouse takes a turn and without words sculpts himself or herself into physical gestures. For example, a blamer points and scowls, a placator gets down on his or her knees and reaches up in supplication. This is acted out and later explored.

[5] Satir's "meditations" are suggestions for group members to close their eyes, go inside, and become calm and clear.

any work she did with groups) and then worked with dissociation in myriad ways. Like Erickson, she believed in experiential processing (she called it "right brain, see–hear–feel learning") and focused on the patient's bodily sensations, weaving back and forth from feeling to thinking to feeling, shifting awareness and the awareness of awareness. She believed that it was important for people to become aware of the unseen shadows of the unconscious, whereas Erickson often reframed these imprints while the client was in trance without ever bringing them into his or her conscious awareness. Both Satir and Erickson worked with early imprints, reframing, installing new patterns, giving suggestions for future growth.

In order to access these unconscious patterns, the subject must move into trance. Kay Thompson, a long-time student of Erickson, employed word play, the rhythm of nursery rhymes, and metaphors to help people move quickly into the special creativity and power of their unconscious worlds, where new patterns can be generated, old imprints transformed. When working with couples, I have found her innovations powerful.

Ernest Rossi worked with Erickson for many years. His research into state-dependent memory, learning, and behavior makes clear the importance of focusing on age regression, early learning, and imprinting. When people shift into trance, their molecular organization also shifts. The imprinted response that is evoked recreates the physiological patterns and informational transfer of the original imprint. People move into the same biochemical state, the same hormonal condition, they were in when they first learned the pattern.

Rossi made use of the breakthroughs in the physiological sciences that occurred after Erickson's death. Recent research confirms that emotional states and imprints are chemically induced states in the body that can be triggered by words, gestures, or images, and that changes in the blood flow in the brain also take place. Erickson anticipated that his work would eventually be supported by such discoveries.

Candace Pert, Ph.D., the pharmacologist who found opiate receptors in the body, which led to the discovery of endorphins, has said: "If you are smoking and drinking coffee when you are studying for an exam, you had better be smoking and drinking coffee when you take the exam." The context in which we learn something is revivified when that learning is accessed. That is probably why Milton Erickson worked with the early-learning patterns of childhood to access the process of movement and thinking in addition to the revivification of the memory itself. Thus the patient is freed from hitherto unrecognized and unwanted behavior.

Rossi utilizes, often in long silences, his hypnotic relationship with the subject by pacing the subject's internal movement on a variety of levels. He sits watching the subject intently, breathing in the same rhythm, sometimes saying "That's right!," nodding his head, although the client with closed eyes doesn't see this. Rossi closely observes as the client shifts from one state of consciousness to another. It is as if he has silently joined with the client and is waiting patiently for whatever happens in the client's unconscious. It is this form of pacing that helps the client go deeper because it communicates unqualified acceptance. His technique and style have been another resource for me.

## CASE STUDY: APPLICATIONS

I always remember that Erickson said: "Hypnosis is a special relationship between two people." When Jim first called for an appointment for his wife, Natasha, and himself, I heard the tension in his voice, paced him, and did my best to create a context of safety and acceptance—acceptance of the negative as well as the positive. (The neglected or split-off parts of the self of each participant are in the most pain, and need most to be invited into the work.) I wrote down any words or phrases or references that could be turned into a metaphor that I could feed back to them in the future. Jim said, "I feel like I'm drowning!" Later, in session, I would talk about being in really deep water, realizing I'm too far from shore, taking a deep breath, and carefully moving with the current, slowly cutting across it and gradually moving toward shore.

Beginning with the initial session, as is the case with any client, I remained aware that I had to operate on two levels simultaneously: the content level and the process level. I was also aware that I had to pace each individual, consciously and unconsciously, as well as track the relationships between them and between each of them and me. The moment they walk into my office, each partner in a couple brings a compromised core self with which he or she may have entered the marriage. They probably started with hopes, wishes, and dreams, now perhaps broken, which they lay at my feet. Each usually comes with the expectation that I, like a good parent, will "fix" the partner.

At their first appointment, Natasha, age 32, could hardly contain her rage, stating that Jim cared more for his ex-wife and his children than for her. She needed desperately to vent the feelings she had been sitting on for a long time. Jim sat frozen. When I interrupted his wide-eyed trance, he shook his head, said he was doing the best that he could, and tried to distract us with a humorous remark. At that moment, I kept in mind how important it was to avoid being hypnotized by the powerful system that had just entered my office. As each person talked, I was noting the shifts from one part of the self to another, change and movement of affect, moments of dissociation, self-interruption. I paced all of these. I was also looking and listening for one or more of those early imprints, not necessarily available to the client's conscious mind, that may be explored in hypnosis. I searched out resources—achievements a couple may not even acknowledge themselves that can be used as a foundation of strength, power, and creativity. I was also listening for what was not said, putting in the back of my mind anything that might lead us to imprints that would need to be explored.

The most important part of the therapeutic relationship is the therapist's use of self. Erickson said to therapists: "Be your own natural self." He also said: "I never saw a dignified, proper neurosis." I create the context by my own self-acceptance, not always an easy thing into which to shift. Being comfortable with my own unconscious made it possible for Jim and Natasha to experience the same comfort. Satir said: "The only time I made mistakes was when I was incongruent." Tracking the process between the two people sitting in front of me requires my whole attention, self-attunement, and communication with the vulnerable self of each. It requires considerable skill and watchfulness not to be put into trance by one or both of the partners. I think the ideal use of yourself as a therapeutic Geiger counter requires a clear flow between your conscious and your unconscious. That flow can communicate with the couple on many levels; it forms the therapeutic hypnotic relationship.

I soon became aware of the underlying respect and caring Jim and Natasha felt for each other and of the fact that neither presented a serious psychological impairment or characterological disorder. Both were bright, witty, and attractive, and they enjoyed being together. They valued their sexual connection. But I began to see a process occurring that was rooted in the mind sets of the couples' respective families of origin. Both had been imprinted by the people with whom they grew up, people for whom they had the deepest feelings.

I did a genogram for each of them in the second and third sessions. I noted historical events, sibling ages, positions, and family coalitions. I also asked for adjectives for each family-of-origin member and anyone else who had played an important role—sometimes as a mentor, a resource. I noted how each client presented the adjectives, and the patterns that appeared when the adjectives were laid out in front of me. I observed the intensity of affect or lack of it in the presentation; the speed, spontaneity, or hesitation evoked by the client's thinking about the people in his or her life. In this way, I learned family myths, rules, and secrets. These questions also tended, as usual, to put each partner in trance. The kinds of questions I ask are: "Who was the most important figure or figures to you as a child?" "What was the relationship between your mother and grandmother?" "What do you know about your father's relationship with his younger sister?"

Jim and Natasha were bringing their unique family trances into the marriage and each was embarking on the unconscious enterprise of getting the partner to answer the unfulfilled needs of childhood.

The partners came from different religious and economic backgrounds. Jim was Jewish, the oldest of five children. He had worked since he was 12, made the *Law Review* at New York University, and was now self-employed. He described his father as uneducated, hard-working, and explosive, who sometimes beat his children, but "had a heart of gold." His mother, "the ice queen," was a frustrated artist who had withdrawn from her husband and children many years earlier. Jim wanted his wife to accept his feelings and do what he said, unlike how his mother had reacted to his father. Natasha had grown up in a Midwestern fundamentalist Christian family. Her father was a successful corporation executive and she, an only child, was "my father's little princess" before she entered puberty. He constantly criticized his placating wife while praising his daughter. She hated her mother's failure to stand up to him, and as she grew up and her father began to criticize her, Natasha felt herself to be the outside member of the triad. Her mother always agreed with her father, and both had little understanding of Natasha's intellectual aspirations and abilities. She wanted Jim to "respect" her as an equal.

Both Jim and Natasha came from families in which the father's word was law and the mother silently feared her husband and/or placated him. Neither Jim nor Natasha wanted that kind of marriage consciously, but they were beginning to create the family patterns. Wanting warmth, he was pushing her away; wanting respect as an adult, she became as demanding as a child.

A major problem that they faced was the continuous pressure that Jim's ex-wife, Sylvia, put on them. She telephoned constantly, took Jim to court every six months, bad-mouthed Natasha and Jim to her children, and repeatedly changed plans for visitation. Natasha complained that Jim never drew the line with Sylvia, although he felt that his ex-wife, a psychologist, was irrational, and he wanted more control over of the children. Jim had divorced six years earlier, and had been married to Natasha for four years.

Jim had encouraged Natasha to stop working and get a graduate degree. But, as she currently is taking only one course, he feels she doesn't have enough to occupy her mind and so obsesses about his ex-wife. This causes him to explode, like his father (although he has never hit his wife). Natasha rages back, determined not to be like her mother. She continually confronts him. She wants to have a baby; he is not sure because he is worried about the resulting financial pressures. This is another painful area for them. Like his father, Jim makes unilateral decisions ("not wanting Natasha to get upset").

As Natasha, tearful, spoke of her helplessness and frustration, I interrupted her flow of thought and asked her, "How old do you feel right now?" In her little-girl voice she replied, "five." Sobbing, she described watching her father scream at her mother and hit her, while the mother did nothing to protect herself. "I vowed always to fight for myself! I felt so alone. It's the story of my life!" We worked with that imprint. While in trance she watched that scene many times, as if it were a film. Then she brought in the adult part of herself, who coached, comforted, and taught the child about all the strengths that she would develop in the future. She freed herself from the power of that scene by taking the child by the hand and leading her out of that room into a safe and beautiful place, where she could, with great compassion, take that helpless and frightened little-girl part of herself and join it with all the strengths she had since developed. By allowing compassion for her own self, she was able to embrace, and so contrive, the fear and helplessness.

Jim was moved to tears as he watched, and he told me he wanted to work on his explosive outbursts. As the sessions continued, Jim limited his contact with his ex-wife by using the lawyer as an intermediary to take her calls, and he instituted a new lawsuit against her. Whatever its outcome, he said, he felt the pressure would be reduced.

As we have continued to work, I have used conversational trance with

Jim and Natasha, often feeding their own language back to them. Humor works well with them, and I use one-liners as a pattern interruption to get them to step back (dissociate from the scene) and break the interaction into smaller parts, introducing a new variable into the pattern, which then changes it. I haven't yet used the strategy of having each partner choreograph a scene in which they are animals and then acting it out. Sometimes I diagram the pattern and get suggestions from them as to what new variable they might introduce. We work with the anxiety of change, and I've taught them to use self-hypnosis, as well.

I often used pattern interruption with this couple as they began to escalate. It shifted them out of the momentum they were building, sometimes going back to family-of-origin experiences.

I use short metaphors reminiscent of Kay Thompson. Here is one example: "I know someone who has a hot tub. When it gets to the point of overflowing, a little gadget shuts off the water and lets the tub drain until the water reaches the right level."

Jim and Natasha are learning new ways to communicate that come from the depths in themselves, which they are beginning to differentiate from what they acquired from their families. I saw how they put each other into negative trances. We identified family trance themes that characteristically always repeat themselves. For example, Natasha has realized how her feeling as an outsider in the triangle with her mother and father was at the root of her irrational feelings about Jim and his ex-wife. The knowledge itself didn't make the change. Experiencing the imprint did.

The more intense the feelings, the deeper is the imprint. Conscious understanding is important, but knowing how to shift out of negative trance is even more important. Because our feelings and our unconscious learnings are experienced throughout our bodies, shifting our physiology out of negative trance states is essential for transforming old patterns.

In addition to joint sessions, I have worked privately with each of them, reframing old imprints, and using self-hypnosis to access resources, to visualize the future, to deal with anxiety, and, in general, to become more creative about life. Jim has been working on his explosive trance, which was his little-boy identification with his sometimes brutal father. He has learned to pinpoint the physiological shifts that lead to his loss of verbal control (he feels hot tightness in his chest), and with practice he has become more able to intervene and shift himself out of that pattern. He now expresses his feelings much more directly. Natasha has worked on separating the helplessness she felt as a little girl and her fear because the mother she loved could not stand up for herself. She has decided to go back to the university and get her Ph.D degree. She is dissolving her guilt, her little-girl fear of loss and her fear that she really does not deserve to be happy. The issue of having a baby has been postponed until after Jim's court case against his ex-wife has been settled.

When two people experience a therapeutic trance together, something new is added to their experience of each other. As Satir said: "I'm not on the side of people divorcing or not divorcing. I'm on the side of people becoming whole."

## CONCLUSION

Milton Erickson defined trance as an everyday natural experience in which the person learns on an unconscious level. Virginia Satir, who was a natural hypnotist, worked with family inductions handed down from one generation to another. Couples bring these unconscious posthypnotic imprints into their relationship, unaware of the limiting effects that their hidden beliefs have on each other—and on themselves.

By working with Ericksonian approaches and the Satir model, therapists can evoke strengths and resources in a couple, access and reframe the early imprints that get in the way of communication between the partners and help them to integrate those imprints, freeing them from unwanted and unworkable assumptions and perceptions.

---

**Points to Remember**

- Contextualization: Create a safe space.
- Access resources: Anchor strengths into awareness.
- Pattern interruption: "Always say the unexpected. When you say the unexpected, the other person has to rearrange his thinking."
  — *M. Erickson*
- Parts model: When in doubt, chunk down the parts.
- Imprint revivification and reframe: Go to the source.

---

## References

Bandler, R., Grinder, J., & Satir, V. (1976). *Changing with families: A book about further education for being human.* Palo Alto, CA: Science & Behavior Books.

Cheek, D. B. (1994). *The application of ideomotor techniques: Hypnosis.* Boston: Allyn and Bacon.

Cheek, D. B., & LeCaron, L. M. (1968). *Clinical hypnotherapy.* New York: Grune & Stratton.

Erickson, M. H., & Rossi, E. L. (1979). *Hypnotherapy: An exploratory casebook.* New York: Irvington.

Haley, J. (1973). *Uncommon therapy.* New York: Norton.

Miller, A. (1981). *The drama of the gifted child.* New York: Basic Books.

Miller, A. (1986). *Society's betrayal of the child: Thou shalt not be aware.* Toronto: Collins Publishers.

Miller, A. (1987). *The roots of violence: For your own good.* New York: Farrar Straus Giroux.

Miller, A. (1990). *The untouched key.* New York: Doubleday.

Nerin, W. F., foreword by V. Satir. (1986). *Family reconstruction: Long day's journey into light.* New York: Norton.

Rossi, E. L. & Cheek, D. (1988). *Mind-body therapy: Method of ideodynamic healing in hypnosis.* New York: Norton.

Rossi, E. L. & Ryan, M. O. (1986). *Mind-body communication in hypnosis: The seminars, workshops and lectures of Milton H. Erickson.* New York: Irvington.

Satir, V. (1972). *Peoplemaking.* Palo Alto, CA: Science & Behavior Books.

Satir, V. (1983). *Conjoint family therapy.* Palo Alto, CA: Science & Behavior Books.

Satir, V., & Baldwin, M. (1983). *Satir step by step: A guide to creating change in families.* Palo Alto, CA: Science & Behavior Books.

Spiegel, H. (1960). Hypnosis and the psychotherapeutic process. *Comparative Psychiatry, 1,* 174–185.

Spiegel, H. & Spiegel, D. (1987). *Trance and treatment: Clinical uses of hypnosis.* Washington, DC: American Psychiatry Press.

# 32

# Three Candies for Five Boys
# and Other
# Strategic and Solution-Oriented Approaches
# for Children and Adolescents

*Bernhard Trenkle*

M ilton Erickson not only was the pioneer of modern hypnosis, but he is also considered the father of strategic family therapy and solution-oriented brief therapy.

His hypnotic techniques have been analyzed in detail and systemized in a number of books and articles (Erickson & Rossi, 1979; Grinder & Bandler, 1975a, 1975b; Lankton & Lankton, 1983). His work had a decisive influence on the development of both strategic family therapy (Haley, 1986; Madanes, 1981, 1984) and solution-oriented psychotherapy (De Shazer, 1985, 1988). However, some aspects of Erickson's therapeutic work have not been so widely noticed or further developed. These include his fascinating efforts in rehabilitation (Rossi, 1980) and children's therapy.

In the area of hypnotherapy with children, Olness and Kohen (1996) describe the state of the art—approaches that were, in part, developed independently of Erickson's work. Erickson's innovative strategic and problem-oriented concepts in working with children and adolescents can be found primarily in his case descriptions, the most important of which appear in Volume 3 of Jay Haley's *Conversations with Milton Erickson* (Haley, 1985). This book contains transcripts from the period in which Haley and John Weakland regularly visited Erickson to learn about his therapy work.

## STRATEGIC PSYCHOTHERAPY

One can speak of therapy as being strategic when the therapist plans an intervention in advance, thinking out a series of steps, like a chess player. Strategic therapy often has elements of staging, as in a stage play, where the pieces usually develop in the course of several acts.

The following story shows the elements of strategic planning and staging (Shah, 1994).

A Muslim was on his way to Mecca and decided to leave a chest containing his valuables with a merchant of repute in Cairo before setting off, and to take with him on the pilgrimage only the few things as he would actually need. He made inquiries and found himself in the shop of a man regarded by his fellows as being of the highest probity. The box was entrusted to him, and the pilgrim set off.

When the pilgrim returned and claimed his property, the merchant denied ever having been given it, and said that he had never seen the man before. Even the neighbors refused to believe that a man with a reputation such as the merchant had could possibly lie.

The pilgrim, with very little money left, without friends, and in a foreign land, wandered down the road in a state of shock and dismay, unable to decide what to do next. At this point, a wise woman dressed in dervish garb noticed him and asked him what troubled him. When he explained what had happened, she asked: "What would you propose to do about this?"

"I can only think that I might resort to force, or go to the police," said the pilgrim.

"The police will not be able to help you, since you can prove no crime," said the woman, "and as for force, that would land you in jail."

"If, however," she continued, "you put your complete trust in me, I can devise a plan that will secure the return of your property."

The pilgrim agreed to do whatever she asked. She helped him to rent, for one day, ten beautiful, valuable-looking chests, which she filled with earth and stones. Then she asked another friend to take the chests on a cart to the merchant's shop. The friend, also a dervish, dressed as a rich man.

When the friend and the cargo arrived at the shop, the man pretended to be a stranger in town and asked the merchant if he would agree to watch the ten chests while he went on a trip. "The chests look as if they are full of valuables," thought the merchant, and he agreed to take them in, for a small fee, and to look after them.

As the boxes were about to be carried into the shop, the pilgrim played his part. He went up to the merchant and the disguised dervish and said: "I have come for my chest of valuables, may I have it now?"

Fearing that he would not be trusted by the owner of the exciting chests of "valuables" if there were any argument, the merchant smilingly handed over the pilgrim's property.

Then the disguised dervish said: "Thank you for your trouble, but I have changed my mind—I think that I shall take my chests with me, after all."

And that was how the pilgrim's difficulty was resolved. He thanked the dervishes for their help, saying, "I cannot imagine how you thought of this ingenious solution."

## SOLUTION, GOAL, AND RESOURCE ORIENTATION

Another characteristic of Ericksonian psychotherapy is its orientation toward solutions, goals, and resources instead of causes, past events, and pathology. De Shazer (1985, 1988), O'Hanlon (1989), and Furman (1992) have described this aspect of Erickson's work. This kind of therapy leads to very pragmatic and often surprising solutions. Change is often possible in a very short time.

A joke I once heard is a good illustration of this (Trenkle, 1999).

A man goes to a psychoanalyst and says, "I think I'm crazy. Every night I see and hear wild animals—lions, tigers, elephants—parading around under my bed."

Analyst:    Lie down on that couch there and tell me more about these animals.
Patient:    Wait a minute. How much does this cost?
Analyst:    One hour costs $150. We can start with 80 hours, and if we need to, we can extend the therapy for another 80.
Patient:    I'm not that crazy.

A few weeks later, the analyst and the patient meet accidentally at the supermarket.

Analyst:    How are you doing?
Patient:    Wonderfully. My brother-in-law cured me in less than an hour.
Analyst:    Oh, your brother-in-law is a therapist?
Patient:    No, he's a carpenter. He sawed the legs off my bed.

Every experienced psychotherapist knows that to accomplish changes in children and adolescents often takes time and patience. However, later I will describe cases in which essential changes were made possible within one hour or less.

First, however, I will briefly describe two basic positions that are important background principles for understanding the case examples.

## THE BASIC PRINCIPLES

### Utilization

Utilization is the most important principle of the Ericksonian approach. Utilization means that all the attitudes, peculiarities, abilities, and values that the patient brings to the therapy can be used for therapeutic purposes. This includes pathological and bizarre characteristics.

A well-known example is that of the patient in a psychiatric ward who thinks he is Jesus Christ. Erickson says to him, "I have heard that you have experience as a carpenter." The patient agrees; after all, if he claims to be Jesus, son of Joseph, he must have some experience as a carpenter. Erickson asks him to build a bookcase for the clinic. This was the beginning of the development of a positive and constructive professional vocation.

### Interrupting Habitual Deadlocked Thought Patterns

Solution-oriented Ericksonian therapy tries to interrupt old habits of thought and to open patients' eyes to new, and often surprising, possibilities. Milton Erickson liked to give clients and colleagues in training puzzles that required them to leave their accustomed mental paths. A well-known example is the puzzle in which nine points arranged in a square must be connected with a single line. This is only possible if the line leaves the frame formed by the points. Another puzzle he liked to use asked how it is possible to plant twelve trees in six equal rows of four.

The following amusing story shows the mental attitude needed to find solutions in Ericksonian therapy:

*Physics Exam*

A candidate failed his oral examination in physics. Feeling that this was unfair as he had given, he claimed, a correct answer, he took the matter to court and won. Because the disagreement between him and the professor had escalated beyond civility, a neutral observer from another university was called in to sit in on the repeat examination.

At the end of the examination, the deciding problem was, "Determine the height of a skyscraper with the help of a barometer." The candidate considered this for a while and then answered: "I would take the barometer and a long string, climb onto the roof of the skyscraper, tie the barometer to the end of the string, and lower it to the ground. Then I would pull it back up and measure how long a length of string was necessary to reach the ground."

The professors consulted. Of course, it is possible to determine the height of a skyscraper in this way, but they had expected something different in a physics test. They asked the question again and specified that the answer must reflect a knowledge of physics. They gave the candidate five minutes to prepare his answer. Three minutes passed, four minutes passed, and the candidate was still sitting there, thinking. The observer became impatient and asked whether or not they might expect to receive an answer. The candidate replied that he was trying to decide which of four answers he should give them.

At last the candidate said, "I would wait until the sun shines. Then I would set the barometer next to the skyscraper and measure the shadow of the barometer and the shadow of the skyscraper. I know how tall my barometer is, and I can determine the height of the skyscraper with the help of a simple proportional calculation."

The two professors had to agree that he had passed the test. The answer reflected knowledge of physics and was correct. The candidate left the room satisfied. The observer caught up to him in the hall, saying, "I have to admit I'm curious. What other answers were you considering?"

The candidate smiled. "I could climb to the roof of the skyscraper again, drop the barometer, time its fall with a stopwatch, and calculate the height of the building. If you want a more demanding answer, I could tie the barometer on my long string again and use it as a pendulum. I could then measure the pendulum movement on the ground and at the top of the skyscraper. With the help of the gravitational constant $g$ it must be possible to calculate the height of the building. But if you hadn't insisted on an answer involving physics, I would have preferred to do something else entirely: I would take the barometer to the building superintendent and say, 'I have a nice barometer here, which I will give to you if you will tell me the height of this building.' "

## Case Histories

The following cases illustrate the use of strategic, solution-, and resource-oriented work and utilization in sometimes surprising and unusual interventions.

### Big Feet

The presenting problem was that of a 14-year-old girl who had developed the idea that her feet were much too large. Initially, her mother came alone to Erickson and described the situation. For three months, the girl had been becoming more and more withdrawn, and she didn't want to go to school or church or be seen on the street. The girl would not allow the subject of her feet to be discussed, and she would not consult a doctor. No amount of reassurance by her mother had any influence, and the girl was becoming more and more reclusive.

Erickson reports: "I arranged with the mother to visit the home on the following day under false pretenses. The girl would be told that I was coming to examine the mother to see if she had the flu. Although it was a pretext, as the mother actually wasn't feeling well, an examination would not be inappropriate. When I arrived at the home, the mother was in bed. I did a careful physical examination, listening to her chest, examining her throat, and so on. The girl was present. I sent her for a towel, and I asked that she stand beside me in case I needed something. She was very concerned about her mother's health. This gave me an opportunity to look her over. She was rather stoutly built but her feet were not large.

"Studying the girl, I wondered what I could do to get her over this problem. Finally, I hit upon a plan. As I finished my examination of the mother, I maneuvered the girl into a position directly behind me. I was sitting on the bed talking to the mother, and I got up slowly and carefully, and then stepped back awkwardly. I put my heel down squarely on the girl's toes. The girl, of course, squawked with pain. I turned to her and in a tone of absolute fury said, 'If you would grow those things large enough for a man to see, I wouldn't be in this situation!' The girl looked at me, puzzled, while I wrote out a prescription and called the drugstore. That day, the girl asked her mother if she could go to a movie, which she hadn't done in months. She went to school and church, and that was the end of three months of reclusiveness. I checked later on how things were going, and the girl was friendly and agreeable. She didn't realize what I had done, nor did her mother. All her mother noticed was that I had been impolite to her daughter when I visited that day. She couldn't connect that with the daughter's return to normal activity."

As Erickson himself said, he gave the girl a suggestion that she couldn't refuse. It wasn't possible to talk about the subject directly, since she refused the discuss it or see a doctor about it. Erickson made a statement primarily about himself. He expressed anger about being in such an embarrassing situation and made the girl's small "things" responsible. The situation had something very "hypnotic" about it. The painful stepping on her foot focused the girl's attention abruptly, the organism was suddenly painfully awake and activated, and the indirect suggestion that "those things" were too small was particularly effective in this condition.

The girl's attitude of withdrawal changed, although no therapeutic conversation was held, no hidden causes were discovered, no homework was assigned, and no family therapy was done. Erickson's procedure had elements of strategic planning and staging. He came as a family doctor making a house call and staged and arranged his examination so that he could conduct this very brief intervention for the girl who was ashamed of the size of her feet.

### The Situation

This case is an example of how unusual solution-oriented and strategic interventions can lead to change in a very short time.

A mother called me about her 11-year-old daughter, Annette, who stuttered. Stuttering was not exactly the reason for the call, though. The daughter was normally a courageous, carefree child, who had not let her speech problem have much influence on her behavior. She even read aloud at church. However, some of the boys at school had begun to tease her, not only about her stuttering, but also because she was slightly overweight. She was in the first stages of puberty and this double attack on her speech and her vanity seemed to be too much for her. She cried and didn't want to go to school and had stopped reading aloud in church.

It seemed to me that fast action was called for, so I gave the family an immediate counseling appointment.

Annette was, in fact, a cheerful, self-assured child, but as we began to talk about the teasing at school, she started to cry, and it was easy to see that she had been badly hurt. Her parents also seemed very moved by the sudden change in mood.

She explained that it was always the same four or five boys who teased her. They called to her on the playground, "Bibibbig fafafat Annannann-ettettette."

A story that I had never used in a therapeutic context occurred to me. Once upon a time, there was a man. He was very curious and was always experimenting. Most of all, he always wanted to know how other people would react when he did something entirely strange and unexpected. Once this man was in a hurry. He ran around the corner of a building and bumped into another pedestrian. Normally people excuse themselves in such situations: "I'm sorry. Did I hurt you? Excuse me. I'm in a dreadful hurry." But this man wanted to see what would happen if he behaved entirely differently. He looked meaningfully at his watch, said, "Yes, it is exactly 10 minutes past 3," and kept on walking. But it was 5:30. He walked on for 30 or 40 steps and then looked back. The other pedestrian was still standing there, frozen in place, because he could not categorize what had happened.

Annette started giggling, as if she knew intuitively what I was thinking. The parents looked at me with a confused expression, as if they wanted to say, "What does this have to do with our daughter's problem and stuttering?"

I said to the daughter, "Wouldn't it be great if you could think of something so crazy, too? Something so crazy that those five guys would never expect it? So crazy and so surprising, that those guys would stand there like stones?"

Annette liked this picture, and we started to develop silly ideas about what crazy things would be totally unexpected for the boys who teased her. Eventually, we came up with the following:

The next time the five boys called "Bibibbig fafafat Anannannette-ttette," she should simply walk up to them, reach into her pocket, and give them three pieces of candy. Of course, because there were three candies and five boys, not everyone would get one. Then she should say: "Sorry, no more today," turn around, and walk away. When she was 40 or 50 feet away, she should turn around and see whether they were still standing there with their candies in their outstretched hands.

Annette was very enthusiastic about this idea. She giggled and the trauma seemed to dissipate. She had suddenly ceased to be the passive victim and had become an actor.

My interns and I were very curious as to whether the gambit would be successful, so we gave Annette an appointment in ten days. We could almost have guessed what happened next. The boys hadn't bothered her at all during that ten days. Annette must have looked so impudent and confident that it didn't occur to anyone to tease her.

So I spent 20 minutes giving her advice about how she must behave in order to get the boys to tease her again. It would be a shame if we never found out whether our ploy had actually worked. I taught her how to look down at the ground, how to avoid meeting the boys' eyes, how to hesitate, how to slip by uncertainly in the schoolyard, and so on. But it didn't help. Unfortunately, the boys never teased her again. Later, Annette came to me for normal stutter therapy. She was really a highly intelligent, quick-witted girl.

## DISCUSSION

Annette's case illustrates solution-oriented and strategic aspects of Ericksonian therapy. She is given a solution directly without addressing causes, reasons, vulnerabilities, or family structures that might be connected with her problem. The intervention is strategically constructed in a number of steps. As in a chess game, it is necessary to think several moves in advance. First, an anecdote that appears to have nothing to do with the problem is told. This anecdote is entertaining and funny. Humor is an excellent antidote to helplessness and shame. Then an aspect of the story is carried over onto the problem: Wouldn't it be super if you could do something so crazy and unexpected that those boys would freeze in their tracks? Then, when the teasing has stopped, Annette is given information about how she can trigger or block the teasing with nonverbal communication under cover of an attempt to get the boys to tease her again.

## The Boy Who Was Teased

About six months later, a 9-year-old boy who was also being teased about his stuttering came to me in therapy. I told him about Annette and said that unfortunately we still didn't know whether this trick would work. The boy was interested in sports and a stopwatch. I assigned him the job of giving the boy who teased him a piece of candy and then starting his stopwatch, so that we could find out how long it would take before the harasser would start again. When my client returned three weeks later, he reported: 40 seconds. I asked if he had given him the candy first. To my surprise, he told me that he still had it. He came from an area where the people are known for their thrift, and he had changed the task a little. He had just called out, "Next time you get a goodie!" and then started the stopwatch.

I attempted to use this technique again, with a 10-year-old boy, but he was too shy and diffident to risk trying it.

### ORDEAL THERAPY, THE GUARANTEED CURE

Ordeals are a technique that Haley developed on the basis of Erickson's work (Haley, 1984). Briefly defined, the client is given a homework assignment that is so unpleasant that it is more advantageous to give up the symptom. A variation is the guaranteed cure, as Haley called the technique. It begins with an announcement that the therapist knows of something that is guaranteed to solve the problem. However, it is difficult and unpleasant to comply with it. This "guaranteed cure" is mentioned again and again, until the patient becomes very curious about it. Then the therapist refuses to reveal the cure unless the client solemnly swears to carry it out.

### The Compulsive Gambler

A case study illustrates this technique: An anxious mother called to make an appointment for her family. She was worried that her hot-tempered husband might harm one of her sons. She explained on the telephone that the 17-year-old son had been gambling compulsively on slot machines for two years. He was in danger of losing his job as an apprentice cook because he had been caught taking money from the cash register, and was told that if he did it again, he would be fired. He had also stolen from his 15-year-old sister and his 20-year-old brother. Now precious metals were missing from his father's dental laboratory, and it seemed clear who must have taken them. The father threatened to kill the son if he caught him stealing from his lab.

The family had already twice seen family therapists concerning this problem, but with no change in the compulsive gambling and accompanying problems. They were desperate, and the mother also saw a connection between the tense family situation and her colitis ulcerosa.

In addition to the parents and the 17-year-old compulsive gambler, the 20-year-old brother and the 15-year-old sister came to the initial appointment. The son stated early in the session—quite annoyed—that the whole family was there again, although he was the one with the problem. Up until now, he said no one had been able to help him get his gambling under control. Every one looked for problems in the family, but it was he who was doing the gambling.

The young man emphasized his desire to stop gambling and intimated that he planned to use the money he would save to move out of the family home and get an apartment with his girlfriend. His statement brought tears to his mother's eyes, so I asked her: "Assuming the alternatives are that he stops gambling and moves out or keeps gambling and ends up a bum, but stays home, which would she prefer?" She ignored the question and changed the subject. When I insisted on an answer, she began to cry. I learned that neither she nor her husband had had a real family life in childhood and that they had built their new house in order to give their children the home that they themselves had always wanted as children. The children, they thought, should stay at home, at least until they married. (At this point, I should mention that it is not uncommon in rural and small-town Germany for adult children to live at home until they marry, or even for married couples to live in an apartment in their parents' house. Thus, her wish not to let her son go did not sound quite as unnatural in our cultural context as it might sound to non-Germans. Nevertheless, it was a problem.)

Remembering the two failed family therapies, I decided to conduct individual therapy with the son in the presence of the family.

I asked the son whether he really wanted to quit gambling, because starting therapy would only make sense if his wish to control his habit was sincere. The young man assured me, somewhat sulkily, that he had already said that he wanted to quit.

Then I told him that there were two possible ways to quit: the quick and easy way and the long and difficult way. Unfortunately, I said I could only see the long and difficult way for him.

The quick and easy way goes like this: A woman came to me to be hypnotized. She wanted to stop smoking. I hypnotized her, and she stopped smoking for a few days, but then started again. Later, when I met her again, she said that she had really quit. I was curious as to how she had managed this. She laughed and explained that she had gone to the doctor for a routine checkup and he had congratulated her on her pregnancy. The cigarette she had smoked before she went into the doctor's office was quite simply her last. She didn't want to do anything that would harm her child, so she just quit. That is the quick and easy way: you just quit. However, in my opinion, the quick and easy way was not an option for him. He was going to have to quit the long and difficult way.

Then I described two cases in which ordeals were used to effect change. First, I told him about a nurse who couldn't get to sleep after a hard day at work. In order to fall asleep at last, she used a little trick. She asked herself what the worst thing was that she could do right now. And she decided that the worst thing would be to do the weekly cleaning of the hall of the nurses' dorm. So she made a contract with herself: "If I see the face of my alarm clock at 11 o'clock, I will get up and mop the hallways and the stairs all the way down to the ground floor." This was really a contract with herself. It is very important that such contracts be kept to the letter. If she had said to herself at 11:00, "Oh, I think I'll wait till 12:00," then there would have been no point to the whole thing. A contract is a contract. And because she honestly intended to get up and mop the halls at 11:00, she never again saw her alarm clock after that time.

Then I told him another story about an ordeal, and again emphasized how important it is to mean the contract honestly. The 17-year-old repeated his serious desire to stop gambling. I asked the father what his son really hated, what would be the equivalent of cleaning the halls for him. The father laughed and named various tasks in the house and garden. There was a lot left to do in the new house: the cellar to whitewash, the fence to paint, the lawn to mow ... I gave the father the job of making a long list of unpleasant jobs in the house and garden.

Now I proposed to the son that he make an ordeal contract with himself. First I provoked him again by repeating that of course there is also a quick and easy way, the possibility of just quitting, but, unfortunately, he was going to have to go the hard road with a lot of work. Then I described the contract: every time he set foot in a video arcade he was to do something on his father's list. The first time, he would work for one hour; the second time, for two hours; and then it was a question of whether he wanted to be free of his gambling quickly or more slowly. If he wanted to progress quickly, I would suggest a geometric progression: one, two, four, eight hours, and so on. However, he and his family had already suffered so long because of his gambling that it wouldn't make much difference whether he stopped quickly or more slowly, so he could just as well make the progression additive: one, two, three, four hours. And so on. A couple of times, I mentioned again that unfortunately he was not the kind of guy to just quit.

At this point, the young man figured out that things were getting serious and that this contract would have a real effect on his gambling behavior and enjoyment. He started to squirm and look for loopholes. He tried to negotiate that the contract should take effect only when he actually gambled, not when he just played pinball or hung around. His older brother intervened with the opinion that this was a trick. After a few minutes of heavy discussion between the brothers, the younger son concluded that it would be better to make entering the video arcade the criterion. But he wanted to start with half an hour and add half an hour each time. I accepted this at once, with the comment that it was his contract that he was making with himself. This slow increase would also lead, sooner or later, to the point where gambling would become "too expensive." I remarked again that this system only strengthened my impression that he was a guy who would have to go the hard road and do a lot of work. Other people take the easy way and just quit.

Our next appointment was seven weeks later. He had not gambled at all and had not had to do a single half-hour task from his father's list. However, the family gave me no chance to show that I recognized his rapid change: The mother attacked her son with reproaches because he had taken his sister's motor scooter without her permission to go to buy cigarettes. The young man, with tears in his eyes, turned to me and said, "You see? I am always the ass in this family. First, it was gambling. Now, it's the motor scooter, or anyway something else. Nothing matters for shit." I was immediately afraid that he would start to gamble again out of disappointment and defiance. I started asking circular questions in the style of the Milan systemic approach: What would the father have to do in order for the son to develop the feeling that he had to gamble again?

What does the brother think the mother could do so that the young man would feel that it was better not to gamble? What could the son do so that the mother would be more likely to do things he didn't like? I tried to name and prevent as many relapse risks as possible with such questions.

About six months later, the mother called me in panic: "My son cleaned out his bank account. Today is his 18th birthday and he has withdrawn all his money, over $1,800!" I asked, "Does he gamble?" She said, "No, he still doesn't gamble, but he can't just take all his money out of the bank. I have no idea what he is planning to do." I tried to make it clear to her that there was no way to stop him, since he was no longer a minor.

More than two years later, I called the family to find out how things had developed. The mother was still complaining. Her son was ungrateful. Shortly after his 18th birthday, he had disappeared, and for nine months she hadn't known where he was. He reappeared at Christmas with presents for the family. He had finished his apprenticeship, was living with his girlfriend, and didn't gamble. He had found a job in a coffee shop in a supermarket, as he preferred the predictable hours of day work to an irregular night job in a regular restaurant.

*Discussion*

The ordeal technique is an ideal addition to a hypnotherapist's repertoire. As in this case, the client often hopes for a miraculous cure or a solution that the therapist would magically bring about through hypnosis. Hypnosis tends to activate such expectations, and the therapeutic utilization of these hopes and expectations often makes it possible to fulfill them. In this case, as with many addictive clients, one of the therapeutic themes is a clear, firm decision that the person really wants to overcome a habit. The client has to take responsibility for his or her behavior. A hypnotherapist can easily end up in a dilemma: The client defines the situation as, "I want to quit, but I can't," and asks to be hypnotized. If the patient repeats the behavior, then the hypnosis was too weak or not deep enough. The responsibility can be pushed onto the therapist. The ordeal technique is an efficient instrument for giving the responsibility back to the client.

## EITHER–OR THINKING

A part of an addictive patient's problem is the series of lost battles against the addiction the person wanted to leave behind. The patient gambles, for example, and then asserts, "This was the last time. Never again!" A few hours or days later, the addiction is stronger than the decision and the addictive behavior is carried out again. The patient sees with shame that he or she has lost again, with an accompanying loss of self-worth. Low self-worth then increases the necessity to distract or stimulate oneself again with the addiction. As a rule, the patient thinks in 0–1 categories: addicted versus not addicted, gambling versus not gambling any more. The ordeal contract described in the above case of the compulsive gambler changes this either–or thinking. Suddenly the patient is allowed to gamble. But gambling has a price, an immediate, unpleasant price. On the one hand, the price gets higher every time he gambles; on the other hand, he has, in a sense, permission to gamble. He just has to pay the agreed-upon price. At the beginning, the price can even be low. The cycle of good intentions and then the shameful realization that he has lost the fight with the addiction has been broken. The addiction seems to have less power and to have become more manageable. The patient also has a transition time in which he can focus on the internal reconstruction of his psyche and the discovery of a new identity without the addiction. In this case, the family interaction was also changed. During the last two years, the addictive behavior had been a constant theme in the family. Other conflicts, such as the necessary separation and individuation of the children, were hidden behind the endless struggle. The ordeal contract changes the rules of this game, too. The father asked who was to check up on all this, and we discovered in the session that no one but the son needed to keep track. He wants to stop gambling, and he has made a contract with himself, which he will keep honestly. If he gambles, then he gambles within the therapeutic contract, and works in the house and garden. The gambling no longer can serve as an occasion for recriminations and insults.

## THE ART OF NEGOTIATING A CONTRACT

It is essential to close all possible loopholes in an ordeal contract. Such contracts also require patients who will keep the contract once they have entered it. This may not be easy for a 17-year-old. Therapist behavior that is too kind can lead to a broken contract, just as can an overly harsh attitude. A rebellious young person can easily be pushed into breaking a contract when someone tries to force him or her to keep it. In the case presented here, I avoided this by describing the two other cases. Scattered throughout both stories were insistent references to the fact that strict honoring of the contract was an absolutely necessary condition in order for the technique to function. The nurse really would have mopped the floor at 11 o'clock. If she had been awake at 11:00 and had postponed the fulfillment of her contract until 12:00, she might just as well have forgotten the whole thing. What was important is that 11:00 means 11:00. It is much easier to fit basic suggestions into a case history about another person than it is to tell a possibly rebellious young patient such things directly.

The success of ordeal therapy usually depends on the therapist's skill in negotiating the contract. He or she must be prepared to spend some time on the matter: of the approximately 100 minutes of this interview, about 40 were devoted to contract negotiations.

### Loopholes in the Contract

The art of ordeal therapy sometimes consists mostly of discovering the loopholes in the contract in time. The contract described above, for example, had a loophole in it, but the patient was honest enough to keep the contract anyway. To explain the loophole more clearly, I will describe another case.

A colleague brought the case of a young gambler to supervision: The young patient was very active politically and very dogmatic in favor of a particular political group. The ordeal contract required him to donate money to his much-hated political enemies. He was to begin with $5 and double the sum every time he gambled: $10, $20, $40, $80 and so on.

When the client came to his next counseling session, he had accumulated a considerable debt to his enemies, far more than the bank would allow him credit for. The loophole in the contract was that no one had thought to specify that the donation was to be made immediately after gambling, before he was allowed to gamble again. I hadn't thought of this either: The 17-year-old could have gambled repeatedly and postponed his tasks until "some other time." It seems to me that it is more difficult to correct such contracts once they are in force than it is to make them watertight to begin with.

## Brief Therapy Can Take a Long Time

Milton Erickson may be the father of solution-oriented brief therapy, and his procedures often make surprising solutions possible, but there are also impressive examples of treatments that extend over long periods. In *Experiencing Erickson*, Jeff Zeig (1985) describes Erickson's work with a psychotic young man whom Erickson saw for more than ten years. He wrote more than 40 therapeutic limericks for this case, and a number of letters that Erickson's dog wrote to the patient's dog still exist. Erickson packed important therapeutic messages into these limericks and letters, which served the purpose of stabilizing the patient enough that he could stay out of the psychiatric ward. A rapid solution, or, in fact, any cure at all was not possible in spite of Erickson's enormous dedication. Ericksonian brief therapy for children, adolescents, and adults lasts as long as is necessary for the individual client.

This kind of solution-oriented and strategic therapy often makes rapid solutions possible, without the necessity for sounding the depths of the problem. Charles Van Riper, pioneer of American speech therapy, gave me an idea that led me to the following picture, which reflects a part of the Ericksonian philosophy of therapy: When a river is high and carries a lot of wood and other debris along, they can get stuck and create a dam. When the water trapped behind the dam threatens to flood the countryside, the therapist doesn't have to jump in and drag all the tree trunks and branches and garbage out. It is enough to keep a good eye on the situation and to loosen a trunk or pull a branch out in the right place. The river will take care of the rest itself.

At a workshop in Heidelberg in 1986, Bill O'Hanlon presented a brief therapy case with a surprisingly rapid solution. A participant with a psychoanalytic background protested that you see only the surface with such procedures! The deeper processes never come into view. You only see the eighth of the iceberg that is above the water; the seven-eighths under the water remain invisible. O'Hanlon answered, "When I treat the tip of the iceberg, and it really is an iceberg, then it floats higher and the next bit becomes visible, and I can go to work on that." Then he added, "My observations suggest, however, that there is often no iceberg there. The tip is just floating alone on the surface of the water."

### References

Bandler, R., & Grinder, J. (1975a). *Patterns of the hypnotic techniques of Milton H. Erickson, M.D., Vol. 1.* Cupertino, CA: Meta Publications.

Bandler, R., & Grinder, J. (1975b). *Patterns of the hypnotic techniques of Milton H. Erickson, M.D., Vol. 2.* Cupertino, CA: Meta Publications.

De Shazer, S. (1985). *Keys to solution in brief therapy.* New York: Norton.

De Shazer, S. (1988). *Clues: Investigating solutions in brief therapy.* New York: Norton.

Erickson, M. H., & Rossi, E. L. (1979). *Hypnotherapy: An exploratory casebook.* New York: Irvington.

Furman, B. (1992). *Solution talk: Hosting therapeutic conversations.* New York: Norton.

Haley, J. (1984). *Ordeal therapy: Unusual ways to change behavior.* San Francisco: Jossey-Bass.

Haley, J. (1985). *Conversations with Milton H. Erickson, M. D., Vol. III: Changing children and families.* New York: Triangle.

Haley, J. (1986). *Uncommon therapy: The psychiatric techniques of Milton H. Erickson.* New York: Norton.

Lankton, S. R., & Lankton, C. H. (1983). *The answer within: A clinical framework of Ericksonian hypnotherapy.* New York: Brunner/Mazel.

Madanes, C. (1981). *Strategic family therapy.* San Francisco: Jossey-Bass.

Madanes, C. (1984). *Behind the one-way mirror.* San Francisco: Jossey-Bass.

O'Hanlon, W. H. (1989). *In search of solutions.* New York: Norton.

Olness, K., & Kohen, D. P. (1986). *Hypnosis and hypnotherapy with children* (3rd ed.). New York: Guilford.

Rossi, E. L. (1980). *Innovative hypnotherapy by Milton H. Erickson: The collected papers of Milton H. Erickson on hypnosis,* Vol. IV. New York: Irvington.

Shah, I. (1994). *The commanding self.* London: Octagon.

Trenkle, B. (2001). *The ha-ha handbook of psychotherapy.* Phoenix, AZ: Zeig, Tucker, & Theisen.

Zeig, J. K. (1985). *Experiencing Erickson.* New York: Brunner/Mazel.

# 33

# "I Want To Treat Him Better Than He Treated Me": Ericksonian and Solution-Focused Interventions in Relation to a Dependent Elderly Parent

*Yvonne M. Dolan*

I n my psychotherapy practice, over the past several years, I have increasingly seen middle-aged adults in the ironic position of being responsible for the care of the elderly parents who abused them in childhood. This chapter illustrates how Ericksonian associational cues (Dolan, 1991, 1994a; Erickson & Rossi, 1979, 1989; Gilligan, 1987) and Ericksonian utilization (Dolan, 1985; Erickson, 1959) can be combined with the "miracle question" (Berg & Miller, 1992; De Shazer, 1988, 1991, 1994; Dolan, 1998) and scaling (Berg & De Shazer, 1993; Berg, 1990; De Jong & Berg, 1996; Dolan, 1994b; Miller, 1997) from solution-focused therapy (Berg, 1990; De Shazer, 1985; De Shazer, Berg, Lipchik, et al., 1989) to provide relief from posttraumatic stress symptoms for clients who find themselves in this challenging role.

During 20 years of working with people who were abused by parents or other significant caregivers, I have noted that the more rarely these victims receive affection or simple kindness from their abusers, the more precious and significant any nurturing experiences become.

Regardless of how pervasive a parent's abusive behavior, it is seldom the sole experience he or she shares with offspring. Perhaps this is one of the reasons, along with a sense of duty or a desire not to replicate the cruelty they experienced, that adult children often want and need to maintain a tenable relationship with a formerly, or even currently, abusive aging parent.

While it might seem reasonable, or even therapeutic, for an adult child simply to cut off a relationship with a parent who continues to be emotionally abusive, this may not be a realistic option for the client. In many cases, the emotional price (grief, anxiety, unpredictability, or temporary disorientation after spending years organizing oneself around coping with the abusive parent) of cutting off the relationship may outweigh its benefits.

Such was the case with Liz. After living an active, fiercely independent life, her widowed elderly father was now dying in a local hospital. Liz was ashamed of the fact that she felt relief when she imagined him as finally being out of her life.

For as long as Liz could remember, her father had told her that her best efforts were not good enough. Her father also had a violent temper, and whenever he did not get his own way in business or in personal relationships, he became rageful and took these feelings out on anyone within hearing range. In her childhood, that person had frequently been Liz. In addition to experiencing her father's unremitting barrage of criticism and episodes of explosive temper, Liz had suffered countless public humiliations because of her father's behavior. In the small Midwestern town where she had grown up, her father had been well-known as a lecherous philanderer, a gambler, and an alcoholic.

Although Liz eventually escaped some of the embarrassment of her father's behavior by moving to a distant city, his criticism and emotional abuse continued to reach her via the telephone and in letters, as well as during her comparatively rare instances of personal contact with him. She explained, "The same emotional abuse from him that made my childhood a living hell didn't stop when I grew up. He continued to criticize me and put me down any time he got the opportunity."

Over the years, Liz had gradually developed ways to minimize the impact of her father's cruelty. She had developed a personal protocol for self-protection that she called her "damage control rules." For example, whenever possible, she would avoid seeing her father alone because his behavior tended to be more equitable when others were present. She had limited any private encounters with him, whether by telephone or in person, to just a few minutes at a time, and had an excuse ready for when she needed to exit.

These "rules" allowed her to avoid emotional escalation into a fight with her father, and to prevent, or at least minimize, the posttraumatic symptoms of anxiety, insomnia, concentration difficulties, and flashbacks that resulted when she was exposed to his aggressive criticism.

However, following these rules had exacted its own price from Liz. She felt guilty about having avoided contact with her father given the fact that he had also done many good things for her. For instance, it had been her father rather than her gentle, passive mother who had encouraged Liz to go to college, and who, upon her graduation, provided her with the funds necessary to establish her own, highly profitable business. Although she resented her father's emotional cruelty, she also was grateful for the help he had given her at various times in her life.

Recently, because of his illness and the knowledge that the next few months were likely to be his last, she had broken her own rules, and had begun spending more time alone with her father in the hospital. During these visits, he often expressed his doubts about her ability to succeed in life. At other times, weak from pain, he only spoke to make his physical needs known. However, even if he said nothing overtly critical, her father's facial expression or voice tone would elicit painful childhood memories in Liz, triggering posttraumatic stress symptoms of anxiety, flashbacks, nightmares, sleep disturbance, and suicidal impulses that lasted for several days. The suicidal ideation was not new. As Liz explained:

> I have thought many times in the past about killing myself just to get away from him. Now that he is finally dying, I find myself overwhelmed by a mixture of rage, sadness, love, and, I guess, mostly relief.

At this point in her life, choosing either not to see her father or to limit the time she spent with him was not an ethical option for Liz.

> He is dying and helpless right now, and I am the only one left in our family to care for him. In order to live with myself after he is gone, I want to have treated him more than decently, with love

and kindness, so that afterward I will know that I did not give in to the patterns of abuse he taught me. And there isn't much time left. I want to put an ending on this relationship that's different from how it's been up until now. This is probably impossible, but after I see him, I don't want to feel suicidal and not be able to sleep for days afterward. I want to be able to function at work and not be totally overwhelmed by all the awful memories of mean things he's said and done to me in the past. I probably want too much. But now that he is finally dying, I want my relationship with him somehow to end better than the way it's been. It's the impossible dream, I guess.

Liz shifted awkwardly in her chair and chewed nervously on a nail. The pain and longing in her voice belied the cynicism of her words.

When clients ask for help with seemingly impossible situations, I like to offer the miracle question from solution-focused therapy. When asked with sensitivity, and after listening carefully to the client's description of the problem, the miracle question invites the client to identify what he or she wants to have happen in therapy while simultaneously empowering the client to develop a new perspective, and to identify potential or previously overlooked resources.

Like all therapeutic offerings, the timing of the miracle question is important. If asked too soon, for instance, before the client has had adequate opportunity to tell why he or she came for therapy, or before the therapist has expressed understanding and compassion, the client may feel trivialized. If asked too late in the session, or not at all, the client may leave feeling needlessly stuck or in despair. In deciding when to offer the miracle question, I have found the Ericksonian concept of the "response attentive moment" (Erickson & Rossi, 1979) very helpful.

The response attentive moment is a naturally occurring state of heightened receptivity to therapeutic communication (Erickson & Rossi, 1979). I have found the effectiveness of the miracle question to be further enhanced if I correlate asking it with the external indications of a response attentive moment. Typically, clients signal this state by becoming quiet, shifting their posture into one of more comfort, breathing in an increasingly deep and relaxed manner, momentarily defocusing their eyes, and then looking expectantly at the therapist. This was true of Liz.

After she had finished speaking, Liz paused. She had settled back further into her chair, shifted into a deeper way of breathing, and with a searching expression, her eyes met mine. This suggested that she had reached a response attentive moment and so I took the opportunity gently to ask her the miracle question. The purpose of asking this question was multifold: to help Liz specify in greater detail what she needed from therapy, to create a context in which she could comfortably explore new possibilities, and to help her to access her hopes, rather than only her fears, before she left the session.

## The Miracle Question

The version of the miracle question that I asked Liz was:

Y.D.: Let's imagine that tonight you go home and go to bed and you fall into a very deep restful sleep, the kind of sleep from which you know you will awaken the next morning feeling very refreshed ...

And let's assume that during that very deep, restful sleep, a change occurs, something changes, and yet you don't know it at the time, because, of course, you are deeply asleep, enjoying all the benefits of a truly restful sleep. And let's suppose that the change that happens is a miracle of sorts, perhaps even something you had never imagined happening before you went to sleep. And in that miracle, while you are sleeping, something shifts in such a way that when you awaken, you find a satisfying and meaningful way to respond to your father, one that allows you to feel all right afterward. But since you were sleeping when the miracle happened, you would not know right away that it had occurred. So what do you suppose you would first notice after you awakened that would begin to let you know that a miracle had happened and that things were different for you?

C: Well, I wouldn't be so anxious when I thought about going to the hospital to see my father. And I wouldn't be worried that I would have insomnia and feel suicidal afterward and not be able to sleep. I'd feel calm.

Y.D.: What would you notice that was different that would let you know that you were calm?

C: I'd be thinking about everyday things like my work, what I was doing at that time of day, focusing on the moment. First thing in the morning, I guess I would be drinking my coffee, and I would be actually tasting it and not worrying about how I was going to feel after I saw my father. If I planned to go to the hospital to visit him that day, I wouldn't be worrying that I would have trouble sleeping or feel suicidal that night when I came home from seeing him.

Y.D.: What would you be doing instead of worrying?

C: It's like I said before, I would be feeling calm, focusing on the moment and knowing that calm feeling would carry over to when I saw my father and that it would continue even after I got home. Of course (laughs cynically), that's a lot easier said than done.

Y.D.: Of course. Let's suppose, miracle of miracles, that you actually did have that calm feeling when you went to see your father. What do you imagine he would notice about you that was different?

C: Well, for one thing I would show up earlier than I usually do. I usually wait until the last half hour of visiting hours because I am afraid of getting stuck spending too long with him and then feeling really upset and out of control afterwards.

Y.D.: So you would arrive earlier, that would be one thing. What else would you be doing differently that your father would notice?

C: Well, I don't know if he would notice it, he's pretty sedated on pain medication these days, but another thing that would be different is I wouldn't be afraid to look him in the eyes. Usually, I try to avoid looking at him. I am afraid that he'll see how vulnerable I am around him and that he'll use it in a bad way against me somehow.

Y.D.: So are you saying you would look him right in the eyes?

C: Yes, but I have a hard time imagining myself really being able to do that.

Y.D.: That's where the miracle comes in. So let's suppose you did look him right in the eyes. What do you suppose would happen next that was different, that would tell you the miracle had really happened?

C: I suppose he might look back at me, and maybe I would see him in a different way, maybe something would change about how I saw him. Of course, maybe he wouldn't look back at me. Maybe his eyes would be closed, or he would look away. It's hard to tell.

Y.D.: That's right, often it's impossible to predict accurately what another person will do. Usually, it's easier to predict your own behavior. Do you find that to be true with yourself?

C: Usually, yes.

Y.D.: So after you looked him in the eyes and he either returned your gaze or not, what would happen next that would allow you to know that this was different, that the miracle had really happened?

C: Well, after really looking at him, I suppose, at least, I hope, I would recognize him for what he is now, this sick old man hooked up to a lot of tubes and monitors lying in a bed by himself in a hospital room, not that powerful dangerous giant that I remember from when I was a kid.

Y.D.: So let's suppose that you really did look right at him and you were able to see him as different from that powerful "giant" you remember from childhood, and instead could see him for who he is now, a sick old man hooked up to a lot of tubes. What do you suppose would happen next?

C: I wouldn't be afraid of him.

Y.D.: What would you be doing instead of being afraid?

C: I would be asking him about his needs there in that room, like if he was being treated all right and if he needed anything.

Y.D.: Let's suppose you really asked him that, how do you suppose he would react?

C: Well, he would probably tell me if he needed anything, and if he needed something, like writing paper, a drink of water, or for me to ask the nurses to do something, I would do what he asked.

Y.D.: So let's suppose that he did tell you he needed you to get something or to ask the nurses to do something and you did it, how do you suppose he would react?

C: I suppose he would like it that I did it for him. Maybe he would appreciate it, maybe not. But, in general, I think his reaction would be positive.

Y.D.: And let's suppose there was something about the way he looked or somehow responded that let you know he liked that you did that for him, how do you imagine you would react?

C: I would feel relieved. I would know that I had behaved decently this time even though he has been a thorn in my side all my life and there is a lot I still really resent about things he did in the past. But those things cannot be erased.

Y.D.: Those things can't be erased. So let's suppose you asked for something on his behalf or got something he needed and he seemed pleased and you felt that you had behaved as you say, "decently," what do you suppose would be the effect of that for you?

C: I suppose, or, at least, I'd like to believe, that after that I would leave and go home and I wouldn't be upset and have flashbacks and trouble sleeping and all that. The problem is that there is a good chance that he would criticize me as usual, if he has any energy.

Y.D.: That's right, because this is your miracle, not his. So let's suppose he did say something mean-spirited or critical as he has so many times before, but this time you had already experienced the miracle. How do you suppose you would know at that point that a miracle really had happened and that something was different, better?

C: I wouldn't feel overwhelmed when he did it. He could say something mean and cutting to me in that sarcastic way he has, and while probably I still wouldn't like it, I would know that what he said about me or seemed to think of me was not the only reality. It was only his reality, not the truth, not who I really am.

Y.D.: What would be happening instead?

C: You mean assuming that this miracle had really happened?

Y.D.: Yes, assuming the miracle had happened and you had a way of, as you said earlier, getting through the time that remains with him in your life in a way that allows you to feel peaceful afterward.

C: Feeling peaceful afterward, that's a big one.

Y.D.: Yes, that sounds like an important part of the miracle. So what would you notice that was different after the miracle in how you responded when he criticized you, assuming that he did?

C: If he's able to talk, it's a pretty safe assumption that he'll be critical of me. He always is.

Y.D.: So given that assumption and the fact that the miracle had happened, what do you suppose you would notice that was different in your reaction to his criticism?

C: I would feel that whatever he said was simply his opinion and not necessarily the God-given truth.

Y.D.: And how would that show up in the way you behaved after he did that?

C: I wouldn't rise to the bait. I wouldn't try to defend myself or explain myself or try to get him to back off from criticizing me.

Y.D.: What would you be doing instead of explaining or trying to get him to back off?

C: I would just stay calm, probably I would be quiet. Maybe I would choose to leave at that point, but not in an angry way. I would say goodbye first. God, that's hard to imagine, I mean the staying calm part. Quiet maybe, but calm is hard to imagine.

Y.D.: Of course, that's part of what would truly make it a miracle. So if you acted calm and quiet, how do you suppose your dad would react?

C: I have no idea. I can't ever remember being that way when I was with him. He always makes me so mad that I either get really hurt and quiet or I tell him off, and either way I feel awful afterward.

Y.D.: So, in this miracle, you would respond calmly and you would perhaps be quieter than usual, and you might choose to leave after saying goodbye when he criticized you?

C: Yes.

Y.D.: So, supposing you did exactly that if he criticized you and you also did the other things you talked about so far in this miracle, what do you suppose would happen next?

C: Well, I think I would go home and I hope I wouldn't have trouble sleeping, or feel agitated and really depressed, and those other reactions I don't want to have.

Y.D.: Since this is a miracle, let's suppose you did go home afterward and you didn't have those reactions you used to have after seeing him. What do you suppose you would be doing instead of having those reactions? How would you be spending your time immediately after seeing him?

C: I would go home, have something to eat, maybe watch television for a while, but I'd really pay attention to what I was watching, I wouldn't be mentally reliving the experience of seeing him.

Y.D.: What would you be doing instead of that, since the miracle had happened? How would you know the miracle had happened when you got home after seeing him?

C: I'd be doing ordinary, everyday things. I'd be watching my favorite television shows, fixing something to eat, getting my clothes washed so I would have something ready to wear to work in the morning, maybe calling a friend to make plans for what I would be doing over the weekend. You know, just normal things.

Y.D.: What difference do you suppose it would make to be doing these ordinary, normal things right after seeing your dad?

C: It would be really different from what usually happens to me. Usually, I come home and I just sort of collapse on my bed and I don't eat usually. And I can't sleep and I feel terrible, and I keep thinking about all the bad experiences I've had with him in the past, and the bad one I've just had with him.

Y.D.: So, in this miracle, you would come home, and you would fix yourself something to eat, and you would watch your favorite television shows like you normally would on other nights, and you'd get your clothes ready for work, and maybe you'd call a friend to make plans for the weekend?

C: That's right.

Y.D.: What difference do you suppose it would make if you came home after seeing him, and you really did those things?

C: I would feel better because I would know that I was in control of my life, not him, that I was acting like an adult and not a helpless little kid like I was when he used to hit me and yell at me and criticize. And I guess that if he died at that point, I would feel I had not given in to the kind of behavior he taught me by the way he treated me. I would have spent some time with him, really treated him decently, but not destroyed myself as a result of doing it.

Y.D.: What would you have done instead of giving in to his kind of behavior?

C: I would have been true to who I really am deep inside.

Y.D.: What difference would that make?

C: I would feel at peace.

Y.D.: Would it be like, as you said earlier today, you had put a new ending onto your relationship with your father?

C: Yes. That's exactly what it would be.

Y.D.: So, if you decide to pretend that this miracle happened and act just as you've described, how confident are you that you can do that when you leave today?

C:      Some parts I suppose I could do, but others I'm not so sure about.

Y.D.:   Which parts do you most suppose you could do?

C:      Oh, I could show up earlier to see him, and maybe I could look him in the eye, but staying calm, that's the big one. I don't ever remember feeling calm around him. And when I'm not calm, I start shooting off my mouth and reacting to his criticizing me, and then we're off and running and I storm out and then afterward I feel like he won again. He got me to behave his way instead of the way I really want to act, the way I value behaving, and the way I am with other people in my life.

Y.D.:   So the acting calm part is important.

C:      Yes, it's probably the most important part and it's the thing that would be hardest to do. I'm really afraid I'm going to blow it, and I'll be so depressed afterward. It's hard to act calm when you don't feel that way.

Y.D.:   Tell me about a time when you felt much calmer than you usually do when you are in your dad's presence.

C:      Almost anytime is calmer than when I am with my dad.

## UTILIZING AN EXISTING RESOURCE

Ericksonian utilization is the process of incorporating a portion of the client's existing experiences, ongoing perceptions, and/or behaviors into the therapeutic change process (Dolan, 1985). Liz's ability to feel calmer "any time" she was not with her dad was an existing experiential resource that could be utilized to help access feelings of calm when she was in his presence. I accomplished this as follows:

Y.D.:   Tell me about an everyday experience in which you feel reasonably calm, maybe not the calmest you've ever been and certainly not the least calm, but somewhere in the middle, or maybe the high middle, range toward being calm.

C:      An everyday experience. It would have to be in my adult life, because I wasn't very calm as a kid, I was always looking over my shoulder, afraid of my old man, or afraid he was going to hurt my mother or my brothers, be really mean to them or tell them they couldn't do something that was really important to them. He always used to make fun of us for liking the things we liked. Anything we liked, he would try to put down to make it feel like nothing, like we were idiots for liking it.

Y.D.: So this would be quite different from that sort of experience. This might be one of those times in your adult life when you feel relatively calm ... maybe just an everyday kind of thing, perhaps one of those ordinary moments that you may have taken for granted when it was happening.

C: The first one that comes to mind is coming home after work, letting myself into the apartment, and locking the door behind me. I still remember the first time I walked into that place after I signed the lease. I remember telling myself, "This is my place. I get to make the rules here. No one comes in unless I let them."

Y.D.: Yes, your place.

C: It's nothing special, but it's all mine, and I love it.

Y.D.: It's all yours, and you love it. In a way, perhaps loving a place is, in fact, what makes it special. (*Client nods.*) I am wondering, where in your apartment do you feel most calm?

C: Well, it would be nice if it were in bed, but I've had so many nightmares there, it isn't exactly the calmest place. Probably the place I feel calmest is sitting or lying on the couch. I just sort of sink into the cushions. They are deep, so I kind of feel like the couch surrounds me.

Y.D.: So if you really imagine yourself on that couch in the way that is nicest for you, and you imagine that familiar comfortable feeling of sinking into those cushions, I wonder what else about that experience you are aware of as that comfortable calm feeling of sinking into the cushions develops ...

C: (*Speaking slowly, somewhat dreamily.*) I notice the mauve color of the cushion where I am resting my arm. There is a pattern of flowers and leaves and a bird; I think the bird is a peacock, but he has different colors from those a real peacock would have.

Y.D.: And I'm going to invite you to notice how that calm feeling continues to develop, maybe even deepen a little more as you think about the flowers and leaves and the peacock that is different from a real peacock. And I wonder what other nice things you might notice as the calm feeling continues ...

C: I hear the people in the apartment above. I think they probably would be fixing supper. They have a cute little baby. I like knowing that they are up there. They are good neighbors. They would come down if something bad happened, if I needed them. Even though the baby cries sometimes and I can hear it, I don't mind. Because I know they are an ordinary family, a family that is kind to each other. They take good care of their baby.

Y.D.: So those sounds are sounds of taking good care.

C: Yes. Good sounds.

Y.D.: Anything else it might be nice to notice that goes along with, or maybe even adds to, that nice calm feeling?

C: Just the feeling of being there on the couch, my back being supported, the texture of the cushions against my skin. The fabric is kind of soft. The covers are washable and I've just washed them again in the last week and so they smell good and they feel that way the fabric feels when it's been in the dryer with one of those little fabric softener sheets. We never had that when I was growing up. I don't think they had been invented yet.

Y.D.: So the calmness has a good smell and a feel that's different from when you were growing up?

C: Yes, and it smells like my home, not just anybody's home, but really mine.

Y.D.: And that's good and that's calm.

C: Yes.

## CREATING AN ASSOCIATIONAL CUE

An associational cue is a word, sound, or sensation that elicits an unconscious response (Dolan, 1985, 1991, 1998). Associational cues can be created to enhance a client's ability later to utilize previously identified resources, such as Liz's calm feeling, outside the therapy session at times when they are most likely to be needed. In order to help Liz create an associational cue, I proceeded as follows:

Y.D.: I'm thinking that this calm feeling, the one you have on the couch, is really good and a really important thing to memorize, really learn by heart so that you can never forget it.

C: Oh, I could never forget it. It's too important.

Y.D.: That's right. You are absolutely right about that. You won't forget it.

C:     Never.

Y.D.:     And I'm wondering, even though you won't forget it, I'm wondering if maybe it might not be nice if you had some special way to remind yourself of it at times when it would be really important to reconnect with the good feelings you have when you are on that couch.

C:     I would like that, but I don't know how.

Y.D.:     Well, it's different for everybody. Some people like to remind themselves with a nice word that somehow reminds them of the experience, like your calm experience. Other people sometimes like to memorize something about how they hold their body when they are having the good experience so that they can assume that position again and relive it in their minds that way. Other people have different ways. I once knew a little girl who carried around a tiny container of ground cinnamon. She sometimes felt anxious at school, and it was a nice thing for her to remember that sooner or later school would be out and she would get to go home, and her mom or her baby-sitter would be there waiting for her and she would get to have her favorite cookies that smelled like cinnamon. They had a funny name, I think they were called Snickerdoodles. (*Client laughs at the name.*) I wonder what way you will use to remind yourself of the calm feeling on that deep mauve couch with the flowers and the leaves and the peacock that's different from a real peacock . . .

C:     The words that keep coming into my mind are "fabric-softener cushions."

Y.D.:     I want to invite you to try it out in your mind. I want you to invite yourself right now to think of those fabric-softener cushions and notice the good feelings that come along with that . . .

C:     (*Smiles.*) It's a good feeling.

Y.D.:     Let's suppose that when you went to see your dad you found that you could bring some of that "fabric-softener cushions" feeling with you. What differences would you notice if you did that?

C:     It would be a lot better. I doubt if I could be perfectly calm, but I would be a lot calmer.

Y.D.:     I wonder what else would be different.

C:     Well, it's interesting because we didn't have the fabric-softener smell when I was living at home. It is something different. Something about my adult life.

Y.D.:   Something about your adult life that is perhaps a reminder that you are an adult now, living your own adult life?

C:      Yes, that's important.

Y.D.:   I wonder what the best way would be really to make sure that you can remind yourself of this feeling when you need to remember it, this nice adult experience of the fabric-softener cushions.

C:      The obvious thing that comes to mind is a sheet of fabric softener, the kind you put in the clothes dryer. They are only about four inches square.

Y.D.:   Would you use a fresh new one or one that had already been in the dryer?

C:      Oh, definitely a used one. It would be softer. More like the couch cushions.

Y.D.:   Your own cushions from your own adult place with your own fabric softener scent on them?

C:      Exactly.

## SCALING THE CLIENT'S CONFIDENCE
## ABOUT THE SOLUTION

Solution-focused scaling is the process of empowering the client to rank potential behaviors according to their level of individual or combined usefulness in reaching an already identified goal (Berg, 1990; De Shazer, 1991). In order to further enhance Liz's ability to succeed in interacting with her father in the way she valued, I offered her scaling to assess her level of confidence, and raise it as necessary. This was done in the following manner.

Y.D.:   If you were to imagine that, on a little scale, 10 means that you are completely confident that you could pretend the miracle happened and act accordingly, and remind yourself of the fabric-softener cushion experience next time you see your dad regardless of what he does, and 0 means you couldn't even imagine the miracle, hadn't even thought of it yet, much less described it, and you had never yet experienced the fabric-softener cushion feeling, what number would you say you are at now in terms of confidence?

C:      8 1/2.

Y.D.:   Is that high enough for you to feel okay about visiting your dad, or does it need to become higher?

C:      I wish it were a little bit higher, but it is high enough that I know I can get through it. I mean I don't feel cocky, not overly confident, but I feel okay.

Y.D.:   I'm curious as to what would make it higher.

C:      The only thing that would make it higher would be to have actually done the "pretending that the miracle happened" behavior in real life.

Y.D.:   So what needs to happen? Realistically, what do you need to do in order for you to know that you are moving in that direction?

C:      I'm going to go home and get my little fabric softener sheet and sit on the couch for a while tonight, and again tomorrow afternoon before I go to see my father. I'm going to put the fabric-softener sheet in my pocket so I can touch it when I am talking to my father, and also so that if I put my hand up near my face, I can smell that good smell.

Y.D.:   So you can take the fabric-softener cushion feeling with you ... take it out and smell it and feel it whenever you need to, anywhere you like, feeling it undeniably any time it's needed?

C:      Yes.

Y.D.:   How confident are you that you can get a fabric-softener sheet and do as you just said you would?

C:      Oh, I know I can do it. I'm going to do it when I get home tonight. And this is a little scary, but I'm really going to try to act as if a miracle really happened when I go see my dad tomorrow. I will really have to concentrate, but I'm going to try, and I think that if I try really hard, I can do it, or at least some of it.

At this point, the session ended.

Subsequently, Liz reported that she had experimented with pretending that the miracle had happened and behaved accordingly as far as possible on visits with her father, and this had been helpful. Understandably, some visits were easier and some more difficult, but acting as if a miracle had happened gave her a different focus, and made the visits less overwhelming.

She carried the little piece of fabric-softener sheet in her pocket on all of her visits to her father, and said that as well as helping her remember what it felt like to be calm, it had also helped her to remember that she was an adult now and no longer under the control of her father or at the mercy of his unreasonable, and often inaccurate, critical responses.

While she still found visits to her dying father draining, Liz no longer suffered subsequent nights of insomnia, prolonged anxiety, and intrusive thoughts, and she felt relieved that she had succeeded in treating her father decently, with the dignity and respect with which she would have wished to have been treated had their roles been reversed. In this way, Liz succeeded in creating a new ending to their relationship, albeit a bittersweet one because she knew she would never have the father she wanted and needed as a little girl. However, most important was the fact that, as Liz observed afterward, she could "live at peace" with the way she had responded to her father in their last encounters.

## DISCUSSION

Imagining the miracle gave Liz a new mental script for how she wanted to behave in her father's presence, rather than for what she wanted to avoid. Once the desired differences and the behaviors associated with the miracle were identified, Liz could decide to enact some of them in real life. The fabric-softener sheet functioned as an associational cue to help Liz reconnect to a recent vivid memory of the familiar, concrete, everyday adult experience of relaxing on her couch. Together, these helped her to add a different dimension to her experience of being with her father in the hospital.

Three basic principles for combining Ericksonian and solution-focused therapy to provide relief for adult children like Liz who experience post-traumatic stress following interactions with formerly or currently abusive parents can be summarized as follows:

1.  Offer the miracle question to help the client specifically identify what he or she wants to have happen, instead of the problem.
2.  Enhance the client's likelihood of success outside the therapy office by utilizing a familiar, and, therefore, undeniable, experience from recent everyday life as an associational cue that the client can later use on his or her own as a way to elicit unconscious resources when and where they are most needed.
3.  Offer solution-focused scaling questions to assess (and, if necessary, raise) the client's confidence and comfort level.

## References

Berg, I. K. (1990). *A solution-focused approach to family based services.* Milwaukee, WI: Brief Family Therapy Center Publications.

Berg, I. K., & Miller, S. D. (1992). *Working with the problem drinker: A solution-focused approach.* New York: Norton.

Berg, I. K., & De Shazer, S. (1993). Making numbers talk: Language in therapy. In S. Friedman (Ed.), *The new language of change: Constructive collaboration in psychotherapy.* New York: Guilford.

De Jong, P., & Berg, I. K. (1996). *How to interview for client strengths and solutions.* Pacific Grove, CA: Brooks/Cole Publishers.

De Shazer, S., Berg, I. K., Lipchik, E., Nunnally, E., Molnar, A., Gingerich, W., & Weiner-Davis, M. (1986). Brief therapy: Focused solution development. *Family Process, 25,* 207–222.

De Shazer, S.(1985). *Keys to solution in brief therapy.* New York: Norton.

De Shazer, S. (1988). *Clues: Investigating solutions in brief family therapy.* New York: Norton.

De Shazer, S. (1991). *Putting difference to work.* New York: Norton.

De Shazer, S. (1994). *Words were originally magic.* New York: Norton.

Dolan, Y. M. (1985). *A path with a heart: Ericksonian utilization with resistant and chronic clients.* New York: Brunner/Mazel.

Dolan, Y. M. (1991). *Resolving sexual abuse: Solution-focused therapy and Ericksonian hypnosis for adult survivors.* New York: Norton.

Dolan, Y. M. (1994a). An Ericksonian perspective on the treatment of sexual abuse. In J. K. Zeig (Ed.), *Ericksonian methods: The essence of the story* (pp. 395–414). New York: Guilford.

Dolan, Y. M. (1994b). Solution-focused therapy with a case of severe abuse. In M. F. Hoyt (Ed.), *Constructive Therapies, Vol. I* (pp. 276–294). New York: Guilford.

Dolan, Y. M. (1998). *One small step: Moving beyond trauma and therapy to a life of joy.* Watsonville, CA: Papier-Mache Press.

Erickson, M. H. (1959/1980). Further techniques of hypnosis—utilization techniques. *American Journal of Clinical Hypnosis, 1* (3–8). In E. L. Rossi (Ed.), *The Collected Papers of Milton H. Erickson, Vol. I.* New York: Irvington.

Erickson, M. H., & Rossi, E. L. (1979). *Hynotherapy.* New York: Irvington.

Erickson, M. H., & Rossi, E. L. (1989). *The February man.* New York: Brunner/ Mazel.

Erickson, M. H., Rossi, E. L., & Rossi, S. I. (1976). *Hypnotic realities.* New York: Irvington.

Gilligan, S. (1987). *Therapeutic trances: The cooperation principle in Ericksonian hypnotherapy.* New York: Brunner/Mazel.

Miller, G. (1997). *Becoming miracle workers: Language and meaning in brief therapy.* Hawthorne, NY: Aldine de Gruyter.

O'Hanlon, B., & Weiner-Davis, M. (1989). *In search of solutions.* New York: Norton.

# 34

# Ericksonian Play Therapy:
# The Spirit of Healing
# with Children and Adolescents

*Joyce C. Mills*

*Play* is the language of children, and *story* is the language of play. With this statement in mind, this chapter focuses on Ericksonian play therapy, a modality of child psychotherapy that has taken me almost two decades to formulate. The basis for a grant written to help the children and families on the remote west side of Kauai, Hawaii, after Hurricane Iniki hit in 1992,[1] it was subsequently presented at the Sixth International Congress on Ericksonian Approaches to Hypnosis and Psychotherapy (1992, 1994). Since then, Ericksonian play therapy has been utilized as a treatment modality with various childhood disorders and as part of different therapeutic philosophies (Marvasti, 1997).

Play therapy in and of itself is not new. Its origins can be traced back

---

[1] The program was entitled: Kauai Westside O'hana (family) Activities Project, sponsored by Child and Family Services of Kauai and funded by Office of Youth Services. It provided opportunities for the youth and their families to move past the focus of PTSD and into a model more focused on "healing and prevention," which I called Posttraumatic Stress Healing (PTSH). The PTSH model was employed in (1) natural healing activities; (2) parent talk-story groups; and (3) the Talk-Story (counseling) Center.

to tribal communities where elders used sticks, stones, shells, sand, clay, masks, and handmade dolls to teach important life lessons and children were encouraged to act out various aspects of life. Today play therapy has grown to include numerous philosophies and modalities. For an extensive historical and theoretical background, see Landreth, 1991; O'Connor & Schaefer, 1994; Oaklander, 1988; O'Connor & Braverman, 1997; Barnes, 1996; Norton & Norton, 1997.

Emphasizing cultural diversity, natural healing abilities, and creative solutions, Ericksonian play therapy is a treatment that can provide children and families who have experienced abuse, adversity, and trauma with the *therapeutic stepping-stones* to rediscovering joy, empowerment, and the inspiration to soar.

A story that best encapsulates the foundational philosophy inherent in Ericksonian play therapy is metaphorically based on an ancient Hawaiian oral tale (Lee & Willis, 1990). I share it as I have heard it told many times since my first reading.

> Every child is born with a perfect Bowl of Light. And with this Bowl of Light the child can swim with the fishes, ride on the backs of sharks, fly with the birds, and know all things. But every once in a while, as the child grows, negativities come into the child's life. These negativities can be hurts, pain, jealousies, and anger. These hurts and angers can become like stones and drop into the bowl. Soon the bowl may have so many stones that you cannot see the light. And pretty soon the child becomes like the stone, he or she cannot grow. But what is wonderful is that all the child needs to learn to do is to turn the bowl upside down and empty the stones, because the light is always there.

Keeping in line with the metamessage of the story, and Dr. Erickson's (1958/1980) belief that "children have a driving need to learn and to discover, and every stimulus constitutes, for them, a possible opportunity to respond in some new way," the job of an Ericksonian play therapist is to focus on the innate light, and help the child empty the symbolic stones that block his or her light. The focus then shifts from being viewed simply as a "survivor" of past traumas to being a "thriving" member of society, reminding us that "scars are markers of where we have been, but not where we are going."

More specifically, in Ericksonian play therapy, it is essential for therapists to recognize and appreciate the innate and unique abilities within each child, to help the child identify his or her struggles or obstacles, and to provide approaches that can help the child learn how to "empty his or her stones," thereby facilitating healing from trauma stemming from a variety of sources—abuse, natural or human-made disasters, divorce, illness, death, violence.

## A PLAYFUL MIND: SHIFTING REALITIES

Maintaining a playful mind is essential when working with children. One needs to be able to see salt shakers as spaceships or seashells as storytellers. Although not noted professionally as a play therapist, or for his work particularly with children, psychiatrist Milton H. Erickson was a master at integrating both play and story into his hypnotherapeutic and psychotherapeutic work. Students who worked directly with Dr. Erickson have described the many humorous antics he employed to help them shift their fixed ways of perceiving situations into more open pathways for the exploration of possibilities and discovery. One such incident is described by Carl Hammerschlag (1988). During a visit, Dr. Erickson picked up a rock-sized piece of turquoise ore. He then looked at Dr. Hammerschlag and threw the rock directly at his crotch. Hammerschlag states (pp. 52–53) that before he could react, the "rock" landed on him, and he realized that it wasn't a rock at all, but a piece of foam rubber. Erickson left him with the message, "Not everything you see is what you see it as. It is only how you see it at the moment."

In line with the philosophy of this important message, the principles of Ericksonian play therapy (1) deemphasize a patient's diagnosis in favor of viewing the uniqueness of each patient, and (2) emphasize the importance of staying in the present moment so that minimal cues can be observed and utilized. In relation to staying in the present moment and not drawing upon the diagnostic labeling of patients, Gilligan (1987) coined the term "experiential deframing," stating:

> Erickson repeatedly stressed that therapeutic communications should be based neither on theoretical generalizations nor on statistical probabilities, but on actual patterns distinguishing the client's present self-expression (e.g., beliefs, behavior, motivation, symp-

toms). This is a truly radical proposition in that it requires therapists to begin each therapy in a state of experiential ignorance. It assumes that the client's expressions are individualized models of "reality" and that the therapy is based on accepting and utilizing these models. To do so, therapists must develop a receptive state of *experiential deframing* in which they set aside their models and become "students" to learn a new "reality" (i.e., that of the client). (p. 14)

This receptive state of experiential deframing was best highlighted by Dr. Erickson's children during a panel discussion, "How Milton H. Erickson Encouraged Individuality in His Children" (1988). One of Erickson's eight children, Lance, shared a time in his younger life when he was feeling a great "worry and concern" over prominent bumps on his forehead. Lance stated that his father: "Let me know what a wonderful thing it was that I had these bumps, these *knowledge bumps* (italics added) that nobody else in the family had developed so well. They would not only stand me in good stead, but someday I would meet a girl who thought they were just delightful, a wonderful physical asset, and they would endear me to her. I am not sure that this is what actually occurred, but his remarks helped me to accept a part of me that I might have rejected."

Lance's story reveals Dr. Erickson's deep appreciation for the ability to shift perception and learn a new "reality." He didn't discount the bumps, or falsify the issue, but instead he *modified* the description by calling them "knowledge bumps." One might tend to view this shift in perception as a quick-fix, clever, manipulative technique. However, this would limit the deeper wisdom being imparted. Dr. Erickson never said that Lance had to see the bumps differently. He just presented him with an opportunity to expand his experience. It was up to Lance's unique unconscious mind to accept or reject the possibilities. Here we see symptoms being transformed into possible solutions.

Providing opportunities for children and adolescents to expand their awareness is essential to their healing process. The following case illustrates this point with a five-year old child who was referred because she was experiencing fears of separation and would have violent temper tantrums whenever either parent tried to leave her in the classroom, and these tantrums ultimately prevented her from participating successfully in kindergarten.

## Seashell Stories

Cinnamon-haired Katie walked into the session holding onto her mother's skirt and gripping her father's hand. She remained somewhat "attached" as all three of them proceeded to sit on the large L-shaped couch. My office was set up like a family play-room, with big fluffy pillows, toys, games, puppets, a play table, miniatures, drums, feathers, and many objects of nature. After a few moments of casual conversation, I noticed Katie eyeing the many items that were on the table in front of the couch: story dolls, rocks, crystals, a piece of blue coral, and a hand-size conch shell. While observing minimal cues, I noticed that Katie's colored eyes remained transfixed on the shell. I leaned forward, picked up the shell, turned it slowly for a few moments, and then handed it to Katie. She let go of her mother's skirt and accepted the shell with both hands.

I then knelt down beside Katie and told her the following short story.

"You know, Katie, this shell reminds me of a time when I was a little girl just about your age and my grandma took me to the beach. I was playing near these great big rocks and there I found a shell kind of like this one. It was sort of stuck between two big rocks that were close together. I quickly ran to tell my grandmother. She was very wise and told me that when you put a shell like that near your ear, you hear the stories of the ocean. I wanted to hear those stories, so I knew that I would have to loosen the shell in order to do so.

"Well, Katie, I tried every way I could, but no matter what I did, the shell stayed stuck there. I sat back on the sand and watched as the tide began to come in. Wave after wave, the ocean washed over the shell and the rocks. [I acted out the sound of the waves by making a "whooshing" sound.] After a time, I don't know how long, the ocean was calm and I decided to try to loosen the shell again. Maybe it was ready to come loose. This time something different happened. When I put my hand on the shell and shook it a little bit [demonstrating a slight movement with my hand], I felt a tiny movement. The shell seemed like it was ready to loosen itself from the rocks. Finally, after a bit of patience, I had the shell in my hand and I rushed to show my grandmother. She smiled and reminded me that when you hold a shell like that close to your ear, you can hear the stories of the ocean." [I moved my hand "as if" holding the shell to my ear.]

When I finished the story, Katie had lifted her hand holding the shell up to her ear. I smiled and asked her to tell me when she was beginning to hear the stories. Katie returned the smile and nodded her head, indicating "Yes." Katie was now completely engaged. She was sitting on the floor with me and talking *to* all the other nature objects on the table, creating a *story world* of her own.

Katie stayed engaged throughout the rest of the session. Her parents were hopeful because this was the first time that she had left their side without a struggle.

In describing Katie's shift, it is helpful to utilize a "braiding process" in which "the child's (client's) presenting problem, the inner resources, and the metaphorical task (the idea or behavior to be learned) are woven into a solution or resolution" (Mills, 1989). All three components are given equal power. Therefore, the symptom/problem is *appreciated, utilized,* and *transformed* rather than *controlled, interpreted,* or *amputated.*

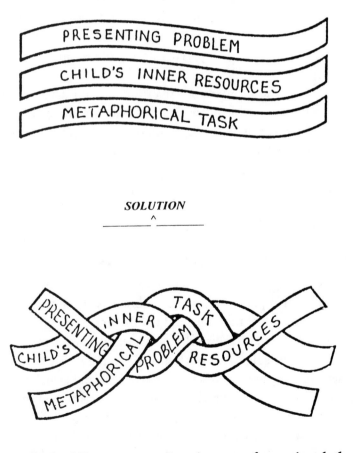

Figure 1. The braiding process: Creating transformational change.

Figure 1 is a diagrammatic view of the braiding process, in which the child's presenting problem, inner resources, and the metaphorical task are woven into a solution.

*The Braiding of Katie's Solution*

| | |
|---|---|
| *Presenting problem* | Frightened, temper tantrums, not able to separate from parents at school. |
| *Katie's inner resources* | Curiosity; ability to focus attention; enjoyment of stories. |
| *Metaphorical task* | Utilization of the shell; Katie's hand holding shell and moving it to her ear and asking if she could hear the stories. |
| *Solution (braid)* | Katie becomes completely engaged; affirms she can hear the stories; actualizes a readiness for change; stays separated from parents during the session. |

As we see in Katie's case, rather than focusing on diagnostic labeling to determine the course of therapeutic intervention, the *braiding process* embraces the Ericksonian theory and philosophy of "utilization." See, in particular, volumes I and IV in Erickson (Erickson, 1966/1980; Erickson & Rossi, 1979), further noting: "Central to the *philosophy* of utilization is a profound respect for the validity and integrity of the child's presenting behavior; central to the *technique* of utilization is a highly skilled ability to observe, participate in, and reframe what is presented" (Mills & Crowley, 1986, p. 48).

While there may be differing views on the subject of diagnostic labeling (Marvasti, 1997), reliance on such categorizations is not a focus when utilizing Ericksonian play therapy approaches in work with children. Furthermore, it is my belief that the child (adolescent or family) too often *is* the diagnostic label, and the disorder or presenting problem becomes the dominant, if not the sole, focus of attention. To the extent that a diagnostic label sets up a preconceived set of expectations and associations, it can become a roadblock to successful therapeutic intervention. Worse, it may even function iatrogenically in a negative direction (Mills, 1989). Moreover, Norton and Norton (1997) warn that "formal categorizations of childhood disorders, such as in the *DSM*-IV [American Psychiatric Association, 1994] or the DRG [Health Care Financing Administration], as well as pop psychology self-help books, have no meaning to them. Children must communicate through their own medium—play" (p. 4). We as therapists must not limit the scope of the vastly creative communications "gifted" to us by the children with whom we work, but instead embrace their breadth and integrity.

## THERAPEUTIC STEPPING-STONES

Whether working with children, adolescents, families, or groups, a variety of approaches can be employed within the Ericksonian play therapy framework. These stepping-stones are summarized as follows:

Storytelling metaphors (Mills & Crowley, 1986, 1988; Mills, 1989, 1992, 1999; Norton & Norton, 1997; Marvasti, 1997).
Artistic metaphors (Mills & Crowley, 1986; Mills, 1989, 1992, 1999; Gregorian, Azarian, DeMaria, & McDonald, 1996).
Living metaphors (Mills & Crowley, 1986, 1988; Mills, 1989, 1999).
Rituals and ceremonies (Mills, 1989, 1992, 1998; Gilligan, 1997; Hammerschlag & Silverman, 1997).

It is important to note that although these techniques can be utilized in brief therapy models as well as in longer-term play therapy models, the emphasis in these techniques is not on quick-fix cure as much as it is on facilitating a deeper level of healing. The philosophy is similar to that of gardening; where "we can't *order* seeds to grow ... they need loving care, nurturance, guidance, and patience in order to take root, sprout, and reach their full blossoming potential."

## THERAPEUTIC PLAY TOOLS:
### GAINING AN EAGLE-VISION PERSPECTIVE

Each of the stepping-stones includes using a wide variety of "therapeutic play tools" in the form of toys, art materials, a sand tray, puppets, and dolls, along with various objects from nature—shells, rocks, sticks, leaves, and the like—to help facilitate unconscious change. In a thorough analysis, Norton and Norton (1997) discuss the symbolic interpretation of using specific types of toys "in order to ascertain metaphors, themes, styles, shifts and direction in the play of children." They wisely remind us to be cognizant of the many possible interpretations that may be inherent in each toy. I like to think of this philosophy as being able to *see with the eyes of an eagle, rather than through the limited vision of a mouse*. By this I mean that whereas it may be important to have "mouse vision" in order to be able to scrutinize details of a specific situation, such as in the case of paying attention to minimal cues, we as therapists must allow ourselves to develop "eagle vision" so that we can not only see what is in front of us, but can gain a greater perspective on possible solutions. In the wonderful imaginative world of a child, a leaf can become a feather, a car, or even a bandage for a wound. Children truly possess the gift of eagle vision.

While the knowledge of interpretations may be essential in many forms of play therapy, they are of less importance in the Ericksonian play therapy model, whereby the toys and nature objects selected are not *analyzed* by the therapist, but instead *utilized* by the child. It is the child who gives meaning and voice to the toy or object chosen, not the therapist. Just as ideomotor movements are signals uniquely relevant for each person in trance (Rossi & Cheek, 1988), so too are the meanings of the toys selected by the child in Ericksonian play therapy. This is a critical difference between Ericksonian play therapy and the psychodynamic modalities of play therapy; that is, a miniature ambulance can mean an accident or danger, or it can be interpreted as healing and rescue. Rather than imposing interpretation from the therapist, it is important to *allow* the meaning to *unfold* as it relates to the particular child and family.

This differentiation is particularly important when working with children or families who come from a multicultural background. Toy police officers may have very different connotations for African American children and Caucasian children because of their personal experiences in the communities in which they were raised. The extensive use of the color "red" by a child can be interpreted as an expression of "anger"; however, in the Asian and Native American cultures red symbolizes "life and the sacred." One needs to allow a process of unfolding of meaning to emerge from the child.

The following example illustrates the use of storytelling, art in the form of *story-crafts*, and a ritual to help the children and families of Kauai to heal from the trauma of Hurricane Iniki. The bowl of light story became a foundation for this multidimensional project encompassed within the Natural Healing Activities program (Mills, 1992). All activities took place in an informal neighborhood center setting. Children of various ages, along with parents, grandparents, and other community members, gathered in a group and were told the bowl of light story. No direct questioning or mentioning of the hurricane ensued at any time.[2] Within the same two-hour session, a *story-craft* was created by giving the children/participants pieces of fast-drying clay the size of a tennis ball and asking them to (1) hold the ball of clay in their hands; (2) close their eyes and take a few, slow deep breaths; and (3) imagine seeing their own bowl of light. The children/participants were then asked to open their eyes when the image was clear, and begin to shape the clay into bowls. The bowls took only a day or so to dry.

The next session began with the telling of the story once again. The children were encouraged to repeat the story as they remembered it. They were then supplied with acrylic paints, shells, feathers, beads, and dried flowers. They were told to hold the now dried bowls in their hands, close their eyes, take a few deep breaths, and allow the images of their bowls to come to their minds. Finally, they were told that after the images were clear, they could open their eyes and begin decorating their bowls. Some children left them unembellished; some painted elaborate designs.

The children then went on a nature walk and were encouraged to gather their "stones." Each child assigned a different meaning to his or her stones. Some children said that the stones represented what they had lost in the hurricane, whereas others talked about fears. Many adolescents identified their stones in relation to drugs and abuse not associated with the hurricane. Some remained silent in the gathering process. The children/participants received no suggestions as to what their stones might represent to them. Their own unconscious minds bridged the associations and gave meanings that were personally relevant for each child.

To expand the healing process, a therapeutic ritual was invoked. After the stones were gathered, the children were told that they could select a special time and place where they could "turn their bowls over" and empty out their stones.[3]

---

[2] Direct approaches, that is, talking in the first person about traumatic memories associated with the hurricane, were viewed by numerous community members as culturally insensitive to the natural healing views held by most. Storytelling and the use of art have been found to be powerful healing tools for working with victims of natural disasters and human-made disasters.

[3] Rituals defined in this chapter are not "homework assignments," nor are they deemed clever

To date, more than a thousand children and their families from various cultural and religious backgrounds on the west side of Kauai have made their own bowls of light and continue to tell the story. It has also been replicated in bilingual classrooms and in residential treatment programs.[4]

## THERAPEUTIC CONNECTEDNESS:
## THE WEB OF RELATIONSHIP

At the heart of Ericksonian play therapy is the relationship between the therapist and child/adolescent. Volumes have been written on the theory of what endows a healing relationship with children (Axline, 1969; Freud, 1946; Gardner, 1971; Gardner & Olness, 1981; Landreth, 1991; Norton & Norton, 1997; Barnes, 1996; O'Connor & Schaefer, 1994; James, 1989; Oaklander, 1978; Gil, 1991; Mills & Crowley, 1986). In referring to "experiential play therapy," psychologist Karen Jordan (1997) tells us that it is "an innovative approach in which the clinician reacts to the child instead of initiating actions of his or her own beliefs and values." Clark Moustakas (1992), a founder of play therapy, states: "The alive relationship between the therapist and the child is the essential dimension, perhaps the only significant reality, in the therapeutic process and in all interhuman growth." These philosophies are remarkably similar to that of Erickson, who believed that the job of the therapist is to enter the world of the client, not to have the client enter the world of the therapist. With regard to his beliefs, Dr. Erickson (1958/1980) stated: "Any therapy used should always be in accordance with the needs of the patient, whatever they may be, and not based in any way upon arbitrary classifications."

Embracing a therapeutic philosophy of connectedness rather than basing therapy on divisive classifications is particularly critical when working with children and families from multicultural backgrounds. Seeing spirits is not something to be feared or labeled as psychotic in the Native American, Hawaiian, African Bushman, and many Indonesian cultures, and talking with trees, birds, insects, and ancestors, or hearing the wind tell stories, is often encouraged among people of these cultures (Barnes, 1996;

---

manipulations to get people to change. Instead, rituals are a means of helping people *reconnect* to a sense of the sacredness and vast natural healing potentials of life.

[4] J. Raniero, M.A., counselor at the Sheridan Magnet School of International Language and Communication, Tacoma, WA; the Christie School, Marylhurst, OR; Hale 'Opio, Kauái, Hawaii.

Keeney, 1994). Such behaviors are not labeled psychotic or dissociative disorders, but instead are viewed as "gifts." Keeping this multicultural framework in mind, the model of Ericksonian play therapy allows for appreciating unique ways of *being in the world*. Once again, we are reminded of Erickson's message, "Not everything you see is what you see it as. It is only how you see it at the moment."

## INTERSPERSED SUGGESTIONS

Another important aspect of Ericksonian play therapy that differentiates it from other child therapy modalities is the use of "interspersed suggestions" (Erickson, 1966/1980; Erickson & Rossi, 1980). Erickson and Rossi (1980) point out that this technique "is the clearest example of two-level communication wherein subject matter of interest to a particular patient is utilized as a general context to fixate conscious attention, while interspersed suggestions are received for their effects on an unconscious level" (p. 447).

Translating the interspersal technique into practical terms, a child's attention can be absorbed in artwork, the sand tray, building with legos or blocks, or working with clay (fixing conscious attention). While the child is playing with any of these media, the therapist can intersperse suggestions for what the child wants to have in his or her life (suggestions given on an unconscious level). The following is an example of utilizing the process of play and art while, at the same time, integrating interspersed suggestions with a group of teenage girls described as having serious emotional problems stemming from abuse, neglect, and substance abuse. It took place in a residential treatment facility where, earlier in the day, we had met for a group story time. Issues of safety and self-protection emerged as the girls expressed themselves during the group exchange.

### Basket Teachings

Upon walking into the large lunchroom, I noticed that the girls had strips of colored construction paper piled on the tables in front of them. The room was very noisy, and most of the girls were running around, throwing their strips of paper, not connected to what they were doing. The instructor tried repeatedly to get their attention. Her attempts would work for a minute or two, but then the energetic teens would become distracted again. Allowing myself to *be in the moment*, I asked one of the

girls what they were making. Without looking up, she replied, "Baskets."
At that point, I thought of a teaching I had learned about basket-weaving
from one of my Native American teachers and decided to share it with
the girls. I began in this way:

"You know, baskets are rather interesting. They can hold some very
special things inside. Some of them even have lids so you can keep treas-
ured secrets locked away ... and you know just how to open it at just the
right time when you want to take out something important ... and you
know just how to close the lid once again so that everything inside stays
safe. What you put into it and what you choose to take out is up to you."

At this point, 15-year-old Jeanette showed me the basket she had been
making. With her fingers opening and closing her basket, Jeanette repeated, "Yes, and sometimes closed ... and sometimes open ... safe inside." As the other girls watched, I repeated, "Yes, and it is up to you to
choose what to put in and what to take out. *And you know a lot about
safety.*"

After a few thoughtful moments, Jeanette said, "Aunty Joyce, it's
kinda like our lives. What we put in and what we take out is up to us."
The art therapist nodded to me and I responded with a smile, saying,
"That's right, baskets are rather interesting ... *And you know a lot about
how you want your life to be.*"

The girls remained wonderfully interactive; however, they were now
focused on weaving their baskets. They continued talking with one another, but their conversation had shifted to talking about what they
would put into their baskets, and how they wanted them to look. Some
of the girls wanted to decorate their baskets with designs; others left them
plainly woven.

## SUMMARY

When utilizing Ericksonian play therapy as a treatment modality for
working with children, adolescents, and families, I believe the most important aspect to focus on asks the question: "If we have one hour with
a child, with what thought do we want to leave that child?" The answer
may be different for each of us. An answer that comes to mind for me is
WINGS: *W*isdom—sharing what is lived in life, not simply knowledge
learned in books; *I*nspiration—imparting a "you can do it" attitude; *N*ur-
turing—feeding the soul by supporting visions, dreams, goals; *G*uidance—

providing a pathway for curiosity and discovery; *Self*—supporting individual uniqueness. When combined with sincerity, integrity, and an authentic sense of caring, the children with whom we work can experience a gift of self-appreciation: the spirit, power, and ability to soar in their world filled with challenges and change.

---

**Five Practical Ideas**

- *Play* is the language of children, and *story* is the language of play.
- Ericksonian play therapy embraces the hypnotic philosophies of Milton H. Erickson; that is, recognizing and utilizing minimal cues, trance phenomena, and interspersed suggestions.
- Maintain a playful mind in order to facilitate a shift in realities.
- Human connectedness is at the heart of successful intervention when using the Ericksonian play therapy modality.
- Focus on the retrieval of inner resources rather than on diagnostic labeling.

---

### References

American Psychiatric Association (1994). *Diagnostic and statistical manual of mental disorders: DSM IV* (4th ed.) Washington, DC: Author.

Axline, V. (1947/1969). *Play therapy.* New York: Ballantine.

Barnes, M. A. (1996). *The healing path with children.* Clayton, NY: Viktoria, Fermoyle & Berrigan.

Erickson, L. (1988). Panel discussion: "How Milton H. Erickson encouraged individuality in his children." In J. K. Zeig & S. R. Lankton, *Developing Ericksonian therapy: State of the arts* (p. 494). New York: Brunner/Mazel.

Erickson, M. (1958/1980). Pediatric hypnotherapy. In E. Rossi (Ed.), *The collected papers of Milton H. Erickson on hypnosis. Vol. IV. Innovative hypnotherapy* (pp. 174–180). New York: Irvington.

Erickson, M. (1966/1980). The interspersal hypnotic technique for symptom correction and pain control. In E. Rossi (Ed.) *The collected papers of Milton H. Erickson on hypnosis. Vol. IV: Innovative hypnotherapy* (pp. 262–278). New York: Irvington.

Erickson, M., & Rossi, E. (1979). *Hypnotherapy: An exploratory casebook.* New York: Irvington.

Erickson, M., & Rossi, E. (1980). Two-level communication and the microdynamics of trance and suggestion. In E. Rossi (Ed.), *The collected papers of Milton H. Erick-*

*son on hypnosis. Vol. 1. The nature of hypnosis and suggestion* (p. 447). New York: Irvington.

Freud, A. (1946). *The psychoanalytic treatment of children.* London: Imago.

Gardner, G., & Olness, K. (1981). *Hypnosis and hypnotherapy with children.* New York: Grune & Stratton.

Gardner, R. (1971). *Therapeutic communication with children: The mutual storytelling techniques.* New York: Science House.

Gil, E. (1991). *The healing power of play: Working with abused children.* New York: Guilford.

Gilligan, S. (1987). *Therapeutic trances.* New York: Brunner/Mazel.

Gilligan, S. (1997). *The courage to love.* New York: Norton.

Gilligan, S., & Price, R. (Ed.). (1993). *Therapeutic conversations.* New York: Norton.

Gregorian, V. S., Azarian, A., DeMaria, M. D., & McDonald, L. D. (1996). The colors of disaster: The psychology of the "black sun." *The arts in psychotherapy, 23*(1), 1–14.

Hammerschlag, C. A. (1988). *Dancing healers.* San Francisco: Harper & Row.

Hammerschlag, C. A., & Silverman, H. D. (1997). *Healing ceremonies.* New York: Berkeley.

Imber-Black, E., Roberts, J., & Whiting, R. (Eds.). (1988). *Rituals in families and family therapy.* New York: Norton.

James, B. (1989). *Treating traumatized children.* Lexington, MA: Lexington Books.

Jordan, K. (1997). Foreword. In C. C. Norton & B. E. Norton, *Reaching children through play therapy.* Denver, CO: Publishing Cooperative.

Keeney, B. (1994). *Shaking out the spirits.* Tarrytown, NY: Station Hill Press.

Landreth, G. L. (1991). *Play therapy: The art of the relationship.* Muncie, IN: Accelerated Development.

Lee, P. J., & Willis, K. (1990). *Tales of the night rainbow.* Honolulu, HI: Night Rainbow Publishing.

Marvasti, J. (1997). Ericksonian play therapy. In K. J. O'Connor & L. M. Braverman (Eds.), *Play therapy: Theory and practice* (chap 10, pp. 285–308). New York: Wiley.

Mills, J. C. (1989). No more monsters and meanies: Multisensory metaphors for helping children with fears and depression. In M. D. Yapko (Ed.), *Brief therapy approaches to treating anxiety and depression.* New York: Brunner/Mazel.

Mills, J. C. (1992). Kauai Westside O'hana Activities Project. Grant sponsored by Child and Family Services of Kauai; funded by Office of Youth Services, Hawaii.

Mills, J. C. (1994). Ericksonian play therapy. Presented at the Sixth International Congress on Ericksonian Approaches to Hypnosis and Psychotherapy. Track Eight: Children & Adolescents.

Mills, J. C. (1999). *Reconnecting to the magic of life.* Kauai, HI: Imagine Press.

Mills, J. C., & Crowley, R. J. (1986). *Therapeutic metaphors for children and the child within.* New York: Brunner/Mazel.

Mills, J., & Crowley, R. (1988). A multidimensional approach to the utilization of therapeutic metaphors for children and adolescents. In J. K. Zeig & S. R. Lankton (Eds.), *Developing Ericksonian therapy: State of the arts* (pp. 302–323). New York: Brunner/Mazel.

Moustakas, C. E. (1992). *Psychotherapy with children.* Greeley, CO: Carron. (Originally published in 1959. New York: Harper & Row.)

Norton, C. C., & Norton, B. E. (1997). *Reaching children through play therapy.* Denver, CO: Publishing Cooperative.

Oaklander, V. (1988). *Windows to our children.* Highland, NY: Center for Gestalt Development.

O'Conner, K. J., & Braverman, L. M. (Eds.). (1997). *Play therapy: Theory and practice.* New York: Wiley

O'Connor, K. J., & Schaefer, C. E. (Eds.). (1994). *Handbook of play therapy: Vol. II. Advances and innovations.* New York: Wiley.

Rossi, E. L., & Cheek, D. B. (1988). *Mind-body therapy.* New York: Norton.

## 35

# Self-Care: Approaches
# from Self-Hypnosis for Utilizing
# Your Unconscious (Inner) Potentials

*Brian M. Alman*

Milton H. Erickson once said to me, "The patient's primary task is to develop their unconscious potential. Everyone is an individual in a process of development. Hypnosis is an experience in which people receive something from themselves. And all hypnosis is self-hypnosis."

Perhaps one of the greatest misunderstandings in the area of self-care, medicine, and psychology is how hypnosis works. Nobody has the power to hypnotize anyone. Only you have the power to hypnotize yourself or to be hypnotized by somebody else—the power is yours.

Are you teaching self-hypnosis to others? You may have already discovered that nearly everyone can learn how to utilize self-hypnosis to make specific changes within themselves: to stop unwanted habits, to manage pain, to reduce stress, to improve self-care. Perhaps you want to help people enhance their relationships at work and to develop their parenting skills, to improve athletic performance, to lose weight and be able to keep it off—even to grow into a healthy, positive self-understanding that improves everyday life in simple ways.

This chapter will help you learn to teach self-hypnosis, as well as provide you with explanations of how to develop your own capacity for self-hypnosis to help others and yourself reach goals.

## Who Can Benefit From Self-Hypnosis?

Self-hypnosis utilizes each individual's belief system and perceptions of his or her own experiences. Dr. Erickson pioneered the idea of integrating each person's unique inner process with suggestions that enhance everyday life and help the person attain his or her personal objectives. His perspective was that self-hypnosis was most likely to be successful if the experiences were bundled with images, symbols, and words to which the individual could relate. He repeatedly reminded the professionals he was training that in order to be an effective teacher of self-hypnosis, above all, one must be a fine observer who can recognize the limitations that bind human potentials. He also encouraged us to make available the means of freeing and facilitating human development. Finally, he suggested that we stand aside to observe, listen, and wonder about its ultimate course.

Dr. Erickson made it very clear that when working with hypnosis, one of our most important responsibilities is to teach individuals self-hypnosis so that they continue in their everyday life to gain self-mastery.

## What Is Self-Hypnosis?

Everyone experiences states of being completely absorbed in an activity—perhaps listening to music, or reading a book—and not noticing what is going on around them. These are self-hypnosis-like experiences. The main difference between them and actual self-hypnosis are the latter's specific motivation and suggestions toward a goal. Self-hypnosis guides you toward a desired result, such as relaxation or pain control.

Self-hypnosis is not a form of sleep, although people practicing the technique often appear to be asleep. Neither are they in their average waking states although they are feeling active within themselves. The experience of self-hypnosis is most similar to daydreaming in that you are creating, relaxing, expressing, and moving inside yourself—although when daydreaming, if you wish to respond to someone talking to you, you can do so by shifting your attention.

To define self-hypnosis is difficult because everyone describes it differently. Most often, people learn self-hypnosis to help themselves integrate and utilize their mindbody potentials for better health and well-being—thus fulfilling their desire to enhance and complement traditional medicine in a scientifically established, safe, and cost-saving way.

Self-hypnosis is an experience of active learning on an unconscious (inner) level when the quality of a relationship (with yourself or someone you trust) is utilized to develop creatively what you already have. It can be defined as a relaxing mindbody interaction in which positive suggestions are responded to with a feeling of empowerment. The continuing suggestions and utilization of self-acceptance enhance self-care potentials. While practicing self-hypnosis, one relaxes the questioning mind and critical opinions. One's focus of attention is much clearer than if one were awake or asleep. During this heightened experience of awareness and acceptance, suggestions can stimulate the bubbling up of ideas from the unconscious mind. The secret of self-hypnosis is that it takes you to the unconscious, and as you nurture the seed of well-being in there, it can grow and blossom in the conscious mind—although the roots will remain in the unconscious. Trust is the foundation of self-hypnosis, which can pose a difficulty because many people do not trust themselves. They decide that tomorrow morning they will get up early, and even while deciding it, they know that it is not going to happen. So, often we need somebody else, someone we can trust, to teach us self-hypnosis. Unless you feel safe enough to cooperate, nobody can hypnotize you—not even yourself.

Unfortunately, most of Western culture has been influenced by Freud's incorrect explanation of the unconscious. He theorized that the unconscious was like a junkyard that the conscious mind uses to store unwanted thoughts, feelings, and memories. The conscious and subconscious minds make up the approximately 10% of ourselves in which we function most of the time. However, Freud confused the subconscious with the unconscious. Some people perhaps wonder whether, if Freud had done more of his own work, he would have realized that the subconscious is like the junkyard in which the conscious mind stores overwhelming stresses, whereas the unconscious is the 90% that we don't use enough and is filled with positive human potentials.

You might think of the conscious mind as the everyday, logical, and rational part of yourself—the part that repeatedly wants you to keep on doing what's familiar. The conscious mind is the part that has helped us survive by making sure that we learn from each experience. The center of the conscious mind is the ego. But the ego is so inflated that it is convinced that it is the center of all of a person instead of only 10%.

If you want to go beyond your conditioning, programming, upbringing, and animal instincts, you must tap into your unconscious mind. You can think of your unconscious mind as the creative, intuitive, and loving part of yourself. This is the part that wants you to see life as an adventure, to be open to new experiences, and to move toward a more total existence. The unconscious mind is about 90% of the mind. Its center is often called the inner voice. And the inner voice is fully aware that it has to be totally patient as you develop your potentials at your own pace. The more you use self-hypnosis, the more you will realize that your unconscious potentials only rise to your conscious mind when you carry out your self-care without judgment.

Most scientists and researchers who work in this area recognize that self-hypnosis has special qualities. In experiencing it, you can develop self-mastery that is normally out of reach of your conscious and subconscious minds. Dr. Erickson recognized that because of the considerable limitations of the conscious mind, the consciousness must be expanded (inner awareness heightened) by learning to relate optimally to the unconscious. For Erickson, this would mean allowing the unconscious to do its own work during self-hypnosis. Then, once the unconscious has done its work, the conscious mind can receive and focus it appropriately in the various moments and sets (circumstances) of life. He taught us that the unconscious is the manufacturer and the conscious is the consumer, and self-hypnosis is the bridge between them.

## All Hypnosis Is Really Self-Hypnosis

We all have the ultimate power to decide how relaxed we want to feel and how open we want to be. Self-hypnosis requires patience. There is no need to go on repeating words or describing images because that becomes a disturbance. You simply let them pass by as if you were watching clouds coming and going. This way, the things that may have distracted or bothered you in the past can actually enhance your experience. A moment will come when all those images will be gone, and for a time, you have invited your unconscious experiences to come to the surface. When you have become capable of this, you are totally your own master. Your self-hypnosis can make you feel relaxed and peaceful.

### When Stage Hypnosis Is the First Impression

Most people learn about hypnosis from watching or hearing about a stage performance. Unfortunately, stage hypnosis perpetuates the myth that during hypnosis, a person gives his or her control to the one who is performing the hypnosis, and will do things that he or she otherwise would not do.

However, when you watch stage hypnotists, you should recognize that they are using tricks to entertain an audience and to deceive people into believing that under hypnosis, one loses the power of volition. They tell volunteers to do something unusual to meet the expectations of the audience; that if they do such things, they will be doing them under hypnosis and so will not be responsible for their own actions; to expect applause and laughter from the audience; and, finally, not to spoil the show.

When you first teach someone self-hypnosis, you may have to cope with an attitude that includes such negative impressions. This issue needs to be discussed before you begin because you want to assure people that they will not do anything that they don't want to do. The truth is that they are totally in control at all times. In more than 20 years of teaching self-hypnosis to thousands of individuals, I have become convinced that when people learn to let go of some control, they gain an even greater control. The unconscious mind protects and cares for us while we are awake, dreaming, relaxing, meditating, and sleeping, and can be supported by our self-hypnosis experiences.

## THE JOURNEY TO SELF-HYPNOSIS

### Selecting a Place in Which to Learn

Some people can relax practically anywhere. Relaxation is a key to self-hypnosis. As you learn how to experience stillness and peacefulness, you can maximize your receptiveness to positive suggestions and the potentials of your unconscious.

Seek out the quietest, most special place you can find. Most important, the place should be as safe, as comfortable, and as free from interruptions as possible. Schedule your self-care time, in which you use self-hypnosis, for as long as it takes you to relax and work on a goal. Usually, people give themselves five minutes to an hour.

Remember, things happen first on the inside and then on the outside. So, pay as much attention to creating a peaceful inner atmosphere (how you are feeling) as you do to the outside environment.

## Opening the Doors to Self-Hypnosis with
## Healthy Breathing and Relaxation

The breathing techniques that I teach to help with self-hypnosis are not about a special system or a particular rhythm. They are about taking breathing as it is. During self-hypnosis, you learn how to accept all the different parts of yourself, and yourself as a whole person, and so the breathing techniques mirror what you are developing within yourself. All you have to do is become aware of certain points in your breathing.

Breathing is the bridge to relaxation, awareness, and self-hypnosis. You can always tell how open or how closed you are by getting in tune with your breathing. In other words, if your breathing is rough and shallow, then you are probably moving tightly and are stressed. On the other hand, if your breathing is full and from your belly, then you are probably feeling open and relaxed.

Your breathing is constantly connecting and relating you to your inner experiences. If you just learn the techniques of breathing, your life will be healthier and you will feel stronger, more filled with energy, more vital, and more alive.

### Awareness and Breathing Technique

Create an opportunity to refresh yourself with this breathing technique whenever you want to relax and begin or complete a self-hypnosis session. Simply focus all of your attention on each breath. With your eyes closed or open, put your hands on your belly as you fix your attention on the movements in your body as you inhale and exhale. Do this for about a minute to slow yourself down and experience your breathing as a continuous flow through any thoughts, feelings, or images.

Then give your attention to the turning points, which are the moments when your inhalation becomes an exhalation and vice versa. Continue this for two or three minutes, or more. By watching and feeling the turning points and giving them your total attention, something magical begins to happen. Experiment. Cooperate. Develop a friendly and relaxing attitude toward your breathing and your whole self. Just be aware of the turning points. It may be helpful to imagine the waves at the beach. The waves roll in and out constantly. So do your breaths. Enjoy and feel the movement—enjoy relaxing breathing many times during each day.

### Self-Hypnosis and Meditation

Most of the techniques of meditation are similar to those of self-hypnosis. The paths are the same but their directions are different: They both begin with a focusing of attention and relaxation, such as breathing and imagery. There is a quieting inside and a refocusing of yourself to your experiences within (thoughts, feelings, imagery, body language). They are linked by the utilization of an observer perspective, which is often included in early learning experiences.

So, the entrances to self-hypnosis and meditation are very similar; the fundamental difference is what you do with them. In meditation, the goal is awareness. In self-hypnosis, you decide on the goal, which can be anything from awareness to pain control to sports performance, to weight loss and maintenance, and the list goes on. Their ways are similar, but what you do within your quiet, empowering relaxation is where they part from each other. There is no need to choose among meditation, relaxation, and self-hypnosis. They are complementary, not contradictory.

## How to Deal with Distractions

Utilize all the sounds outside, as well as all the thoughts and feelings inside, to go deeper into your self-hypnosis experience. Consider them and let them go. If a plane flies by, imagine putting all of your stresses into the baggage compartment. When you hear a dog barking, imagine a beautiful park where all the dogs run free and where you are relaxing on a rock by the lake. When you feel a worry building up inside, imagine that you are watching clouds in the sky and that all of your worries are also temporary, just like the clouds. If you are thinking too much, imagine a train that is going down the tracks. Then imagine yourself getting off the train and sitting on a hill, watching your thoughts go by like the train. As you learn to watch your own thoughts and your ego, a profound level of relaxation results instead of the usual tensions that come with overidentifying with your ego.

Accept the distractions. Be aware of them, too. Express the feelings you have about them within yourself, watch them turn into pleasing situations, and then let them go. Be relaxed and friendly toward all the distractions and utilize them as opportunities to help you go deeper.

## Increase Your Motivation to Reach Your Goals

There's a saying, "The definition of an adult is somebody who does something even though they know they're supposed to." Most people know what they need to do to be happier and healthier, but few actually do it. This is true of losing and keeping weight off, quitting smoking, improving relationships, dealing effectively with stress, exercising, and many other challenges. Some experts say all you need to do is find the right button (the motivating factor for each person). Others say that if you find out what caused the problem, it will disappear. Still others say that if you show people more effective ways of living, they will learn. There are many theories about what helps people change. But the how-to's seem always to come back to the same point: For long-term and successful changes, the process must be customized to fit each individual's unconscious resources and potentials. And relationships motivate people, including our relationship with ourself. Clearly, self-hypnosis can be that bridge from old forms of self-care to the new skills of self-care. It's simply a matter of devotion and patience in learning how to take better care of yourself. As Dr. Erickson taught, change not only is possible, it's inevitable.

## THE POWER OF POSTHYPNOTIC
## SUGGESTIONS AND CUES

A posthypnotic suggestion is a suggestion given, while the individual is practicing with self-hypnosis, for an action or other response to take place during the course of everyday life. During self-hypnosis, your unconscious mind understands your intent. This develops easily over time as you learn to have more trust in yourself.

Posthypnotic cues are any thoughts, actions, words, images, symbols, or events that initiate or trigger your posthypnotic suggestion. For example, the sound of the train that passes your house can become the cue to remind you to take a deep, satisfying breath and relax. The posthypnotic suggestion was seeded during a previous self-hypnosis session.

According to Dr. Erickson, the most important posthypnotic suggestion relates to being able to reinstate the self-hypnosis experience whenever and wherever we wish. Once you recognize the power of this self-care tool, you can feel calmer and more relaxed any time you choose.

Posthypnotic suggestions and cues are a powerful extension of your self-hypnosis work. They enhance your abilities to change or improve your actions and feelings at will, not just while you are practicing self-hypnosis. It's often helpful to give a variety of posthypnotic suggestions and cues in order to maximize the likelihood of success.

## How to Utilize Imagery and Positive Visualization

Aristotle said, "The soul never thinks without a picture." But there is more to imagery than just visualization. You have five senses plus a sixth sense, intuition, and your sense of humor. That's seven senses that can help you with your imagery, positive intentions, and self-hypnosis.

All of us enjoy some sort of imagery, but we have varying degrees of experience and skill. Here is a process that can help you develop your imagery skills (spend one minute or more on each of the following steps).

1. Gaze at an object and observe it as if you have never seen it before (look at the details, size, parts, the whole, dimensions, location, colors): *be your eyes.*

2. Listen to all the sounds around you (inside and outside, your breathing, and all the sounds that may have distracted you before, but can now become part of your experience): *be your ears.*

3. Feel all the feelings that you can be aware of from your toes to the top of your head, and let the tensions rise up from your feet to the top of your head (accept the tensions, the posture of your feet, legs, back, neck and head—without judgment, criticism, or filtering): *be your feelings.*

4. Smell all the fragrances in your environment (the time of day, the season, even life itself is said to have a fragrance): *be your nose.*

5. Taste all the tastes in your mouth, lick your lips, move your tongue around and taste (something you ate or drank earlier, the moisture, the dryness): *be your tastebuds.*

6. Allow your intuition to come to the surface (accept all images, feelings that are light and easy, decisions that come from rising above a situation and allow you to see everything with different eyes): *be your highest self.*

7. Giggle a little with yourself (about the awkwardness of learning something new, the silliness of giving your attention to your senses, amused at any resistances that are arising): *be your funny, light self.*

8. Now be open to all of your seven senses for at least a few minutes (one at a time, two at a time, or all seven at the same time): *be your whole self.*

What makes this imagery so powerful is that it comes from within you.

You have created it. You are using the language of your unconscious to be open, to relax, and to create positive changes.

### Results and Process Imagery

You can utilize your imagery to work toward specific goals. One approach is to use the imagery techniques to jump forward into the experience of having achieved your goal. This result imagery is the process of imagining yourself and your life situation as it can be once your goal has been accomplished. The process imagery is when you imagine the many steps that may be needed to reach that goal. During these experiences, you are seeding posthypnotic suggestions and cues. For example, if you wanted to lose weight, you would follow these three steps:

1.  Develop your self-hypnosis experiences with breathing, relaxation, and imagery techniques. Be comfortable inside and out. Keep your eyes closed and yet feel totally open within. Give yourself the time you need each day (even five minutes) to be total in your devotion to achieving inner and outer success.

2.  Results imagery: Utilize the openness of your self-hypnosis experience to imagine with all seven of your senses what you will feel like when you weigh and look the way you want. Be specific about how your clothes fit, exercising easily, socializing with confidence, and being unconditionally accepting when you're by yourself. Imagine yourself totally free of the old, unwanted problem and in the flow with your self-care, inside and out. You can create such posthypnotic suggestions as watching the sunset and feeling satisfied in all ways, just as every sunset will be an opportunity to accept change.

3.  Process imagery: Utilize the openness of your self-hypnosis experience to imagine with all seven of your senses each of the steps that you may need to take in order to reach your goal of weight loss and weight-loss maintenance. Be specific about the movements you need to make. For example, use your senses to be present and proactive on your journey into self-discovery and self-improvement. Remember to practice breathing more slowly, eating more slowly, and evolving at your pace. Imagine first (in your self-hypnosis) how you want to rest each night and even what you want to dream about. Another step may be to offer yourself

posthypnotic suggestions on waking up in the morning relaxed
and confident about your desire to lose weight and keep it off.
Next, you can use all seven senses to rehearse walking; eating
lunch, dinner, and snacks; self-hypnosis; and letting go of tensions
with every exhalation.

This is only one of many self-hypnosis approaches for weight loss, but
you will find that if you practice it every day, you will feel a subtle
change within seven days; you can feel your self-care improving. Then try
another experiment. Take the same five or ten minutes every day to begin
your self-hypnosis experience and, in addition to utilizing your senses and
posthypnotic suggestions, integrate this mindbody communication and repeat these phrases: "Thank you for working so well for me all these
years. I'm sorry if I've been ignoring you. If there's anything you're trying to tell me, I'm totally open right now." Repeat this for the same
amount of time you practiced self-hypnosis for the first week. You will
find that self-hypnosis is an invaluable tool for self-care. As Dr. Erickson
might add, "You'll be pleasantly surprised to find out that your unconscious mind is even smarter than you are."

## FURTHER TECHNIQUES FOR ENTERING
## INTO SELF-HYPNOSIS

Learning self-hypnosis and self-care approaches is rather like learning the
ABCs, learning to ride a bicycle, learning to type, or being in a healthy
relationship. It takes devotion and patience, but the benefits are enormous
and can positively affect everything you do. And it can work for everyone.
First, begin your self-hypnosis with your breathing and relaxation
techniques. The following techniques demonstrate what it feels like to
experience this self-caring opportunity to create positive changes.

1.    Counting for going deeply and naturally into self-care experiences:
      Self-hypnosis is a very soft method, like mellow music. It can hap-
      pen when you are just sitting quietly in silence. It can happen just
      by listening to someone so intently that all your worries and ten-
      sions disappear. As this happens, you naturally start moving
      deeper into yourself.
         Write down how long you would like to spend practicing self-

hypnosis. Choose five minutes or whatever you wish. Then write down your goal. This may be to reinstate self-hypnosis later on or to be more relaxed during a presentation at work or to control pain. In a minute, begin counting to yourself from zero up to 100 and then back down from 100 to zero. After you finish with the counting, just stay within yourself for the remaining time. The time you spend after finishing the counting and just being is the self-hypnosis experience. When you finish your practice session, repeat it twice more in the same day. After one week of doing it three times a day, you will be enjoying the experience of self-hypnosis.

2. Relaxing: Focus your conscious mind on a spot on the wall. Don't be concerned with anything else in the room or outside. Lie down or sit down to be the most relaxed you can. Be open to trusting the person in whom you already have or want to have total trust—yourself. This is a most important message because the conscious mind will not relax unless there is trust. It will keep itself alert because it wants to guarantee you are safe. As you become more comfortable and are relaxing, give your attention to your body, starting with your toes. If there is any tension near the foot, or near the knee, or the stomach, or anywhere else, relax it by touching the area with one of your hands and saying, "Please relax." You can say this silently or quietly and directly to that part of your body with any tension. Continue this until you've gone through your entire body. Bring the relaxation up to your head—and keep your eyes focused on the spot on the wall. It's easy to recognize when you are at the border between your conscious and your unconscious: your face changes; it feels and looks sleepy, relaxed and calm, and at that moment you know deep inside yourself that relaxation and self-hypnosis are like being in the middle of a sunset or a colorful sunrise. In the outer world, the moments of dusk and dawn are magical, transforming, and happen every day.

Similarly, in your own inner world, you can create the experience of self-hypnosis whenever you wish, and thus you design your own inspirations and changes, mirroring the potentials of nature in action. You express to yourself in words: "Dreams are coming ... calming dreams are coming ... I am flowing into a restfulness I have rarely flowed into before." This may go on for two, three, or, at most, five minutes, and then your eyes start wanting to close. That means you are crossing the border. And you say within yourself, "I am flowing into dreams and I will count up to seven. With each number I will be going deeper into dreaming." And you start counting, "One ..." and go on repeating, "The dream is becoming deeper. Two ... the dream is becoming deeper. Three ..." And at seven, you stop and say, "I have slowed into a dreamy consciousness. Now I will be available to myself and nobody else or anything else. Now the only communication with the world is through me, myself, and I only need to hear me and answer to me ..." You settle into your experience. Then, after a few seconds, begin describing to yourself in detail where you are. Perhaps you are on a journey through time, perhaps you are somewhere beautiful that you have never seen before, perhaps you are by yourself or with others doing something you truly enjoy. And answer yourself in detail describing where you are. This can be tape-recorded so that you can listen to it whenever you want.

The process has to be repeated many times because this is the proof; your unconscious will continually create dreams for you that will help you understand yourself in important ways. You will be learning how to be a fine observer and the master of your human development. Then you can wisely observe and wonder about your ultimate course. Perhaps the most important message about your self-hypnosis and the positive changes you are working on in your life is that the journey itself is the goal.

3.   Adding more light to your path: Close off your room from outside things as much as possible. Turn off the lights, close the curtains, and make it completely dark. Light a small candle so that it is in front of your eyes. Then, without blinking, stare at the flame and just go on thinking you are drifting into a dream, you are dreaming. A dreamy relaxation will arise within you—just let this thought be floating within (as you go on staring at the candle and letting this thought be there as a puffy white cloud hovering over you). You are flowing into dreaming, you are becoming your dream. When you do it, you say within yourself, "I am flowing into a dream. Dreaming is approaching. My limbs are relaxing." You will immediately feel a subtle change, and within

three minutes, you can feel that your body has become more relaxed. Any moment you can flow into your dream. The lids of your eyes get heavy and it becomes very difficult to keep on staring at the flame. Your eyes want to close. Everything becomes relaxed and heavy. Now, you can feel what self-hypnosis is like; being more dreamy, falling into a safe unconscious awareness and becoming very comfortable within yourself. Feel the movement. Feel what is happening. Within seven days, you will come to a point where you will feel more relaxed and in harmony with yourself, as your relaxing breaths become a continuous part of your experience.

You will know whether you have succeeded when you notice how much easier it is to relax: when your body feels warm, light, and calmer during your self-hypnosis, and in your everyday life, when you stop caring about how much time passes when you are giving yourself opportunities for self-care, when your mind feels clearer, when you feel you can count on yourself more often, and when you feel more able to participate in self-development. So, whatever your goals may be, remember that things happen first on the inside, and then on the outside.

## THE MOST IMPORTANT SELF-HYPNOSIS TECHNIQUE FOR CREATING CHANGE

The self-hypnosis approach that I recommend for working with conscious, subconscious, or unconscious resistance is as follows: Write on a piece of paper the issue that you are working on right now. Then write down and encircle one word or one phrase describing how you feel about that issue. For example, you might write "frustrated" in the circle. Then, you might write the word "confused" in a second circle. Then, you might write "hopeful" in a third circle. Keep going until you have as many circles as you have feelings, or thoughts, or concerns about your problem. Finally, write the word "observer" at the top of the paper. At this point, you are almost ready to begin your self-hypnosis experience. This will be different from your previous experiences in a number of ways: (1) you'll be spending from 30 to 60 minutes completing it; (2) you'll be writing with your eyes closed and with your nondominant hand, if you wish; (3) you'll be keeping your eyes closed most of the time and opening them very briefly, as needed, to read the feeling that you wrote in each of the circles; and (4) you'll be coming up with solutions during the self-hypnosis experience that will help you immediately and in the future.

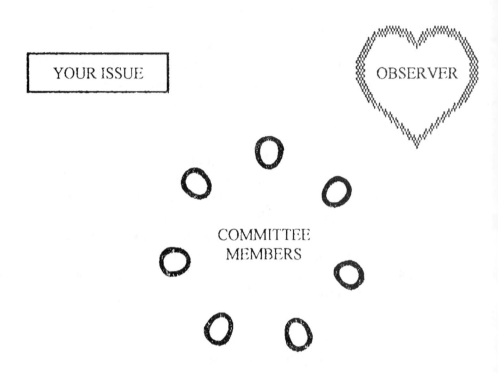

This approach will be carried out in six steps.

1. Write your issue on a sheet of paper.
2. Write down—in a word or phrase—how you feel about your issue (I call these committee members).
3. Write down how you experience your observer perspective (I call this the chairperson or inner voice).
4. Utilize breathing and relaxation techniques.
5. Write, with your eyes closed, everything each of your committee members feels about the issue (with your dominant hand and with your nondominant hand). The intention here is to accept and express each committee member's feelings without any judgment or desire to change.

6. After each one of your committee members has expressed itself totally and with a feeling of openness and acceptance, then, from your observer perspective, you will be able to come up with your best solution to the issue.

After you've completed steps 1 and 2, you are ready to move on to step 3 (the most important step). Next, adjacent to the word "observer," create your version of the observer perspective. Close your eyes and do the following. You may draw a hill or a mountain, or an airplane, or a deck or a balcony, or anything that would give you the experience of watching and observing from a comfortable distance. With your eyes still closed, write with your dominant hand a description of what it's like to be observing things from a safe and comfortable perspective. Go back and forth between your dominant and nondominant hands, drawing and writing whatever you wish about your experience as the observer. Take your time, because this is going to be very useful now, and probably for the rest of your life in the areas of self-care and self-hypnosis. You can never practice it too often.

Be intelligent, diligent, and open with all of your self-hypnosis committee work because you will soon discover that most people stay stuck in their committees. Very few ever learn what you are learning now, and during any attempt to resolve their own issues, they bounce from one committee member to another. And whichever has the biggest mouth wins. Other people are so cool and removed that they get stuck in the observer. But you are learning how to be whole and healthy, and total with this approach, to be accepting and open as you express your committee members (feelings), and then move into the perspective of the observer in order to resolve any issue to the best of your potential. You may think of this as the bridge between your conscious and unconscious minds.

When you're ready for step 4, you can begin your breathing, relaxation, and imagery. Do this until you feel relaxed and open within yourself.

The fifth step is to begin writing, with your eyes closed, how each of your committee members feels about the issue which which you are dealing. It's very important to always know that if you want to slow down or stop, simply go back to your observer perspective and look down on things from a safe perspective. This will give you the self-mastery you need to enter or exit the committee meeting whenever you wish. You can picture a committee meeting as a circle of friends sitting around expressing themselves, one at a time, with the observer looking down from the hill with compassion and open to giving you the best resolution possible after hearing from everyone. The hearing is actually the writing that you are doing for each one.

My experience in teaching this technique is that we don't get rid of any of our committee members. They've been with us for years, trying to help us cope with our issues the best we could. Plus, we wouldn't want to get rid of them because each has an opposite side that can be very good to know. Once you learn how to be aware and accept which committee member needs to express itself, then when you go to the observer perspective, you'll be able to enjoy your own best solutions every day and wherever you go.

The sixth and final step comes after you've expressed each committee member's feelings with your dominant and nondominant hands. Then you imagine yourself as the observer, and you are relaxed and friendly with all of the committee members. From the observer perspective, you are ready to write down your best solution to the issue that troubles you. It may help to read all of the committee members' feelings, or you may remember them. Most important, after expressing the feelings, move up to the observer and, with your eyes closed, and with your dominant and nondominant hands, write down your best solution to the problem. You can utilize this self-hypnosis problem-solving approach with any issue and you can learn to do it without paper, in your mind. Without question, you will be pleasantly surprised at yourself!

We are all capable of different emotions. They come and they go, like clouds in the sky. We do not get rid of our emotions and committee members. You could waste a lot of time, even a lifetime, trying not to feel something or trying to suppress feelings you don't want to have. The solution is to accept those feelings, express them, and then go to your observer perspective and come up with your own best solution(s).

If you've wondered where your self-sabotaging comes from, or your addictive self, or your sexually frustrated self, or your need to run away from things, these are all committee members. The people you read about who do cruel or crazy things are people who are stuck in committee. We all have crazy, and even cruel, parts of ourselves—and suppression of these parts makes them stronger. Trying not to feel them makes them more difficult to manage. The solution is acceptance, expression, and your own best solution from your observer perspective. Naturally, the healthier our self-care becomes, the more manageable our committee members are, and they actually become positive, helpful aspects of our daily lives.

### BASIC STEPS IN LEARNING TO TEACH SELF-HYPNOSIS

- Study Milton Erickson's utilization strategies.
- Study Dr. Erickson's approaches that emphasize individualizing the techniques to fit the person.
- Continue learning about different relaxation, meditation, self-care, and self-hypnosis techniques for experiencing peace.
- Continue practicing the approaches described in this chapter so that you can teach from your experience as you encourage the people with whom you work to gain knowledge from their own experiences.

---

**How to Utilize Self-Hypnosis**

- Relax yourself with self-hypnosis for moments every day.
- Focus your attention on your breathing as a posthypnotic cue to re-instate your relaxation and self-hypnosis.
- Develop your ability to be the observer of your moods, your thoughts, and your body.
- Hold "committee meetings" whenever you need to problem-solve.
- Continue developing unconditional acceptance of yourself and others.
- Enjoy the present with a positive view of the future.
- Remember, the journey itself is the goal.

---

### Suggested Readings

Alman, B. (1994). *Thin meditations.* San Diego: International Health Publications.

Alman, B. (1996). *The six steps to freedom.* San Diego: International Health Publications.

Alman, B., & Lambrou. (1992). *Self-hypnosis.* New York: Brunner/Mazel.

Erickson, M. H. (1967). In J. Haley (Ed.), *Advanced techniques of hypnosis and therapy.* New York: Grune & Stratton.

Erickson, M. H. (1983). In E. L. Rossi, M. O. Ryan, & F. A. Sharp (Eds.), *Healing in hypnosis* (Vol. 1). New York: Irvington.

Erickson, M. H. (1989). *The February man*. New York: Brunner/Mazel.

Erickson, M. H., Rossi, E., & Rossi, S. (1976). *Hypnotic realities*. New York: Irvington.

# 36

# Utilization of the Relationship in Hypnotherapy[1]

*Dirk Revenstorf*

## LEVELS OF HYPNOTIC TRANCE

Cognitive changes take place in different states of trance. Some of these cognitive changes are *active* processes, such as waking, imagery, and search processes to retrieve memories that are related to the problem in some way. Others are *receptive* processes, such as scanning suggestions without evaluating them critically. Moreover, nonspecific healing may take place when the individual responds in a holistic and adaptive way to an unstructured, perhaps even nonverbally induced, trance experience. Finally, sometimes the individual feels overwhelmed by suggestions that contradict his or her values and so may become *passive resistant*. Even this state can be utilized to facilitate trance experiences and create solutions.

To understand hypnotherapy, it is helpful to distinguish among several aspects of trance, some of which are related to one another, hierarchically, that is, they are based on one another (Hall, 1989).

[1] The author wishes to thank Carmela Latham and Isa Zalaman for reading this chapter and helping with the translation.

1.  *Physiological relaxation* may be induced by tape, autogenic train-
    ing, or meditation. A therapist is not necessary. Relaxation can
    lead to a harmonious internal state with positive effects on the im-
    mune system and, therefore, is healthy in and of itself.
2.  *Focusing* on a specific stimulus (e.g., visual fixation) or theme
    causes dissociation from other parts of the environment. If the fo-
    cus is internal, the images are usually more vivid than in a normal
    state of wakefulness.
3.  *Regression* easily occurs because of the pronounced asymmetry of
    the roles of therapist and patient. The therapist speaks in the em-
    pathic manner of a mother and with the suggestive authority of a
    father, while the patient typically says nothing for a long time.
    Therefore, the patient can easily project a parental figure onto the
    therapist. In this transference situation, he or she gives up control
    to the therapist and becomes more childlike; that is, more suggest-
    ible, flexible, and fantasy-prone.
4.  *Transcendental* activation is possible when the patient partially
    leaves superego and ego-control functions to the therapist, thereby
    activating dissociated parts of the personality that transcend every-
    day consciousness. These may be traumatic situations or unac-
    cepted parts of the personality, such as the shadow or animus/
    anima described by Jung.
5.  *Transpersonal* activation refers to the fact that the patient becomes
    aware of contents that are not based on direct personal experi-
    ence, but on the unconscious collective knowledge (archetypes)
    that, according to Jung, each individual possesses.

That last point might sound somewhat mysterious and could be clarified by a case example.

The girlfriend of a 32-year-old man with Hodgkin's disease asked
him to marry her. He was undecided as to whether or not he
should accept. He was not sure that he should burden his girlfriend
with a such a seriously ill husband. On the other hand, he was uncertain whether or not he would be able to find another girlfriend
after recovery. In trance he was asked to visualize an inner counsel-
or whom he could ask for guidance. He visualized an old man with
a bishop's crosier. The patient said he could not relate to this

image, because he was an atheist. Neither he nor the therapist could make sense of this image. However, during the following night he dreamed of the same image again. The next day, while discussing the dream the patient had the idea that this was the Apostle Peter, who became the first pope. Peter, of course, was the man who doubted Jesus ("Before the cock crows you will deny me three times"). At the same time, Peter was the rock on which the Christian church was later founded. With this wisdom, the patient decided to marry his girlfriend immediately.

Most important is that the therapist must be aware of the transference that can occur in hypnosis as a result of the patient's rapid regression. A transference may take various forms. During hypnosis, the patient may project onto the therapist a loving parent, an authority figure, a person with magical powers, or a superego-like moral figure. According to Roustang (cited in Zindel, 1996), a distinction must be made between the induction phase and the trance state itself. Transference takes place only during induction, whereas a genuinely close relationship between the patient and therapist is established during trance. Moreover, by using the patient's regressive mechanisms, the therapist can become a potent agent of change—by suggesting behavior and attitude changes (direct suggestion), by helping the patient to overcome failures in relational experiences in the past (e.g., by not making the patient feel helpless when he or she abandons control), and by correcting false indoctrinations, such as missing or ambiguous values not adequately conveyed by the parents. The therapist also may serve as a role model for the patient, who can participate in the therapist's projected abilities. Such projections may include erotic components, which should not be misinterpreted.

The therapist should be aware of the possibility of negative projections, such as fear, masochistic submission, and passive-aggressive resistance, that arise when, for example, the patient is unable to enter trance or to come out of trance. Both situations necessitate special interventions by the therapist.

## DECISIONS IN SOLUTION-ORIENTED HYPNOTHERAPY

### Symptom-Oriented Treatment

The therapist has to decide on the treatment that will be most efficient in the case of a particular symptom. For one thing, he or she has to ascertain whether or not secondary gain is an important factor in maintaining a symptom. If this is not the case, the therapist may proceed and treat the problem on the symptom level. This means facilitating change in such somatic phenomena as pain, warts, herpes, or circulatory problems (e.g., Renaud's syndrome) by using specific visualization techniques that promote relevant healing processes. For example, the patient may imagine activating the immune system by having his or her leukocytes approach the infection site.

## Conflict-Oriented Treatment

The procedure is different when the symptom seems to serve a psychological function—be it primary gain, secondary gain, or a well-established interactional style that makes the individual feel at home in a social setting. The patient may have chronic pain, for example, originating from an accident, which was later compounded with shame, guilt, or anger also originating from the accident. If the patient had no way of expressing these feelings, he or she may now express them through pain. The same may be true of hysterical paralysis. In these cases, hypnotherapy can uncover the original trauma or conflict and provide a solution, such as adding something by hypnotic reconstruction that was lacking in reality. This may be a fantasy in which some of the anger, sadness, or whatever emotion was blocked at the time of the traumatic event is released. It may also be a reframing of a seemingly overwhelming situation by adding self-comments, comments from the adult self or by a respected third party.

## Explicit Procedure

Whether treating the symptom or the conflict, the hypnotherapist has to decide whether or not there is some explicit procedure that can be used to reach the desired treatment objective. For example, a phobia may be treated on the symptom level by reassociating a resource; that is, by recalling a memory, which enables the patient to cope with the phobic situation. This can be done by utilizing a technique called "collapsing anchors," a procedure similar to desensitization. Or the treatment may proceed on the conflict level: flashbacks of a traumatic scene that cause the phobic response may be treated by reactivating the traumatic event and then by ameliorating the emotional impact through the implementation of corrective reconstruction. For example, a woman who, as a child, was abused by her grandfather in a chicken coop invented the following hypnotic fantasy while reconstructing this event. She visualized her grandfather as exposing his genitals to her in the chicken coop while her grandmother stabbed him with a pitchfork.

## Implicit Procedure

In some cases, no clear-cut goals or procedures are available. For instance, when confronted with decision-making problems ("Shall I quit smoking or not?"), or poorly understood healing processes (e.g., in a reactive depression or cancer), the therapist may resort to the unconscious wisdom of the patient. There are two approaches that might be utilized: divergent and convergent. In the divergent approach, the therapist uses metaphors, which initiate internal search processes. For example, the metamorphosis of an insect from caterpillar to pupa to a butterfly may be described to an overweight person. The way in which he or she uses this image is left to the patient's unconscious information processing. The precise effect of the metaphor is unknown to the therapist, but it most likely launches associative thought processes in the patient, which may be followed by an attitude or behavior change. The effectiveness of metaphors depends to a large extent on the preparedness of the patient and his or her state of heightened receptivity, which the therapist provides by trance induction.

In a convergent approach to the problem, the patient might be guided to use his or her tacit knowledge by means of ideomotoric movements. For example, the patient may be asked a number of questions concerning information relevant to the problem using Rossi's "hand approach" technique. Table 36.1 summarizes these strategy options.

## ANALYSIS OF THE RELATIONSHIP

The most distinct feature of hypnotherapy is its combination of solution-oriented and relation-oriented approaches. As mentioned, hypnotherapy establishes a strong transference situation in which the patient is allowed to project various paternal and maternal aspects onto the therapist. The projection also may be of an abusive figure, and thereby cause negative transference and reactivate traumatic experiences (as sometimes unwittingly happens in stage hypnosis). The therapist must be aware of this possibility and take proper precautions.

---

**Table 36.1**
**Intervention Decisions**

---

**A. Strategies**

Symptom-oriented (e.g., eliminating pain, warts)

or

Function-oriented (e.g., uncovering the traumatic cause of chronic pain)

**B. Form**

Explicit-direct (structured procedure)

or

Implicit-indirect:

Metaphoric-suggestive (giving analogous information)

or

Using tacit knowledge (asking the unconscious)

**C. Tactics**

1.  Imagining a healing process (e.g., blood flowing to warts).
2.  Dissociation (e.g., changing sensations of pain).
3.  Association (e.g., offering a resource for a phobic situation).
4.  Reframing (e.g., giving new meaning to a symptom).
5.  Reconstruction (e.g., "editing" a trauma).
6.  Initiating internal search (e.g., by anecdotes).
7.  Direct suggestions of change.

---

When negative transference or resistance is expected, the therapist may use a trance induction as proposed by Zindel (1996). Zindel suggests to the patient that his or her arm has to learn to levitate. Like a child who needs the help of a parent in order to learn how to stand, the arm (child) needs the help of the voluntary, conscious mind (parent) to learn to levitate. If the parent provides too much help, the child will never have the feeling that he or she accomplished anything by himself or herself and won't learn to be independent of the parent. The same is true regarding the arm and support by the conscious mind in the process of arm levitation. If the parent provides insufficient support, the child will not learn how to stand and consequently will give up. Therefore, the patient must gently reduce conscious support of the arm, until the arm finally supports itself. This procedure guides the patient to experience his or her resistance or overdependence, not in relation to the therapist, but between the arm and the conscious mind (as a parent). Thus, he or she can reactivate his or her own experience as a child and, at the same time, experience the parental response as well. The therapist is freed from negative transference and can act as the good parent, giving appropriate instructions to either lessen or heighten conscious support until the levitation succeeds.

On the relationship level, the therapist analyzes the interactional patterns the patient unconsciously tries to establish (R1 in Table 36.2). To achieve this, the therapist may use a variety of models: nonverbal styles, communication types, or character structure. In the *nonverbal style*, the therapist may begin by observing the preferred modes of perception used by the patient (visual, auditory, or tactile): whether his or her attentive processes are focused or diffuse; whether the patient is mostly a repressor, a sensitizer, or a container when expressing emotions; whether he or she prefers to give away or take over social control, is defiant, or compliant, and so on (Zeig, personal communication).

With regard to *communication type*, the therapist may begin by identifying which of four types of self-esteem regulation the patient shows, as proposed by Satir, who found that individuals may be distinguished by patterns of accusing, harmonizing, rationalizing, or diffusing in relationships. These communication categories are derived mostly from the observation of nonverbal behavior without direct questioning.

Another system the therapist can use to analyze interaction patterns involves the *character structures* elaborated on by Reich (1969), Pierrakos (1990), Kurtz (1983), and other body therapists. These character structures are largely based on the observation of body posture and provide such diagnoses as schizoid, oral (dependent and compensated), masochistic, psychopathic (seductive and aggressive), and rigid structures (phallic and hysteric). The therapist may also use the Axis II classification of personality disorders of the fourth edition of the *Diagnostic and Statistical Manual of Mental Disorders* (*DSM*-IV).

These observations may lead to pacing responses by the therapist. For example, a patient with a diffused attention style should not be forced to focus his or her attention. A patient who wants social control should be

### Table 36.2
### Two Levels of Communication
### in Hypnotherapy (General Scheme)

**Problem Presentation**

| Solution Level | Relation Level | |
|---|---|---|
| S1: Problem analysis | Interaction analysis (observation) | R1 |
| S2: Anamnesis (in trance) | Pacing Establishing rapport (indirect suggestion) | R2 |
| S3: Defining goal | Defining (observation) Developmental deficit | R3 |
| S4: Intervention (in trance) for change | Utilizing transference (in trance) | R4 |
| S5: Maintenance | Dissolving transference (in trance) | R5 |

**Termination of Therapy**

given choices. The defiant patient should receive a paradoxical suggestion ("You probably will not succeed immediately"). On the communication level, the therapist can pace the accusing type, for example, by being impressed by his or her critical capacity, or the rationalizer can be met in the factual arena, leaving his emotional vulnerability untouched. On the character level, the schizoid will be given secure distance but reliable contact, the oral dependent will be given support, the seductive psychopath can be given to understand that the therapist is charmed, and so on. By pacing the patient in this way, the therapist establishes rapport and facilitates regression and transference, while avoiding countertransference.

## HYPNOTHERAPY ON THE SOLUTION AND RELATION LEVELS

Being aware of transference patterns, the hypnotherapist may proceed on two levels, working toward mobilizing change in the patient. On the solution level, he or she may analyze the problem together with the patient (S1), take a history (S2), and define a goal (S3). The therapist then decides which type of hypnotherapeutic strategy (see Table 36.3) should be used (S4) and takes care that the patient is able to maintain behavioral changes (S5).

Table 36.3 shows an example of how these two levels of communication are interrelated. The patient is a 35-year-old woman presenting with dysparenuria, that is, pain and burning during sexual intercourse that are not attributable to lubrication. Her history reveals emotional abuse by men during her adolescence (S2): her father and elder brother frequently teased her about the size of her breasts, telling her that they were much too small to need a bra. She did not become submissive or depressed, but instead developed a hatred of men and unconsciously looked for opportunities for revenge. The case is somewhat analogous to the story of the princess Turandot. (Turandot condemned men to death when they didn't live up to her expectations. One of her ancestors had been raped by invading soldiers.) The patient engaged in many relationships, and after a time would despise her lover, find him boring, and refuse to have sexual intercourse. This left the men helpless and hurt. The therapeutic goal (S3) was to help her overcome her hatred of men. The intervention (S4) was a hypnotic reconstruction of her emotional abuse by her father and her brother.

The analysis of communication (R1) leads to an interactional diagnosis of a developmental deficit (R3). For example, the schizoid type suffered from a lack of relational stability; the oral type experienced emotional deprivation; the masochistic type felt unaccepted for his achievements; the psychopath was impeded in proper identity formation owing to overwhelming parental pressure; or the rigid type became obsessive/compulsive as a result of demands for achievement and lack of emotional bonding. On the basis of this personal history, individuals develop various coping mechanisms: the schizoid uses dissociative strategies; the oral-compensated type becomes undemanding whereas the oral dependent be-

**Table 36.3**
**Two Levels of Communication**
**in Hypnotherapy: A Case Example**

**Problem Presentation:** *Pain During Intercourse*

| Solution Level | Relation Level | |
|---|---|---|
| S1: Problem analysis<br>*Men become boring after*<br>*a while, loss of libido*<br>*(many partners).* | Interaction analysis<br>*Flirtatious–dominating.* | R1 |
| S2: Anamnesis<br>*Father and brother*<br>*humiliated her.* | Pacing<br>*Accept the flirtation;*<br>*Resist dominance.* | R2 |
| S3: Goal<br>*Overcoming hatred of men.* | Developmental deficit<br>*Seductive–psychopathic*<br>*(overcoming and avenging*<br>*male dominance).* | R3 |
| S4: Intervention<br>*Reconstruction of trauma*<br>*catharsis of affect.* | Utilizing transference<br>*Being a "good father."*<br>*Dominance without abuse*<br>*(during the trance).* | R4 |
| S5: Maintenance<br>*Revising present sexual*<br>*relationship.* | Dissolving transference<br>*Facilitating dominance*<br>*without contempt (by*<br>*metaphor in trance).* | R5 |

**Termination of Therapy**

comes overly demanding; the masochistic type endures; the psychopath utilizes aggressive and seductive tactics to overcome dependency; the rigid type avoids emotional contact.

In this case, during trance, the male therapist would deliver interventions aimed at solving the problem (S4). At the same time, he might use positive transference to help the patient to revise interactional schemata. Based on the assumption that the patient's presenting problem and communication style are two sides of the same coin, the therapist can shape the hypnotic interaction by allowing the patient to work on the solution while the therapist's behavior compensates for the patient's developmental deficits (R4). For instance, the therapist may introduce, in the voice of a benevolent (better) parent, the distinction between love and abuse to a patient who was an abused child. Or the therapist may create a surrogate parental figure in the patient's imagination, who nurtures the patient in such a way as to make up for what the patient missed during childhood. An example can be found in the case of Erickson's "February Man" (Erickson & Rossi, 1979).

On the interactional level, the therapist experiences flirtatious approaches by the patient (R1). He responds by enjoying them, but, at the same, time avoids becoming dependent on her approval, while maintaining interest (R2). When viewed as a developmental deficit, her behavior could be diagnosed as a seductive type of psychopathology, a coping strategy used by the patient to prevent feeling overwhelmed by men (R3). Utilizing the transference (R4), the therapist tries, both in and out of trance, to be a supportive and respectful father figure.

One intervention strategy on the relationship level was to ask her to experience a trance induction with her eyes open and to close them when she felt safe. To make further surrender possible, the therapist proposed that she turn her palms upward—but only if she really felt safe and was certain that she would not be abused. Once she had turned her palms upward, he proposed that she slide down in her seat—but only after she felt truly safe. This should enable her to tolerate a vulnerable position without needing to defend herself. To dissolve the transference (R5), the patient was given opportunities to resist the therapist's decisions. This was done in such a way that she could experience independence while still respecting the therapist, for example, by learning to terminate the trance state on her own.

The therapist uses his own emotional response to the patient's behavior to determine the type of relationship the patient is unconsciously trying to establish. Thus, he may recognize the character structure and sense the underlying emotional needs that resulted from developmental deficits. In order to use this information, the therapist must be able to distinguish between his own developmental deficits and those of the patient as the source of his response.[2]

## CASE TRANSCRIPT: THE INDEPENDENT SMOKER

In the following case, hypnotic communication on the two levels discussed is described in more detail. The patient, a 43-year-old physician, is married and has one child. He wants to quit smoking. Although he is not a heavy smoker (10–16 cigarettes per day), he finds his habit incompatible with his job as a health professional, and also complains about coughing. In addition, his wife wants him to quit. He smokes after breakfast, during lunch with colleagues, after work, and in the evening at home. He smokes primarily to reduce stress, to become more tranquil, and possibly to annoy his wife. The patient is a friendly and overtly cooperative man who is interested in using hypnosis.

The hypnotic intervention used was based on a procedure developed by Ulrich Freund (personal communication). Hand levitation was employed as a metaphor to demonstrate the independence of the patient's body and mind. The left hand was levitated first as a symbol of the patient's now being "half a nonsmoker" (as is done with those who hold their cigarettes in their right hands) and to represent health and the will to live. The mother–child projection method mentioned earlier was used in order to introduce the idea that the therapeutic goal of independence (as opposed to cigarette dependence) needs the caring support of the conscious mind. After levitating the nonsmoking hand, the therapist suggested to the smoking hand that it prove its independence as well. Because the levitation of the right hand was slow, the "resistance" method was used, in which the patient was asked to press the back of his hand upward against the tip of the therapist's index finger in order to achieve a balance of power between the two of them. Slowly, the therapist released the pressure, so that the patient involuntarily provided the necessary support to maintain the levitation by himself.

---

[2] The author wishes to thank Ria Schnell for an enlightening discussion of this point.

After the right-hand levitation was established, a cigarette was put between the patient's fingers with the suggestion that his fingers would release the cigarette involuntarily when he was unconsciously ready to stop smoking. During this time, the patient was given a number of common direct suggestions.

Smoking is good for you, but it is toxic for your body. You have to respect your body as long as you want to live. Your left hand represents your desire to live and be healthy and your right hand represents your desire to enjoy, relax, and communicate with others. And the left hand will extend the light feeling to the right hand, when your unconscious mind has a solution for how you can combine both wishes without smoking.

He also was given a series of embedded metaphors, as proposed by Lankton and Lankton (1989). These metaphors were:

1.  An anecdote was told about a woman who recalled during trance that she started smoking after her husband died in an accident (confusion metaphor).

    The prisoner Papillon on a rocky island was a metaphor for addictive behavior (pacing metaphor). Papillon observed that every seventh wave did not hit the rocks and, therefore, offered him a chance to escape from the island.

    There was an old Indian on the island, whom Papillon consulted (similar to the therapist, having some features in common). This was done to pace the dependency needs of the patient (resource metaphor).

    Papillon managed to escape from the prison (addiction) by waiting for the right time and having the support of the (Indian) consultant (solution metaphor).

2.  A story was told about an eagle that was raised as a chicken on a farm. Later a stranger visited the farm and taught the eagle to fly. After overcoming some resistance, he flew away, but who knows, perhaps in the end he will marry a chicken (maintenance metaphor with an element of humor to distract the patient from the previous stories).

The patient was diagnosed as a dependent personality. Therefore, after rapport had been established, he was given suggestions of independence (e.g., independence of the arm, independence in terminating trance, independence of the fingers in letting go of the cigarette, independence from the therapist's suggestions). The patient had a difficult time going into trance, but when reoriented after 45 minutes, he refused to come out. He was told to take his time and was informed that the therapist, after a while, would count to 100 to deepen the trance. (This was meant to provoke resistance and to help to terminate the trance in due time.) Without the therapist's intervening any further, the patient fell into a deep trance, levitating his right hand again, and finally dropping his cigarette without any suggestions. It was not a problem to reorient him (counting from 3 to 1) afterward.

In general, the trance was induced in such a way as to allow the patient to resist the induction, the suggestions, and the reorientation in order to do it on his own, enabling him to gain more independence. As a posthypnotic suggestion, the therapist proposed to the patient that he would remember the stiff feeling in his right hand as a sign of independence whenever he desired a peaceful state of mind. In terms of ratification, the patient reported that the left hand was numb, while the right hand felt as stiff as a board. He estimated that the first part of the trance had lasted 30 minutes, instead of 45, and that the last 15 minutes felt like 30 minutes. He remembered the stories only dimly, except for the first one. After the trance, he felt well, although a little tired. This was explained as being the result of all the mental work he had done.

The next day, he reported that he had smoked only half as much as usual. His homework was to practice one hand levitation per day after work with a cigarette in his right hand and to let a "stiff as a board" feeling develop in that hand. The therapist explained that he could check his hypnotic ability by using Spiegel's eye-roll test. Because the patient showed only the whites of his eyes shortly before his lids closed while the eyes were turned upwards, he proved to be a good hypnotic subject.

## DEVELOPMENTAL DEFICIT AND HYPNOTIC REPARENTING

The goal of this chapter is to discuss the idea of hypnotic interventions aimed at reparenting a patient with regard to his or her particular developmental deficit. According to bioenergetic theory, basic frustrations in early childhood make an individual vulnerable to certain types of stress. In order to protect himself or herself, the child generates specific responses which are usually called defenses. The resulting character structure or personality (disorder) can be described in terms of specific interactional schemes that govern one's social behavior in an often competent, but also restrictive, way. This character structure can be detected in the body posture, facial expression, and communication style exhibited by the individual.

While in a regressed state, presupposing a positive transference, the patient is receptive to the therapist's suggestions, which may supplement his or her interactional scheme. In order to create therapeutic suggestions, the therapist has to consider the patient's basic defense pattern, the typical response the patient creates in others (countertransference), and the resources provided by the specific character structures predominantly shown by the patient. On the basis of this information, the therapist may proceed to construct pacing strategies. Another strategy is to take over the patient's defenses and thus provoke an otherwise inhibited impulse. He or she also may give hypnotic reparenting suggestions aimed at some of the deficits the patient has experienced in previous relationships.

For example, the schizoid personality perhaps experienced rejection very early in life, leaving him or her with no space of his or her own and a feeling of having no right to exist. Unconsciously, he or she decided to deny his or her needs. This personality type may be recognized by its disintegrated and dissociative style of communication. Schizoids are extremely sensitive to information overload and exhibit a tendency to withdraw from social contact. Basic survival strategies are impulse suppression, social avoidance, and detachment. The countertransference this behavior evokes is confusion. On the other hand, a vivid imagination and good abstract thinking are some of the resources of this type of personality.

Using this information, the hypnotherapist may pace the patient by allowing the patient to take his or her time and maintaining the distance the patient needs to feel comfortable. Having established rapport in this way, the therapist then may propose to the patient that he or she go into trance by using the patient's natural tendency to go inward, as well as his or her vivid imagination. At first, the therapist may suggest that the patient close his or her eyes (pacing the avoidance of eye contact), and later gently propose that he or she stay in trance while keeping his or her eyes open (leading the patient to stay in touch). The therapist should avoid information overload and too much physical closeness. When the patient is not in trance, the therapist may ask permission to cover the patient's eyes or restrict his or her arm movement, in order to take over the patient's defenses, thus evoking and strengthening the desire to regain eye contact and to reach out. In constructing reparenting suggestions, the therapist can use a direct approach, such as giving the patient such affirmations as, "You are welcome to take as much time as you need," during the trance. Or he or she may use an indirect approach by mentioning anecdotes or metaphors that depict the situation of being welcome.

The seductive personality, as another example, was supposedly impeded in developing his or her own identity. In the case of the woman briefly described above (see Table 36.3), the identity impediment was caused by being scorned by her father and her elder brother, who belittled her femininity—possibly to protect themselves against their own sexual impulses. In other cases, pampering can result in a negation of the child's identity. But in both instances, the child or adolescent feels unaccepted and has to pretend to be someone else in order to be accepted by his or her surroundings. By pretending, the person maintains a certain degree of independence but gives up the feeling of belonging. This patient had to disguise her needs and hide her anger toward those who abused her emotionally. This personality structure often is characterized by a communication style that avoids commitment. The survival strategy consists of hiding one's true intentions. By doing this, she seduced her partners into giving in to her demands. The vulnerable side of the seductive personality is the challenge to be honest. Its resource is an entertaining and fascinating charm.

A pacing strategy could be to assure her that her needs and intentions, especially her need to be in control, are acceptable and will not be denied or punished. Out of trance, taking over the patient's defenses, the therapist might suggest to this patient that she be more skeptical and secretive about her intentions. A therapeutic use of the relationship could be to let her experience safety in trance to the point that she leaves control to the therapist. Specifically, the therapist may suggest how relaxing trust can be, that she is all right the way she is, that she herself can decide to take each step of commitment or acceptance. The therapist has to be particularly careful that the patient experiences the therapist as a respectful and benevolent companion.

A third example would be the masochistic structure. Supposedly, this person's achievements were not reinforced, although he or she was pushed to achieve. Because open aggression was censured, he or she learned to resort to passive resistance in order not to risk belonging. The person's overt decisions were for acceptance and security instead of liberty and open protest. His or her communication style appears cooperative. The survival strategy is passive resistance, for example, saying. "Yes, but ..." Partners feel easily frustrated and tend to be pushy. This is exactly the vulnerable point that the therapist should avoid. His or her resource is loyalty: the person can be relied on as long as he or she is not pushed.

The pacing strategy is to suggest that the person take his or her time and proceed at his or her own pace. One way of taking over such a person's defenses would be to overload the person by applying pressure on his or her shoulders from above, so that the person feels the impulse to stand up openly and discharge his or her feelings. The therapeutic use of the relationship would be to suggest to the masochist that he or she express criticism, resist openly, and fight to feel free to reject undue demands. Specifically, in the receptive state of trance, the therapist might suggest that it is all right to do things his or her own way.

In summary, the use of the hypnotic relationship necessitates different intervention strategies for different interactional types. In a similar vein, Mende (1998) points out the different types of transference that the patient may have for the hypnotist according to his or her personality structure (Axis II, *DSM*-IV). He assumes that the following personages are projected onto the therapist by the depressive, borderline, schizoid, narcissistic, and compulsive, respectively: savior, angel, surgeon, magician, and dictator. The basic principle of using the hypnotic trance on a relationship level is to tailor the therapist's response and the suggested supplements to the interactional scheme of the patient. This can be done by detecting the patient's specific vulnerability, taking over his or her defenses, nurturing his or her specific needs, and allowing him or her to express his or her suppressed impulses. These methods of tailoring hypnotic communication are independent of interventions on the solution level, such as anchoring, reconstruction, or disassociation.

## CONCLUSIONS

All therapy proceeds on two levels: the problem or symptom level and the personality level, the structure that supports the problematic behavior or symptom. Psychoanalysts believe that the personality can be healed when patients reexperience aspects of past relationships with the therapist and work through this transference. In other words, within the framework of the patient–therapist relationship, attempts are made to revise parts of the interactional scheme that patients use to restrict themselves.

Hypnotherapy offers a special opportunity for such revision. While in trance, the patient tends to regress to a childlike state simply by deciding temporarily to relinquish partial control to the therapist. The patient also can be led to regress to childhood experiences that were critical to the formation of his or her interactional scheme. On the solution level, the therapist may, for example, suggest elements that alter a traumatic experience during the reconstruction of these key scenes. In this way, the patient can reexperience the scene in fantasy, adding behaviors and reframing events and actions, which can reactivate unexpressed emotions and thus help complete an affective Gestalt, for example, abreaction of rage in an abusive or traumatic situation.

At the same time, the therapist may supplement the value system with elements that were missing during the formative period, such as the idea that an abusive parent was sick. On the relationship level, the therapist generally has the opportunity to use regression to remold the patient's interactional schemes, in addition to providing solution-oriented interventions. Because of his or her heightened receptivity in trance, the patient may accept specific suggestions that facilitate a change in typical defenses by being allowed to experience himself or herself differently during the hypnotic relationship. This is assumed to aid in repairing some aspects of the patient's interactional schemes.

### References

Erickson, M. H., & Rossi, E. (1979). *Hypnotherapy. An exploratory casebook.* New York: Irvington.

Hall, J. A. (1989). *Hypnosis. A Jungian perspective.* New York: Guilford.

Kurtz, R. (1983). *Hakomi therapy.* Boulder, CO: Hakomi Institute.

Lankton, C. H., & Lankton, S. R. (1989). *Tales of enchantment. Goal-oriented metaphors for adults and children in therapy.* New York: Brunner/Mazel.

Lenk, W. (1993). Krebserkrankungen. In D. Revenstorf (Ed.), *Klinische Hypnose* (pp. 358–375). Berlin: Springer.

Mende, M. (1998). Hypnotherapeutic responses to transference in the face of therapeutic change. *Hypnos, 25,* 130–149.

Pettigrew, L. S. (1979). The paradox game. Identifying and overcoming untenable interactions. *Simulation & Games, 10*, 359–383.

Pierrakos, J. C. (1990). *Core energetics. Developing the capacity to love and heal.* Mendocino, CA: Life Rhythm Publications.

Reich, W. (1969). *Charakteranalyse. Technik und Grundlagen für Studierende und Analytiker.* Amsterdam: De Munter.

Satir, V. (1972). *People making.* Palo Alto, CA: Science & Behavior Books.

Spiegel, D. (1988). Dissociation and hypnosis in PTSD. *Journal of Traumatic Stress, 1*, 17–33.

Zindel, J. P. (1996). Eine hypnoanalytische Methode zur aktiven Introjektion des Therapeuten bei tief gestörten Patienten. *Imagination, 18*, 29–47.

# Index